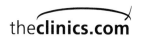

SURGICAL CLINICS
OF NORTH AMERICA

Soft Tissue Sarcomas

GUEST EDITORS
Matthew T. Hueman, MD
Nita Ahuja, MD

CONSULTING EDITOR
Ronald F. Martin, MD

June 2008 • Volume 88 • Number 3

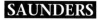

An Imprint of Elsevier, Inc.
PHILADELPHIA   LONDON   TORONTO   MONTREAL   SYDNEY   TOKYO

W.B. SAUNDERS COMPANY
A Division of Elsevier Inc.

1600 John F. Kennedy Blvd., Suite 1800, Philadelphia, PA 19103-2899

http://www.theclinics.com

SURGICAL CLINICS OF NORTH AMERICA   Volume 88, Number 3
June 2008   ISSN 0039–6109
Editor: Catherine Bewick   ISBN-10: 1-4160-5805-2
                                                                              ISBN-13: 978-1-4160-5805-2

The ideas and opinions expressed in *The Surgical Clinics of North America* do not necessarily reflect those of the Publisher. The Publisher does not assume any responsibility for any injury and/or damage to persons or property arising out of or related to any use of the material contained in this periodical. The reader is advised to check the appropriate medical literature and the product information currently provided by the manufacturer of each drug to be administered to verify the dosage, the method and duration of administration, or contraindications. It is the responsibility of the treating physician or other health care professional, relying on independent experience and knowledge of the patient, to determine drug dosages and the best treatment for the patient. Mention of any product in this issue should not be construed as endorsement by the contributors, editors, or the Publisher of the product or manufacturers' claims.

Surgical Clinics of North America (ISSN 0039–6109) is published bimonthly by Elsevier Inc., 360 Park Avenue South, New York, NY 10010-1710. Months of publication are February, April, June, August, October, and December. Business and Editorial Offices: 1600 John F. Kennedy Blvd., Suite 1800, Philadelphia, PA 19103-2899. Customer Service Office: 6277 Sea Harbor Drive, Orlando, FL 32887-4800. Periodicals postage paid at New York, NY and additional mailing offices. Subscription prices are $238.00 per year for US individuals, $382.00 per year for US institutions, $119.00 per year for US students and residents, $292.00 per year for Canadian individuals, $466.00 per year for Canadian institutions, $309.00 for international individuals, $466.00 per year for international institutions and $154.00 per year for Canadian and foreign students/residents. To receive student/resident rate, orders must be accompanied by name of affiliated institution, date of term, and the *signature* of program/residency coordinator on institution letterhead. Orders will be billed at individual rate until proof of status is received. Foreign air speed delivery is included in all *Clinics* subscription prices. All prices are subject to change without notice. POSTMASTER: Send address changes to *Surgical Clinics*, Elsevier Journals Customer Service, 6277 Sea Harbor Drive, Orlando, FL 32887-4800. **Customer Service: 1-800-654-2452 (US). From outside of the United States, call 1-407-563-6020. Fax: 1-407-363-9661.** E-mail: JournalsCustomerService-usa@elsevier.com.

The Surgical Clinics of North America is also published in Spanish by McGraw-Hill Interamericana Editores S.A., P.O. Box 5-237 06500 Mexico D.F. Mexico; and in Portuguese by Interlivros Edicoes Ltda., Rua Comandante Coelho 1085, CEP 21250, Rio de Janeiro, Brazil; and in Greek by Paschalidis Medical Publications, Athens Greece.

The Surgical Clinics of North America is covered in *Index Medicus, EMBASE/Excerpta Medica, Current Contents/Clinical Medicine, Current Contents/Life Sciences, Science Citation Index,* and *ISI/BIOMED.*

Printed in the United States of America.

CONSULTING EDITOR

RONALD F. MARTIN, MD, Staff Surgeon, Marshfield Clinic, Marshfield; and Clinical Associate Professor, University of Wisconsin School of Medicine and Public Health, Madison, Wisconsin; Lieutenant Colonel, Medical Corps, United States Army Reserve

GUEST EDITORS

MATTHEW T. HUEMAN, MD, Surgical Oncology Fellow and Instructor of Surgery, The Johns Hopkins University School of Medicine, Baltimore, Maryland

NITA AHUJA, MD, Assistant Professor of Surgery, The Johns Hopkins University School of Medicine; and Assistant Professor of Oncology, The Sidney Kimmel Comprehensive Cancer Center at Johns Hopkins, Baltimore, Maryland

CONTRIBUTORS

NITA AHUJA, MD, Assistant Professor of Surgery, The Johns Hopkins University School of Medicine; and Assistant Professor of Oncology, The Sidney Kimmel Comprehensive Cancer Center at Johns Hopkins, Baltimore, Maryland

MICHAEL A. CHOTI, MD, MBA, Professor of Surgery and Oncology, Jacob C. Handelsman Professor of Surgery, The Johns Hopkins University School of Medicine, The Sidney Kimmel Comprehensive Cancer Center at Johns Hopkins, Baltimore, Maryland

DEBORAH CITRIN, MD, Tenure Track Investigator, Section of Imaging and Molecular Therapeutics, Radiation Oncology Branch, National Cancer Center, National Cancer Institute, Bethesda, Maryland

DALIA FADUL, MD, Instructor, The Russell H. Morgan Department of Radiology and Radiological Science, The Johns Hopkins University, Baltimore, Maryland

LAURA M. FAYAD, MD, Assistant Professor, The Russell H. Morgan Department of Radiology and Radiological Science, The Johns Hopkins University, Baltimore, Maryland

JOSEPH M. HERMAN, MD, MSc, Assistant Professor of Radiation Oncology and Oncology, The Sidney Kimmel Comprehensive Cancer Center at Johns Hopkins, Baltimore, Maryland

MATTHEW T. HUEMAN, MD, Surgical Oncology Fellow and Instructor of Surgery, The Johns Hopkins University School of Medicine, Baltimore, Maryland

LISA JACOBS, MD, Assistant Professor, Department of Surgery & Oncology, Johns Hopkins Hospital, Baltimore, Maryland

ARADHANA KAUSHAL, MD, Staff Clinician, Radiation Oncology Branch, National Cancer Center, National Cancer Institute, Bethesda, Maryland

GUY LAHAT, MD, Fellow, Department of Surgical Oncology, Sarcoma Research Center, University of Texas MD Anderson Cancer Center, Houston, Texas

ALEXANDER LAZAR, MD, PhD, Assistant Professor, Department of Pathology, Sarcoma Research Center, University of Texas MD Anderson Cancer Center, Houston, Texas

STEVEN D. LEACH, MD, The Paul K. Neumann Professor in Pancreatic Cancer, Professor of Surgery, Oncology and Cell Biology, Johns Hopkins Medical Institution, Baltimore, Maryland

DINA LEV, MD, Assistant Professor, Department of Cancer Biology, Sarcoma Research Center, University of Texas MD Anderson Cancer Center, Houston, Texas

DAVID M. LOEB, MD, PhD, Assistant Professor, Oncology and Pediatrics, and Director, Musculoskeletal Tumor Program, Sidney Kimmel Comprehensive Cancer Center, Johns Hopkins University, Baltimore, Maryland

YING WEI LUM, MD, Resident, Department of Surgery, Johns Hopkins University School of Medicine, Baltimore, Maryland

ELIZABETH MONTGOMERY, MD, Associate Professor of Pathology, The Johns Hopkins University, Baltimore, Maryland

CATHERINE E. PESCE, MD, Surgery Resident, Department of Surgery, The Johns Hopkins University School of Medicine, Baltimore, Maryland

RICHARD D. SCHULICK, MD, Associate Professor of Surgery and Oncology, The John L. Cameron Professor of Alimentary Tract Diseases, The Johns Hopkins University School of Medicine, Baltimore, Maryland

ORI SHOKEK, MD, Instructor, Radiation Oncology and Molecular Radiation Sciences, Sidney Kimmel Comprehensive Cancer Center, Johns Hopkins University, Weinberg, Baltimore, Maryland

KATHERINE THORNTON, MD, Assistant Professor of Oncology, Musculoskeletal Oncology, The Sidney Kimmel Comprehensive Cancer Center at Johns Hopkins, Baltimore, Maryland

JULIE M. WU, MD, Resident, Pathology, The Johns Hopkins University, Baltimore, Maryland

JACQUELINE M. GARONZIK WANG, MD, Resident, Department of Surgery, Johns Hopkins University School of Medicine, Baltimore, Maryland

CONTENTS

> Sarcomas are a heterogeneous group of tumors that may have many etiologies. The incidence of histologic subtypes differs significantly between children and adults. The increase in incidence may be due to improved registry systems, diagnostic tools, and pathologic definitions. Environmental causes may contribute to increased incidence. Genetic alternations may play a role in sarcoma development. As a result of rapidly evolving genomic and proteomic technologies, increased knowledge of the oncogenic mechanisms underlying sarcomagenesis is being generated. Understanding the mechanisms involved in sarcomagenesis is rudimentary. Insight into the molecular basis of sarcoma inception, proliferation, and dissemination hopefully will lead to more effective therapies.

> Soft tissue tumors are a heterogeneous group of benign and malignant processes. Some are assumed to be reactive; others are clearly neoplastic. Because of their rarity, they frequently pose diagnostic problems for surgical pathologists. Accurate diagnosis

of these tumors is enhanced by knowledge of the clinical features of the given lesions and, at times, by application of immunohisto-chemical and molecular techniques. In this article the lesions are described essentially in accordance with the World Health Organization classification.

recommendations regarding optimal treating are lacking. A multi-disciplinary approach to these entities therefore is critical to select appropriate therapeutic strategies for individual patients.

Retroperitoneal sarcomas present a therapeutic challenge based on their location, extent of invasion at diagnosis, and propensity for local recurrence. Surgical therapy remains the only potentially curative treatment option; however, even with aggressive surgical approaches, local recurrence remains a common type of failure. For patients who have high-grade lesions, distant metastatic disease may also limit survival. Optimizing disease control while minimizing the morbidity of therapy remains the primary goal of management. In this article, the authors describe the presentation, evaluation, and management of patients who have retroperitoneal sarcoma.

A gastrointestinal stromal tumor (GIST) is a rare mesenchymal malignancy of the gastrointestinal (GI) tract. Malignant GISTs were first defined as a separate entity from a collection of nonepithelial malignancies of the GI tract in the 1980s and 1990s based on pathologic and clinical behavior. The discovery of activating KIT mutations as a near-uniform occurrence in these tumors greatly influenced the classification [1] and revolutionized therapeutic management of these tumors. To meet the next challenges, newer tyrosine kinase inhibitors and targeted agents are being developed with the goal of providing improved response rates or alternative therapies for patients progressing on established agents. In this article, the authors describe the management of GISTs, concentrating on surgical management and targeted therapies.

Soft tissue sarcomas in children are rare. Approximately 850 to 900 children and adolescents are diagnosed each year with rhabdomyosarcoma (RMS) or a non-RMS soft tissue sarcoma (NRSTS). RMS is more common in children 14 years old and younger and NRSTS in adolescents and young adults. Infants get NRSTS, but their tumors constitute a distinctive set of histologies. Surgery is a major therapeutic modality and radiation plays a role. RMS is treated with adjuvant chemotherapy, whereas chemotherapy is reserved for the NRSTS that are high grade or unresectable. This review discusses the etiology, biology, and treatment of pediatric soft tissue sarcomas.

FORTHCOMING ISSUES

August 2008

Familial Cancer Syndromes
Ismail Jatoi, MD, *Guest Editor*

October 2008

Minimally Invasive Surgery
Jon Gould, MD, *Guest Editor*

December 2008

Biliary Surgery
J. Lawrence Munson, MD, *Guest Editor*

RECENT ISSUES

April 2008

OB/GYN for the General Surgeon
Charles Dietrich, III, MD, *Guest Editor*

February 2008

Advances in Abdominal Wall Hernia Repair
Kamal FMF Itani, MD, and Mary Hawn, MD,
Guest Editors

December 2007

Benign Pancreatic Disorders
Stephen W. Behrman, MD, *Guest Editor*

The Clinics are now available online!

www.theclinics.com

ELSEVIER
SAUNDERS

Surg Clin N Am 88 (2008) xi–xii

SURGICAL
CLINICS OF
NORTH AMERICA

Foreword

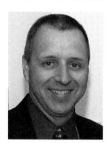

Ronald F. Martin, MD
Consulting Editor

There are few words in surgery that grab your attention quite like sarcoma. No matter what one's specialty or subspecialty, once one finds oneself dealing with sarcoma, the game seems to be afoot. Thoughts of large complex operations, detailed imaging studies, meticulous planning, and maybe looking for a bit more help creep into one's mind fairly quickly—and if those thoughts don't occur they probably should.

Sarcoma as a clinical entity provides surgeons with a great many opportunities: a chance to apply detailed knowledge of complicated anatomic relationships, a chance to participate in complex multi-team operations, a chance to participate in poly-disciplinary care, and a chance to be humbled. This is not to say that other clinical challenges are not humbling as well—they all can be. Sarcoma, though, is probably the closest thing to an oncologic knuckleball there is, and as such has a unique opportunity to lure us into pitfalls.

For those who have read these Forewords for the past few years, it may be apparent that I try (with varying degrees of success) to explain why a topic is chosen as an issue for the series and where it fits into the larger objectives of the series' educational goals. Some topics are chosen because of significant changes in our understanding or approach. Some are chosen because we need to review in detail a mainstay of general surgical practice. Some are picked because it seems as if the topic is important and not easily covered by other means.

One of the objectives of every issue is to make sure that the topic is important and relevant to the general surgeon. Some topics are relevant

0039-6109/08/$ - see front matter © 2008 Elsevier Inc. All rights reserved.
doi:10.1016/j.suc.2008.04.008   *surgical.theclinics.com*

because most general surgeons are directly involved in the definitive management of patients with those problems, while some topics are relevant for the nearly opposite reason: that very few general surgeons provide the definitive care. Sarcoma is an excellent example of the latter. To make it even a bit more interesting, a significant fraction of these patients will be initally referred to a surgeon who does not routinely manage these patients. As a result, even those who do not routinely manage patients with sarcoma still need to be very well versed in the appropriate (and inappropriate) initial evaluations and principles of care.

The surgeon who does manage patients with sarcoma needs to be very fluent in the topics discussed in this issue, as well as be able to work effectively in teams of varying size and complexity. In addition, institutional support well beyond operative facilities is mandatory to manage many of the "unintended consequences" of eradicating these tumors from those so inflicted. The surgeon historically has and will most likely continue to have a significant leadership role in these teams.

Drs. Hueman and Ahuja have assembled a group of talented and varied contributors to this issue. The have emphasized, and rightly so in my opinion, the intrinsic need to approach the patient with sarcoma as a comprehensive team. Furthermore, the authors in this issue consistently relate the need for making clinical decisions in an orderly fashion based on the facts as they unfold. Whether one is considering limb salvage versus amputation or neoadjuvant therapy versus primary resection, there is no one-size-fits-all solution for any given patient with any given tumor. All factors must be considered early, as it is very easy to burn bridges in these situations.

As always, feedback from our readers is welcome and sought after. Please enjoy this issue and let us know if there are topics that you feel are important that we are not addressing.

Ronald F. Martin, MD
Department of Surgery
Marshfield Clinic
1000 North Oak Avenue
Marshfield, WI 54449, USA

E-mail address: martin.ronald@marshfieldclinic.org

SURGICAL
CLINICS OF
NORTH AMERICA

Surg Clin N Am 88 (2008) xiii–xvii

Preface

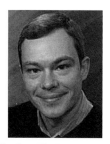 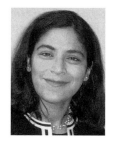

Matthew T. Hueman, MD   Nita Ahuja, MD
Guest Editors

Sarcoma is a heterogenous collection of over 50 different histologies derived primarily from a variety of mesenchymal tissues, including muscle, skin, nerves, blood vessels, bones, fat, and connective tissue. While often discussed as a single entity, the label of sarcoma describes a heterogeneous set of tumors with differing biology, aggressiveness, patterns of spread, propensity for local and distant recurrence, location, and ultimately, management. While the optimal treatment for most soft tissue sarcomas can be summarized as wide, local margin, negative surgical excision with the use of radiotherapy to control local recurrence, the heterogeneity of the manifestations of this collection of diseases, because of factors such as age, histology, tissue origin, grade, and location of the sarcoma (even among similar biology and histology), adds a significant layer of complexity to attempts to provide local control. The seemingly unpredictable response of sarcomas to toxic chemotherapy has made defining the timing and utility of systemic therapy challenging and adds to this complexity. This astounding level of heterogeneity has tremendous implications for treatment and prognosis. We believe that because of these issues, the management of sarcoma deserves an in-depth review. Our understanding of the disease is often limited by the rarity of sarcomas and, unfortunately, by bleak outcomes because of limits in our ability to control the disease.

We personally have become fascinated by this complexity and have attempted to invite several experts within their fields to help provide an up-to-date overview of sarcoma. Accordingly, this issue of the *Surgical*

doi:10.1016/j.suc.2008.04.009   *surgical.theclinics.com*

Clinics of North America covers a wide spectrum of sarcomas and is geared not only towards the general surgeon who is often called on to evaluate patients with masses in a variety of locations and origins, but also to the practicing surgical oncologist, who is commonly called upon to offer expert opinion in this uncommon disease. Much of our understanding and management of sarcoma is extrapolated from successful studies of patients with extremity sarcomas, perhaps because local recurrence as a result of failed therapy can more "easily" be salvaged (eg, amputation, resection of recurrence) without impacting on more vital, central organs—allowing us to best study the natural history of disease.

Despite our preconceived notions of the surgeon's view of their ability to eradicate disease with surgical precision, generally the biology—or aggressiveness—of the primary tumor, and not the local therapy, impacts on the occurrence of systemic disease for sarcomas. This initially counterintuitive principle is shown in the Rosenberg and colleagues' landmark National Cancer Institute trial of limb-sparing, function-sparing surgery versus amputation in the treatment of extremity sarcoma [1]. This previously heretical notion has allowed us to apply this principle increasingly to other diseases, most notably breast cancer, where breast preservation has become the standard of care. Nonetheless, aggressive surgical therapy for local and limited metastatic disease remains—and should remain—as the mainstay of treatment for sarcoma. The aggressiveness of the surgical approach for primary, recurrent, and metastatic tumors at all locations should be determined in the context of an understanding of the unique biology of sarcoma itself as it relates to each unique patient we encounter.

Despite the deceptively simple presentation of sarcoma as a single disease with a single treatment and a uniformly bleak future—surgery with radiation with high rates of recurrence, systemic disease unaffected by local treatment, and toxic, partially effective systemic treatment—we learn in this issue of *Surgical Clinics of North America* that much hope for a brighter future for patients with this disease remains. Perhaps most importantly, our increased understanding of the biology and natural history of this disease has led to a better appreciation of our limitations. Despite the amazing advancements in nearly all aspects of diagnosis and management of sarcoma, long-term survival for the majority of these patients remains at a disappointing 30% to 50%. We continue to gain more by understanding of where we need to improve to spur future generations to help gain a stronger foothold in the control of this deadly disease.

For those of you who are, like us, amazed by the complexity of sarcoma, this issue only scratches the surface but provides a broad overview. In the first article, Drs. Lahat, Lazar, and Lev's "Sarcoma epidemiology and etiology; potential environmental and genetic factors," for example, we learn that sarcoma represents only 1% of solid tumor cancers in the United States but that it is more common than small bowel cancer, Hodgkin's lymphoma, or testicular carcinoma (of "livestrong" and Lance Armstrong fame) and account for up to 15% of pediatric malignancies. Most interestingly, this article highlights that the most common genetic alterations associated with sarcoma are nonrandom chromosomal translocations that produce fusion genes. These fusion genes represent ideal targets for potential anticancer therapy, development of which would be based on the ability to inhibit the fusion genes' transcript product or its downstream mediator.

In the next article, Drs. Wu and Montgomery's "Classification and pathology of sarcoma," we get insight into the broad spectrum of classification and of biology of the variety of manifestations of soft tissue tumors; but at the same time recognize that we are limited in our ability to understand the disease by what we are able to observe. Histology, based on morphology alone, characterizes much of our classification systems for sarcomas, but molecular pathology, and genetics in particular, will likely dictate our future understanding. Drs. Fayud and Fadal's article "Advanced modalities for the imaging for sarcoma," provides an excellent overview of our current use of computed tomography and magnetic resonance imaging in the evaluation of the management of primary and recurrent sarcoma. This outstanding article also highlights our increasing understanding of the use of positron emission tomography to evaluate for staging, recurrence, and the response to therapy (in particular in the face of the growing sense of utility of neoadjuvant therapy).

Drs. Hueman, Thornton, Herman and Ahuja's article "Extremity soft tissue sarcoma," provides the backbone of our understanding of the management, sequence and timing of adjuvant therapy, and relationship of local therapy to systemic disease for the entire spectrum of extremity sarcomas. Drs. Lum and Jacobs' article "Breast sarcomas," covers an uncommon presentation of a possibly increasing problem: with the advent of increasing longevity in the thousands of women treated annually in the United States with radiation for breast cancer, despite the low incidence, it is a malignancy we may see with more frequency (at least in absolute number). The next article, Drs. Garonzik and Leach's "Truncal sarcomas," is quite intriguing as it covers a broad spectrum of locally benign to locally malignant disease with variable predilection for systemic spread; especially for intra-abdominal desmoids, we are reminded of our first obligation: *primum non nocere* (first, do no harm). Depending on the size, relationship to symptoms, and location, tamoxifen and nonsteroidal anti-inflammatories may be the best, and at the very least first, prescribed treatment of intra- or transabdominal desmoids.

In Drs. Hueman and Ahuja's article "Management of retroperitoneal sarcomas," we learn of the importance of sequencing adjuvant therapy in relationship to toxicity, the importance and difficulty in achieving margin-negative resection, and the continued challenge we face in the management of this disease not just because of its rarity but to the preconceived notions as to what is the best therapy. In Drs. Hueman and Schulick's article "Management of gastrointestinal stromal tumors," we gain new hope in the development of molecularly targeted therapy, but also new perspective. Imatinib has prolonged disease-free intervals in high-risk gastrointestinal stromal tumor (GIST) patients, but as of yet has not provided proven overall survival benefit. Targeted therapy offers new hope for patients with unresectable or metastatic disease; however, determining optimal and sustainable treatment in the face of imatinib-resistant, sunitinib-resistant disease remains our next challenge.

In the article by Drs. Loeb, Thornton, and Shokek, "Pediatric Sarcoma," we are amazed at the ability of the pediatric sarcoma teams to perform national cooperative group studies in rare diseases to determine optimal treatment and outcomes. The success of pediatric sarcoma trials in defining a standard of care impresses upon us that the rarity of these tumors does not preclude completion of well-designed randomized trials. In Drs. Kaushal and Citrin's article "The role of radiation in the management of sarcomas," the authors expertly highlight the controversies, limitations, and effectiveness of radiation therapy in relationship to its timing, sequence, and delivery. The future of sarcoma management, in fact, may lie (at least in the near short term) in our ability to use molecular pathology or proliferation markers instead of histology and grade to predict the benefits and risks of adjuvant radiotherapy, thus defining the population who would most benefit from the inclusion, or exclusion, of radiotherapy in preventing local recurrence. This article, in combination with the several other articles of this issue (in particular Drs. Hueman and Ahuja's "Management of retroperitoneal sarcomas"), helps highlight the importance of local control balanced by toxicity. In doing so, this article reinforces in those of us who may tend to be nihilistic, the need to strongly question the notion that any therapies that do not provide overall survival benefit in the treatment are not worthwhile.

The next article, Dr. Thornton's "Medical management of sarcoma," highlights the successes and limitations of therapy and of randomized trials of systemic therapy for sarcoma in the establishment of doxorubicin, ifosfamide (with mesna), and darcabazine (or imatinib and sunitinib in GIST) as standard of care, in combination or even as single agents. This comprehensive article also highlights the exciting prospect of future therapies, in particular new therapies such as Ecteinascidin-743, or ET-743 (Yondelis), which was originally derived from the Caribbean sea squirt, *Ecteinascidia turbinate*. ET-743 is a novel chemotherapeutic that has shown promise by yielding impressive response rates (up to 51% responders in early studies). Finally, Drs. Thornton, Pesce, and Choti's article "Metastatic sarcoma," highlights the difficulty but also promise of using multimodality therapy to treat patients with metastatic sarcoma.

In all, we are indebted to the countless hours of work from our coauthors who have labored to help make this final product. In particular, we would like to thank Dr. Ronald Martin, who proved invaluable, not only in the initial crafting of the table of contents (while in a Combat Support Hospital in Mosul, Iraq), but for his continued guidance through the process of creating this issue. And, lastly, the enduring patience, commitment, and support of our Publisher, Catherine Bewick, who has spent countless hours helping generate this final product. We greatly appreciate her tireless and enormous behind-the-scenes effort on our behalf.

Acknowledgments

I would personally like to thank Dr. Ronald Martin, in his efforts at helping me make a junior attempt at meeting the lofty aspirations to be a surgical oncologist and committed combat Army trauma surgeon. I have a long, but well-paved and enjoyable, road ahead of me. Secondly, I want to personally thank Dr. Nita Ahuja, who has been a friend and mentor during times I needed help the most; she has helped me not only produce this issue but help guide me at an overwhelmingly humbling, awe-inspiring institution. Closest to my heart is my deepest gratitude to my wife, Deborah Citrin, who has been an invaluable partner not just in life but in the crafting of this issue; and to my newly born son, Ethan Alexander Hueman, in the hopes that he will one day be able to read this thank you and understand the depths of my commitment to, and love for, him.

Matthew T. Hueman

Matthew T. Hueman, MD
The Johns Hopkins University School of Medicine
Division of Surgical Oncology
Department of Surgery
Blalock 665
600 North Wolfe Street
Baltimore, MD 21287, USA

E-mail address: mhueman1@jhmi.edu

Nita Ahuja, MD
The Johns Hopkins University School of Medicine
Division of Surgical Oncology
Department of Surgery
Osler 625
600 North Wolfe Street
Baltimore, MD 21287, USA

E-mail address: nahuja@jhmi.edu

Reference

[1] Rosenberg SA, Tepper J, Glatstein E, et al. The treatment of soft-tissue sarcomas of the extremities: prospective randomized evaluations of (1) limb-sparing surgery plus radiation therapy compared with amputation and (2) the role of adjuvant chemotherapy. Ann Surg 1982;196:305.

SURGICAL
CLINICS OF
NORTH AMERICA

Surg Clin N Am 88 (2008) 451–481

Sarcoma Epidemiology and Etiology: Potential Environmental and Genetic Factors

Guy Lahat, MD[a], Alexander Lazar, MD, PhD[b], Dina Lev, MD[c],*

[a]*Department of Surgical Oncology, Sarcoma Research Center, University of Texas MD Anderson Cancer Center, 1515 Holcombe Boulevard, Unit 1104, Houston, TX 77030, USA*
[b]*Department of Pathology, Sarcoma Research Center, University of Texas MD Anderson Cancer Center, 1515 Holcombe Boulevard, Unit 1104, Houston, TX 77030, USA*
[c]*Department of Cancer Biology, Sarcoma Research Center, University of Texas MD Anderson Cancer Center, 1515 Holcombe Boulevard, Unit 1104, Houston, TX 77030, USA*

Although somatic mesenchymal origin tissues account for more than two thirds of total body weight, sarcomas, which are tumors of putative mesenchymal origin, represent less than 1% of adult solid malignancy. The histologic and biologic spectrum of this disease is remarkable in comparison to the more prevalent epithelial-based malignancies. Comprising a family of more than 50 distinct histologic subtypes, which can occur at any age and at any location in the human body, sarcoma represents a multitude of malignancies rather than a single entity. Although as a group sarcomas exhibit unique clinical behaviors that differentiate these tumors from epithelial tumors, individual sarcoma subtypes widely differ in comparison to each other. This diversity makes it challenging to evaluate and analyze the epidemiology and etiology of sarcoma. Only via better knowledge of the clinical and molecular determinants underlying sarcoma inception, proliferation, and dissemination, however, will it be possible to improve outcomes for patients suffering from these malignancies.

It is difficult to undertake the study of sarcoma as a laboratory proposition in that the rarity of this disease can impair the ability of investigators to secure requisite sarcoma biologic resources. Nonetheless, progress must be made in order to achieve the molecular understanding necessary to

* Corresponding author.
E-mail address: dlev@mdanderson.org (D. Lev).

0039-6109/08/$ - see front matter © 2008 Elsevier Inc. All rights reserved.
doi:10.1016/j.suc.2008.03.006
surgical.theclinics.com

ultimately drive personal therapeutics in this disease entity. As more is learned about the relevant molecular determinants, the interaction between tumor, host, and environment becomes ever more important. Although at this juncture most sarcomas seem sporadic, it is clear that the host-environment interaction does have a role in sarcomagenesis at macro and molecular levels. A systematic biologic understanding of these interactions ultimately will enable identification of populations at risk and "risky" environments. Armed with this knowledge, clinicians will be optimally positioned to better prevent and treat patients who can and do develop this all too devastating malignant disease.

Epidemiology

Sarcomas are a diverse group of malignant tumors that arise predominantly from the embryonic mesoderm and can be categorized as tumors arising primarily from the bone (eg, osteosarcoma and Ewing's sarcoma [ES]) and those that arise from soft tissues. The World Health Organization has defined approximately 50 soft tissue sarcoma (STS) histologic subtypes [1]. There is overlap, however, between certain tumors and the differences between subtypes are not always distinct. STSs are subcategorized according their apparent line of differentiation, which also may be etiologically relevant (eg, liposarcoma [fat], leiomyosarcoma [smooth muscle] and rhabdomyosarcoma [skeletal muscle], and fibrosarcoma [connective tissue]) (Fig. 1).

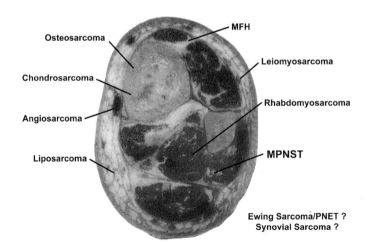

Fig. 1. Cross-section of lower leg showing sarcoma differentiation patterns. Many sarcomas show recognizable differentiation from normal mesenchymal tissues. This lineage of differentiation may be indicative of etiology, but as the cell of origin is not known for most sarcomas, this remains speculative. Some sarcomas lack recognizable differentiation from any mesenchymal tissue, such as ES and synovial sarcoma. PNET, primitive neuroectodermal tumor. (*Courtesy of* Dr. Brian Rubin, Cleveland Clinic, Cleveland, OH.)

The specific histologic subtype may be an important determinant of specific treatment (ie, gastrointestinal stromal tumor [GIST] and imatinib therapy). The Surveillance, Epidemiology, and End Results (SEER) database (1978–2001), which is maintained by the National Cancer Institute, is an authoritative source of information on cancer incidence and survival in the United States. SEER data demonstrate that leiomyosarcoma accounts for 23.7% of all cases and, therefore, is the most common STS subtype [2]. Other major histologic subtypes include malignant fibrous histiocytoma (MFH) (17.1%), liposarcoma (11.5%), dermatofibrosarcoma (10.5%), and rhabdomyosarcoma (4.6%); these five histologic subtypes account for slightly more than two thirds of all SEER database STS cases [2]. Comparable subtype rates have been observed in a large cohort of patients who had STS and were evaluated in The University of Texas M. D. Anderson Cancer Center (UTMDACC); however, the most common histopathology in the author's series is MFH, as in other large series, rather than leiomyosarcoma, perhaps pointing to the inherent difficulties in rigid application of light microscopic diagnostic criteria for this complex disease cluster (Table 1) [3]. Determining the exact numbers of patients diagnosed with sarcoma also is problematic, mainly because of inconsistencies in disease classification. Per the SEER database, the annual United States incidence of bone sarcoma and STS is approximately 15,000 cases, of which 9220 are adult STSs. As such, STS constitutes 1% of all new solid tumor cases in the United States annually with a projected incidence of 2.5 to 3.5 cases per 100,000 United States inhabitants per year and an overall mortality rate of 30% to 50% [4–7]. This STS incidence level is comparable to that of chronic lymphocytic leukemia

Table 1
Percentage distribution of sarcomas and soft tissue sarcomas according to histologic type in a series of 7765 patients evaluated at The University of Texas M. D. Anderson Cancer Center between 1990 and 2003

Histology	Percentage
MFH	28%
Liposarcoma	15%
Leiomyosarcoma	12%
Unclassified	11%
Synovial sarcoma	10%
MPNST	6%
Rhabdomyosarcoma	5%
Fibrosarcoma	3%
Angiosarcoma	2%
Extraosseous ES	2%
Epitheloid sarcoma	1%
Chondrosarcoma	1%
Clear cell sarcoma	1%
Alveolar soft part sarcoma	1%
Malignant hemangiopericytoma	4%

or uterine cervical carcinoma and renders STS more frequent than small bowel cancer, Hodgkin's disease, or testicular carcinoma [8,9].

Currently, the median age of diagnosis for STS is 56 years of age; approximately 10.4% are diagnosed in patients under age 20, whereas 52.2% are found in patients over age 55 (Fig. 2). According to the SEER database, the incidence of STS currently is 3.7 per 100,000 men versus 2.6 per 100,000 women (Table 2), and there is an increasing number of STSs diagnosed in the United States annually. The diagnosis of sarcomas among the United States black population decreased between 2000 and 2004 for reasons that are not clear.

Sarcomas as a group, in particular STS, are more frequent in the pediatric population where they account for up to 15% of all malignancies. The most common pediatric STS is rhabdomyosarcoma, which accounts for 5% to 8% of all childhood cancers. The incidence of rhabdomyosarcoma is twice as high in white compared with black children; almost two thirds occur in children under the age of 10 [10]. Nonrhabdomyosarcoma pediatric STS constitutes a heterogeneous group of malignancies that account for 3%

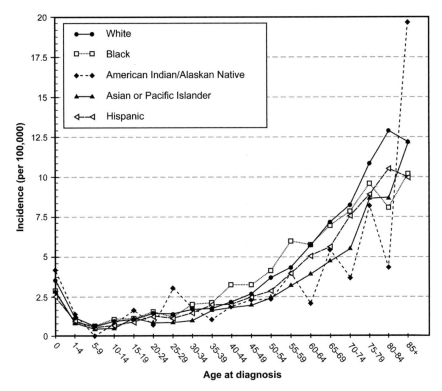

Fig. 2. Age-specific SEER incidence rates categorized by race for STS. This data indicate increased sarcoma incidence in early childhood, which diminishes by age 10 and is followed by a slow rise throughout adult years, accelerating in the sixth and seventh decades of life.

Table 2
Incidence of soft tissue sarcomas by race and ethnicity according to the Surveillance, Epidemiology, and End Results database

Race/ethnicity	Male (per 100,00)	Female (per 100,000)
All races	3.7	2.6
White	3.7	2.6
Black	3.6	3.0
Asian/Pacific Islander	2.7	1.8
American Indian/Alaska Native[a]	1.9	1.3
Hispanic[b]	3.0	2.5

[a] Incidence data for American Indian/Alaska Natives is based on the contract health service delivery area counties.

[b] Incidence data for Hispanics are based on Hispanic Identification Algorithm and excludes cases from Alaska native registry and Kentucky.

of all childhood neoplastic disease [11]. Osteosarcoma and ES account for 3.5% and 2% of all pediatric sarcomas, respectively. Most ESs arise from bone, but some originate from soft tissue. ES is an extremely rare tumor in black children with at least a ninefold higher incidence observed in white children [12]. In contrast, osteosarcoma occurs in both races and is slightly more prevalent in black children. Osteosarcomas arise mainly in the metaphyses of long bones whereas ESs typically arise within the diaphyses of long bones and flat bones.

ES and osteosarcoma are 1.5-fold more common in boys than girls [11,13]. The peak incidence of osteosarcoma is in the second decade of life during the adolescent growth spurt, suggesting a possible association between rapid bone growth and malignant transformation [8]. Sarcomas are a major cause of cancer-related death during the first two decades of life and account for the fifth leading cause of cancer-related deaths in men under age 20 and the fourth leading cause of cancer mortality among women in that same age group [14].

STS can arise in virtually any anatomic site within the human body; anatomic distribution and site-specific STS histologic subtype of the more than 5000 patients who have STS presenting to UTMDACC from 1996 to 2005 is presented in Fig. 3. Most STSs originate in the extremity, 32% in the lower and 13% in the upper extremities. Almost one third of the STSs are retroperitoneal or intra-abdominal. Thoracic (9%) and head and neck locations (6%) are rarer [15]. The incidence by location patterns of 26,758 STSs in the SEER database (1978–2001) is shown in Table 3 [2]. In contrast, pediatric STSs have a different distribution of anatomic loci. Rhabdomyosarcomas, which account for the majority of pediatric STSs, are found most often in the head and neck (40%), genitourinary tract (20%), extremities (20%), and trunk (10%). In the pediatric population, approximately half of all nonrhabdomysarcoma STSs arise in the extremities but may also occur in the trunk, head and neck, and intrathoracic/intra-abdominal regions [11].

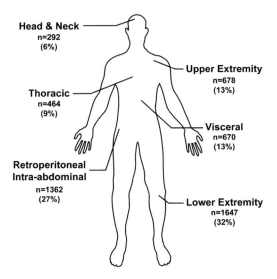

Fig. 3. Anatomic distribution of sarcomas from UTMDACC Sarcoma Surgical Database, 1996–2005. Sarcomas can arise anywhere in the human body. This may indicate that potential precursor cells are widespread but also complicates interpretation of incidence data, which usually categorize tumors by site of origin.

Pediatric STSs comprise approximately 4% of childhood malignancies [11]. Primary retroperitoneal STSs are rare in childhood. These differences in STS anatomic sites when comparing adults and children may reflect differences in the underlying biology of the various histopathologies that predominate within each age group.

Etiology

Most STSs are etiologically indeterminate; however, several etiologic factors are identified, which can be divided into environmental and host/genetic considerations (Box 1).

Environmental etiologies

Radiation exposure

Certain environmental factors are associated with the development of sarcoma. For example, exposure to radiation has long been recognized to induce sarcomas, with published reports from the 1920s documenting the development of sarcomas in workers manufacturing radium watch dials [16]. Since then, it has been shown that the risk for sarcoma development is increased in patients in whom radiotherapy is used to treat lymphoma, breast, testicular, ovarian, prostate, lung, or other cancers [6,17–19]. Current estimates suggest that radiotherapy-induced sarcomas account for

Table 3
Anatomic sites of soft tissue sarcomas diagnosed during 1978–2001 in the ninth Surveillance, Epidemiology, and End Results program

	Cases	Percent
Soft tissue, including heart	12,818	47.9
Skin	3758	14
Uterus	1861	7
Retroperitoneum	1777	6.6
Stomach	1002	3.7
Small intestine	715	2.7
Lung and bronchus	410	1.5
Breast	330	1.2
Peritoneum, omentum, and mesentery	289	1.1
Other male genital organs	281	1.1
Colon and rectum	276	1
Oral cavity and pharynx	234	0.9
Nose, nasal cavity, and middle ear	226	0.8
Kidney and renal pelvis	205	0.8
Liver and intrahepatic bile duct	202	0.8
Urinary bladder	177	0.7
Cranial nerves and other nervous system	176	0.7
Trachea, mediastinum, and other respiratory organs	169	0.6
Ovary	119	0.4
Testis	105	0.4
Eye and orbit	102	0.4
Other	1526	5.7
Total	*26,758*	*100*

Attributed to the Surveillance, Epidemiology, and End Results database.

approximately 0.5% to 5.5% of all sarcomas [20,21]. This estimate is based on series of patients operated on for sarcoma; however, large population-based studies of long-term outcomes for patients radiated for various reasons report lower overall incidence rates in the 0.03% to 0.8% range [22,23]. In a Swedish Cancer Registry population-based analysis of 122,991 patients who had breast cancer, the postradiation risk for developing sarcoma was 0.13% at 10 years [24]. There is a dose-response correlation between radiation dose and the development of sarcoma, with a very low risk for individuals who are incidentally exposed to less than 10 Gy [25]. Sarcomas typically arise in the margins of radiation fields, suggesting that the mutagenic effect may be maximal at the periphery where scatter radiation could lead to a dose sufficient to induce mutations but insufficient to kill the mutated cells [15]. There usually is an interval of several years between radiation treatment and the subsequent development of sarcoma. In 1947, Cahan and colleagues [26] initially defined the criteria for postradiation sarcoma induction, which included an interval of at least 5 years between radiotherapy and the development of disease. More recent data have shown that a shorter latency period is possible [20,27]. Radiation-associated sarcomas usually are aggressive high-grade tumors. In a large

---

Box 1. Potential sarcoma etiologies

Environmental
Radiation
Chemicals
    Polyvinyl chloride (PVC)
    Thorotrast
    Inorganic arsenic
    Androgenic-anabolic steroids
    Hemochromatosis
    Copper exposure
    Dioxins
    Chlorophenoles
    Benzophenone
    O-nitrotoluene

Host related
Immune suppression
AIDS
Transplantation
Chronic irritation of tissues
    Chronic inflammation
    Foreign body
Genetic alternations
    Genetic syndromes (Table 4)
    Discrete genetic alternations-fusion genes
    Complex nonspecific genetic alternations

---

series of 160 radiation-induced sarcomas from the Memorial Sloan-Kettering Cancer Center, the most common histologic subtypes were extraskeletal osteosarcoma (21%), MFH (16%), and angiosarcoma/lymphangiosarcoma (15%); 87% percent of these tumors were high grade [17].

Exposure to chemicals

Sarcomas also are associated with exposure to certain chemicals. Exposure to PVC, thorotrast use in angiography, exposure to inorganic arsenic, and treatment with androgenic-anabolic steroids all are associated with hepatic angiosarcoma (HAS) [28]. Epidemiologic studies of PVC polymerization workers exposed to vinyl chloride monomer have demonstrated high relative risks for the development of HAS [29,30]. Thorotrast is a colloidal suspension of thorium dioxide with prolonged radiologic and biologic half-life that was used for carotid angiography and liver-spleen scans from 1930 to 1955. Thorium dioxide is sequestered by the reticuloendothelial system, primarily in Kupffer's cells of the liver; radiation injury to adjacent cells is the presumed carcinogenic mechanism. Epidemiologic studies of thorotrast recipients show high relative risks for the development of HAS and other hepatic malignancies [31,32].

The association between arsenic and HAS is based on data from several small autopsy series of German vintners from the 1940s and 1950s, demonstrating an increased incidence of liver disease (including HAS) as an occupational hazard [33,34]. These workers were exposed to inorganic arsenical pesticides during application of the pesticide and by drinking beverages prepared from the skins of the inorganic arsenic–sprayed grapes. Cases of HAS also are reported after long-term ingestion of Fowler's solution (potassium arsenite) [35,36] and arsenic-contaminated well water [37]. Individual cases suggesting associations between HAS and hemochromatosis [38] resulting from copper exposure [39] also are reported. Other chemical exposures leading to subsequent development of STS are reported anecdotally [40–42], including androgenic-anabolic steroids, which are implicated in the development of HAS [43].

Additional agents also receiving mention in the STS etiology literature include dioxins and chlorophenoles; however, their association with sarcoma development is less certain [44–46]. Chemicals, such as benzophenone and o-nitrotoluene, also are proposed as causative agents that can be shown to induce sarcoma in animal models [47,48].

A history of trauma not uncommonly is associated with the diagnosis of sarcoma. STSs, in particular intra-abdominal/retroperitoneal masses, usually are asymptomatic until quite large. Trauma may cause painful intra/peritumoral bleeding that may first prompt a patient to seek medical attention. A second possible explanation for this association may be related to the liberal use of abdominal imaging in trauma patients. Such imaging may demonstrate asymptomatic intra-abdominal tumors whose discovery after trauma is temporally but probably not causatively related to the etiology of STS.

Host-related etiologies

Most host-related etiologies are genetic and are discussed later. There are several additional nonspecific possible STS etiologies, however, including chronic irritation of tissues and host immune suppression. Chronic inflammation is well established as an etiologic factor for many epithelial cancers (eg, squamous cell carcinoma). Chronic upper extremity lymphedema after mastectomy with radiation increases the risk for subsequent sarcoma development, primarily angiosarcoma (Stewart-Treves syndrome) [49,50]. Limited (primarily experimental) data suggest a possible association between foreign body–induced chronic irritation and subsequent development of sarcoma; for example, unplasticized vinyl chloride vinyl acetate copolymer implanted into mice is associated with sarcomagenesis, where the incidence of

STS increased in direct proportion to the size of the copolymer that is implanted [51].

Chronic immunosuppression increases the risk for developing many different malignancies. The incidence of certain epithelial cancers is increased several hundred–fold compared with the general population. The association of AIDS and Kaposi sarcoma (KS) is well established. Given that KS typically is associated with human herpesvirus 8 (HHV8) infection and tends to regress with improvement of host immunosuppression, its inclusion as a mesenchymal-derived STS remains controversial [52]. Despite its name, many consider KS a virally induced endothelial proliferation rather than a genetically driven malignant process per se [52]. This perception is underscored by the recent development of a mouse model where KS growth was shown dependent on the presence of the HHV8 viral genome within the tumor cells, with regression of KS when the viral genome was lost [52]. Solid organ transplant recipients also demonstrate an increased incidence of KS, particularly in geographic locations where exposure to HHV8 is endemic [53,54]. According to the Cincinnati Transplant Tumor Registry, up to 6% of all de novo cancers after solid organ transplantation are KS, and the risk for developing KS in renal transplant recipients is approximately 500-fold greater than that of the nontransplant population at large [55].

In a review of 8724 de novo malignancies that occurred in 8191 organ allograft recipients, sarcomas accounted for 7.4% of the cases, of which KS was 5.7% and non-KS 1.7%, the latter presenting a nearly twofold higher STS incidence than in the general population [56]. In addition to this single retrospective study, several case reports describe the development of non-KS sarcomas in transplant organ recipients. Overall, the causative association suggested by these anecdotal reports remains inconclusive.

Epstein-Barr virus (EBV)-driven leiomyosarcomas have been increasingly reported during the past decade in immunocompromised patients, in particular the pediatric AIDS population [57]. Multiple tumors commonly are seen in individual patients suffering from this disease entity and can be shown to arise from different progenitor clones, supporting the view that multifocal tumors arise from serial multiple infections rather than from metastasis per se [57]. Previous studies have shown that EBV has a direct role in the development of smooth muscle tumors and that Epstein-Barr nuclear antigen (EBNA)-2 protein is consistently expressed in smooth muscle cells of immunocompromised individuals [58]. Decreased immune surveillance, increased expression of the EBV receptor, and high plasma EBV levels all may contribute to the pathogenesis of this process [59]. Observed tumors typically are well differentiated with little atypia and a low level of mitotic activity; unlike classic leiomyosarcomas, these tumors lack significant pleomorphism. In the largest series of EBV-associated smooth muscle tumors, strain typing by analysis of the EBNA-3C gene confirmed the presence of EBV type 2 [57]. Moreover, several tumors demonstrated positivity for a 30-bp deletion in the LMP1 gene. Although it seems that EBV-2 can transform smooth muscle cells independent of LMP1 deletion, this latter alteration is associated with enhanced tumor virulence [57].

Molecular genetics and sarcoma development

It has been known for decades that persons who have certain genetic syndromes are predisposed to develop sarcoma. The most well known are Li-Fraumeni syndrome (LFS) and neurofibromatosis type 1 (NF-1) (von Recklinghausen's disease). Table 4 lists the inherited diseases predisposing to sarcoma development.

The reported genetic alternations associated with sarcoma fall into three major categories: (1) genetic diseases (germline) that are associated with predisposition to sarcoma development; (2) discrete somatic genetic alternations, including fusion genes resulting from reciprocal translocations (simple karyotypes) that seem to initiate sarcomagenesis; and (3) complex genetic alternations reflected by multiple genetic losses and gains (complex karyotypes).

Genetic syndromes associated with sarcoma

Familial gastrointestinal stromal tumor syndrome. GIST is the most common mesenchymal neoplasm of the gastrointestinal tract and is highly resistant to conventional chemotherapy. A leading hypothesis is that GISTs arise from the interstitial cells of Cajal or that they share a common stem cell [60]. Approximately 75% to 80% of GISTs have c-kit mutations [61,62]. Most of these mutations involve exon 11 and consist of in-frame deletions, insertions, missense mutations, or combinations thereof. Mutations also occur in exons 8, 9, 13, and 17. Advances in understanding the molecular biology of these tumors have facilitated the development of targeted therapy using imatinib mesylate and its derivatives. Causative factors have not been identified, although NF-1 confers an increased risk for developing GIST as do as two other tumor syndromes: Carney's triad [63,64] and familial GIST syndrome [65–67]. Only familial GIST syndrome is associated with

Table 4
Inherited diseases that commonly predispose to development of sarcoma

Disease	Gene	Location	Function
BS	BLM(RecQL3)	15q26.1	DNA helicase
Familial GIST	KIT	4q12	Receptor tyrosinase kinase
FH leiomyosarcoma and renal cell carcinoma syndrome	FH	1q43	FH
LFS	P53	17p13.1	DNA damage response
Neurofibromatosis	NF1	17q11.2	GTPase-activator
Rb	RB1	13q14.2	Cell cycle checkpoint
RTS	RTS (RecQL4)	18q24.3	DNA helicase
WS	WRN(RecQL2)	8p12-p11.2	DNA helicase Exonuclease activity

Abbreviations: BS, bloom syndrome; FH, fumarate hydratase; LFS, Li-Fraumeni syndrome; Rb, retinoblastoma; RTS, Rothmund-Thompson syndrome; WS, Werner syndrome.

activating mutations in *KIT* or *PDGFRA*. Several inherited mutations in exon 8, exon 11, exon 13, and exon 17 of *KIT* and in exon 12 of *PDGFRA* have been identified [65,66].

These mutations result in constitutive kinase activation and tumorigenesis. Affected individuals can develop many GISTs originating from the stomach and the small bowel during childhood and early adulthood. Diffuse hyperplasia of the interstitial cells of Cajal often is evident in the adjacent gut wall. The molecular basis of GIST and all other aspects of the disease is discussed elsewhere in this issue.

Li-Fraumeni syndrome and germline mutations in p53. LFS is one of the first familial cancer syndromes to have been described. After the initial description, based on four families in which siblings or first cousins had a pediatric sarcoma and a parent who had early-onset cancer [68], the authors defined the classical LFS as follows: a proband who had a sarcoma diagnosed before 45 years of age and a first-degree relative who had any cancer under 45 years of age and a first- or second-degree relative who had any cancer under 45 years of age or a sarcoma at any age [69]. Germline mutations in the p53 tumor suppressor gene are observed in LFS; somatic mutations in the p53 gene are observed in 30% to 60% of STSs [70,71]. In addition to sarcomas, these patients tend to develop a variety of tumors, including breast, brain, and adrenocortical tumors, and leukemias. The p53 protein is a transcription factor that normally inhibits cell growth and stimulates cell death when induced by cellular stress [72,73]. After DNA damage, p53 up-regulates p21, which binds to cyclin complexes, transiently arresting cell division [74]. In cases of severe damage to DNA, p53 activation is prolonged and induces cellular apoptosis [75]. Most of the described mutations in p53 are loss of function mutations that block this important pathway to apoptosis, but certain mutations may induce gain of function, although this is not well understood [76].

Aberrations in multiple regulators and effectors of p53 have been found to play a role in sarcoma development. One of the better-known regulators is the mouse double minute 2 (MDM2), a nuclear phosphoprotein that is a key regulator of cell growth and death and plays a pivotal role in the transformation of normal cells into tumor cells [77]. The MDM2 gene is located at 12q13-q14. The MDM2 protein can inactivate p53 by binding to pRB. MDM2 itself is up-regulated by p53 and can act in a negative feedback manner, blocking the activity of p53 by causing it to be ubiquinated and degraded; MDM2 also can decrease the levels of p53 at the transcriptional level. Overexpression of MDM2 is observed in a variety of sarcomas [78]; significant amplification of the MDM2 locus with subsequent protein overexpression is a hallmark of well-differentiated liposarcomas and has diagnostic implications [79,80]. MDM2 also is overexpressed in osteosarcomas and its overexpression correlates with recurrence and metastasis [81].

Neurofibromatosis. Patients who have neurofibromatosis are prone to develop malignant peripheral nerve sheath tumors (MPNST), with a cumulative lifetime risk of up to 10% [82]. Although a variety of clinical subgroups are described, type 1 and type 2 account for 99% of cases. NF-1, or von Recklinghausen's disease, is an autosomal dominant process that can disrupt the function of the *NF1* gene located at 17q11.2. Neurofibromin, the gene product, acts as a tumor suppressor via stimulation of guanosine triphosphatase (GTPase) activity of the proto-oncogene Ras. Loss of neurofibromin is postulated to lead to functional up-regulation of the Ras pathway. *NF-1* neurofibromas and neurogenic sarcomas, compared with non–*NF-1* schwannomas, have markedly elevated levels of activated Ras. Moreover, increased Ras activity is associated with increased tumor vascularity in the *NF-1* neurogenic sarcomas, perhaps related to an increased vascular endothelial growth factor (VEGF) secretion [83]. Tumor progression often results from loss of heterozygosity at the wild-type *NF1* allele. Mutations in p53 often are seen in MPNST, leading to increased cell survival and genomic instability that likely work cooperatively with increased Ras activity in promoting tumor progression.

Retinoblastoma. Survivors of hereditary retinoblastoma (Rb), a rare childhood cancer of the eye, have an elevated risk for developing sarcomas (in particular osteosarcomas), brain cancer, or melanoma, whereas survivors who have nonhereditary Rb do not seem prone to secondary malignancies [84–87]. Secondary malignancies are particularly prevalent in prior radiation treatment fields for this disease, and this likely is a strong predisposing factor. Rb is caused by inactivating germline mutations in one allele of the *RB1* tumor suppressor gene; tumors emerge with loss of heterozygosity at the wild-type allele. Loss of *RB1* also commonly is found in sporadic osteosarcoma, which is the second most common tumor in Rb survivors; the incidence of osteosarcoma in Rb survivors is increased 500-fold compared with the general population [88].

RB1 is located at chromosome 13q14. The Rb protein, pRb, negatively regulates progression from G0/G1 into the S phase and is dysregulated in most human cancers [89]. During the G1 phase of cell cycle, pRb binds to E2F1, E2F2, and E2F3 transcription factors. Sequential hypophosphorylation of pRb by cyclin-dependent kinases results in release of the E2F and transcription of genes required for cell progression to S phase [89]. pRb also plays an important role in normal development. Transgenic mice lacking the Rb gene die early in utero, with defects in neurogenesis, erythropoiesis, myogenesis, and lens development. Surprisingly, no skeletal phenotype abnormalities have been observed in these mice. To date, there is no mouse model involving knockout of the RB gene that results in osteosarcoma. Although much is known about the role of Rb in cell cycle biology, some of its functions in cancer development are yet to be determined.

Werner syndrome. Werner syndrome (WS) is a rare autosomal recessive disease. Patients seem normal until the second decade of life, when they develop pathologies that mimic many aspects of normal human aging, including ischemic heart disease, alopecia, osteoporosis, bilateral ocular cataracts, type 2 diabetes mellitus, and hypogonadism [90]. Patients who have WS also experience an increased risk for developing rare nonepithelial cancers, especially mesenchymal tumors, such as sarcomas [91]. Death usually occurs in the fourth decade from cardiovascular compromise or cancer. Fibroblasts isolated from patients who have WS characteristically senesce prematurely in culture [92] and display increased chromosomal aberrations [93]. WS is caused by mutation of a single gene, *WRN* (8p12-p11.2). *WRN* encodes a protein containing a highly conserved 3' to 5' DNA helicase domain of the RecQ family [94]. The RecQ helicase family members are involved in diverse biochemical processes, including DNA recombination, replication, and repair, and *WRN* is implicated in all of these processes [95]. *WRN* also interacts with many factors that participate in diverse aspects of DNA metabolism that are beyond the scope of this review. Sarcoma (20%), melanoma, and thyroid cancer constitute 57% of all cancers in WS [91]. When the *WRN* gene was disrupted in mice, the human disease phenotype was not observed; these mice did not age prematurely and were not predisposed to cancer, thus do not represent a good model of the human disease [96]. When these mice were crossed with p53 null mice, tumors grew remarkably faster in the p53 null/Wrn mutant mice compared with p53 null mice. These crossed mice also were distinguished by the variety of tumors they developed compared with those that developed in p53 null mice [97]. Unusual sarcomas of the mouth, including the salivary glands, were noticed in the p53 null/Wrn mutant mice. Such tumors included rare pericytoma, spindle cell sarcoma, and chondrosarcoma.

Two other intriguing members of the RecQ helicase family are Bloom syndrome (BS) gene (*BLM*) and Rothmund-Thomson syndrome gene (*RTS*). Mutations of *BLM* and *RTS* result in BS and Rothmund-Thomson syndrome (RTS), which are associated with genomic instability [98] (discussed later). The spectrum of sarcomas seen in these syndromes includes those sarcomas associated with complex cytogenetics, as might be expected from their underlying genetic mechanisms.

Bloom syndrome. BS is a rare human autosomal recessive disorder characterized by marked genetic instability associated with a greatly increased predisposition to a wide range of cancers, including sarcoma [99]. BS occurs most commonly in the Ashkenazi Jewish population as a result of an apparent founder effect. The *BLM* gene on chromosome 15q26.1 was identified as encoding a RecQ DNA helicase. Multiple mutations have been identified, with Ashkenazi Jewish patients who have BS almost exclusively homozygous for a complex frameshift mutation [100]. Cells from patients who have BS have a mutator phenotype and display many cytogenetic abnormalities, including increased chromosome breaks, symmetric quadriradial chromatid interchanges between homologous chromosomes, and sister chromatid exchanges (SCEs). The hallmark of BS cells and the standard criterion for BS diagnosis is the approximately 10-fold higher frequency of SCEs seen in BS cells as compared with normal cells [101]. *BLM* also interacts with topoisomerase III alpha (TOP3A) located on chromosome

17p12-p11.2, a region amplified in 68% of high-grade osteosarcomas [102]. Blm^{m3}/Blm^{m3} (a mutant variant of the mouse homolog of human *BLM*) is prone to a wide variety of cancers. Cell lines from these mice show elevations in the rates of mitotic recombination. The increased loss of heterozygosity rate resulting from mitotic recombination in vivo may constitute the underlying mechanism causing tumor susceptibility in these mice [103].

Rothmund-Thompson syndrome. RTS is a rare autosomal recessive disease associated with an increased risk for developing skin cancer; osteosarcoma is the second most frequently reported malignancy in this syndrome [104–106]. Children who have RTS typically present with a characteristic skin rash (poikiloderma), small stature, and skeletal dysplasias. Mutations in the *RecQ4* gene, encoding a RecQ DNA helicase, are reported in a few patients who have RTS. The *RecQ4* gene is located at chromosome 8q24.3, a frequent site of amplification in osteosarcoma adjacent to the *MYC* gene. RecQ4 does not seem to be a frequent target for somatic mutations in sporadic osteosarcoma. Transgenic mice homozygous for loss of RecQ4 gene function display defects of skin and skeleton and have a predisposition to lymphomas and osteosarcomas [104].

Fumarate hydratase leiomyosarcoma and renal cell carcinoma syndrome. Heterozygous germline mutation in fumarate hydratase (FH), a tumor suppressor gene that encodes the Krebs cycle and is located at 1q43, is known to cause hereditary leiomyomatosis and renal cell cancer (HLRCC) [107]. This rare syndrome is characterized by leiomyomas of the skin and uterus and less frequently occurring renal cell carcinomas [108,109]. These patients also are predisposed to developing leiomyosarcoma at various sites, most often the uterus [110]. Most HLRCC tumors overexpress hypoxia-inducible factor (HIF) 1α and its target genes, such as VEGF and BNIP3, and have increased vascularity in comparison to their sporadic counterparts [111,112]. It recently was shown in a mouse model that pseudohypoxic drive, resulting from HIF1α (and HIF2α) overexpression, is a direct consequence of Fh1 inactivation [113]. This model may be useful for testing future therapeutic interventions that target angiogenesis and HIF-prolyl hydroxylation.

Discrete genetic alternations-fusion genes

Nonrandom chromosomal translocations comprise the majority of currently recognized discrete genetic alternations associated with sarcoma (Table 5). As a result of such translocations, two genes are fused and a chimeric protein is formed (ESs as the paradigm of this process) (Fig. 4). These translocations often, but not always, involve genes encoding transcription factors in one or both of the breakpoints, often with one gene contributing a DNA-binding domain and the other providing an activation domain. Therefore, the fusion proteins often are aberrant transcription factors that dysregulate gene expression [114]. This results in various alternations in key cellular pathways, such as cell cycle control, apoptosis, and

Table 5
Cytogenetic and molecular alternations in sarcoma

Complex molecular/cytogenetic profile	Cytogenetic alternations	Molecular alternations
Angiosarcoma	Complex	
Chondrosarcoma	Complex	
Leiomyosarcoma	Complex (frequent deletion of 1p)	
MPNST	Complex	
Osteosarcoma	Complex	
Pleomorphic rhabdomyosarcoma	Complex	
Pleomorphic sarcoma, NOS (MFH)	Complex	
Simple molecular/cytogenetic profile		
Alveolar rhabdomyosarcoma	t(2;13)(q35;q14)	*PAX3-FOXO1A* fusion
	t(1;13)(p36;q14), double minutes	*PAX7-FOXO1A* fusion
	t(2;2)(q35;p23)	*PAX3-NCOA1* fusion
	t(X;2)(q35;q13)	*PAX3-AFX* fusion
Alveolar soft part sarcoma	t(X;17)(p11;q25)	*TFE3- ASPSCR1* fusion
Angiomatoid fibrous histiocytoma	t(12;16)(q13;p11)	*EWSR1-CREB1* fusion
	t(12;22)(q13;q12)	*FUS-ATF1* fusion
	t(2;22)(q33;q12)	*EWSR1-ATF1* fusion
Embryonal rhabdomyosarcoma	Trisomies 2q, 8 and 20	*Loss of heterozigosity at 11p15*
Clear cell sarcoma	t(12;22)(q13;q12)	*EWSR1-ATF1* fusion
	t(2;22)(q33;q12)	*EWSR1-CREB1* fusion
Desmoids fibromatosis	Trisomies 8 and 20 and loss of 5q21	*CTNNB1 or APC mutation*
Desmoplastic small round cell tumor	t(11;22)(p13;q12)	*EWSR1-WT1* fusion
Dermatofibrosarcoma protuberans	Ring form of chromosomes 17 and 22	*COL1A1-PDGFB* fusion
Endometrial stromal sarcoma	t(7;17)(p15;q21)	*JAZF1-JJAZ1* fusion
	t(6;7)(p21;p15)	*JAZF1-PHF1* fusion
	t(6;10)(p21;p11)	*EPC1-PHF1* fusion
Epitheloid hemangioendothelioma	t(1;3)(p36;7p25)	*Unknown fusion*

ES/primitive neuroectodermal tumor	t(11;22)(q24;q12)	*EWSR1-FLI1* fusion
	t(21;22)(q12;q12)	*EWSR1-ERG* fusion
	t(2;22)(q33;q12)	*EWSR1-FEV* fusion
	t(7;22)(p22;q12)	*EWSR1-ETV* fusion
	t(17;22)(q12;q12)	*EWSR1-E1AF* fusion
	inv(22)(q12;q12)	*EWSR1-ZSG* fusion
	t(2;22)(q31;q12)	*EWSR1-SP3* fusion
	t(16;21)(p11;q22)	*FUS-ERG* fusion
	t(2;16)(q33;p11)	*FUS-FEV* fusion
Extraskeletal myxoid chondrosarcoma	t(9;22)(q22;q12)	*EWSR1-NR4A3* fusion
	t(9;17)(q22;q11)	*TAF2N-NR4A3* fusion
	t(9;15)(q22;q21)	*TCF12-NR4A3* fusion
	t(3;9)(q11;q22)	*TFG-NR4A3* fusion
Fibrosarcoma, infantile	t(12;15)(p13;q26)	*ETV6-NTRK3* fusion
	Trisomies 8, 11, 17 and 20	
GIST	Monosomies 14 and 22	*KIT* mutation
	Deletion of 1p	
Inflammatory myofibroblastic tumor	t(1;2)(q22;p23)	*TPM3-ALK* fusion
	t(2;19)(p23;p13)	*TPM4-ALK* fusion
	t(2;17)(p23;q23)	*CLTC-ALK* fusion
	t(2;2)(p23;q13)	*RANB2-ALK* fusion
Low-grade fibromyxoid sarcoma	t(7;16)(q33;p11)	*FUS-CREB3L2* fusion
	t(11;16)(p11;p11)	*FUS-CREB3L1* fusion
Myxoid/round cell liposarcoma	t(12;16)(q13;p11)t	*FUS-DDIT3* fusion
	(12;22)(q13;q12)	*EWSR1-DDIT3* fusion
Myxofibrosarcoma (myxoid MFH)	Ring form of chromosome 12	
Synovial sarcoma		
Biphasic	t(x;18)(p11;q11)	Predominately *SS18-SSX1* fusion
Monophasic	t(x;18)(p11;q11)	*SS18-SSX1*, *SS18-SSX2* or *SSX4* fusion
Well-differentiated liposarcoma	Ring form of chromosome 12	Others

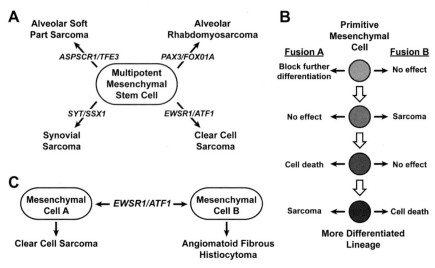

Fig. 4. The cytogenetics of ES. (*A*) Simple karyotype demonstrates the translocation between chromosomes 11 and 22 that is characteristic of ES. (*B*) This idiotype shows the breakpoints and derivative chromosomes. The active fusion transcript is produced from the derivative chromosome 22. This can be exploited diagnostically using fluorescent in-situ hybridization (FISH) to demonstrate re-arrangement of the 22q12 *EWSR1* (22q12) locus. Red centromeric probes and green telomeric probes appear yellow because of spectral overlap when the locus is intact; two yellow signals are present in an intact nucleus as demonstrated in the DAPI-stained nuclei (black background). Upon re-arrangement, the red probe is retained on the derivative chromosome 22 and the green probe is translocated to the reciprocal chromosome, derivative 11 in this example. Thus, a re-arranged locus leads to a nucleus generating three signals: yellow, red, and green. This approach can be used to detect reciprocal translocation involving the *EWSR1* locus but does not provide information regarding the identity of the reciprocal chromosome.

differentiation. Fusion proteins are considered oncogenic as they are able to transform cells in culture [115–117]. This is supported by the fact that specific fusion genes are required for in vitro growth of corresponding cell lines. Moreover, subcutaneous injection of transfected cells into immunodeficient mice can result in tumor formation [118,119]. There is a caveat, however; it seems that only specific cell types are susceptible to the transforming effects of fusion proteins. Gene fusions may modify the phenotype of a specific particular mesenchymal cell or precursor (Fig. 5A). This phenomenon could represent a type of lineage-dependent oncogenesis, as described by Garraway and Sellers [120]. It may explain the difficulty of creating a transgenic mouse model using fusion genes. Although it does not clearly replicate the human disease completely, the recently reported transgenic mouse model for synovial sarcoma [121,122] was predicated on the precise expression of the fusion gene in a specific myogenic precursor cell compartment present at a specific time in development. Thus, it seems that the fusion gene must be present in a particular place and time for tumorigenesis to occur (Fig. 5B). Others have shown that mesenchymal progenitor cells can be

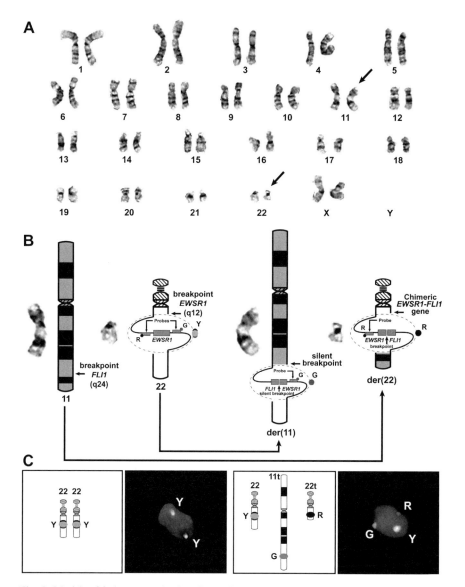

Fig. 5. Models of fusion transcript function. It is unclear how fusion transcripts cause sarcomas and whether or not these are sufficient for tumorigenesis. (*A*) A primitive mesenchymal cell could be capable of producing multiple sarcoma types given the right genetic events. Cell culture data indicates that this conception may be too simplistic. (*B*) It is possible that only specific cells types are susceptible to transformation via a fusion transcript within a mesenchymal lineage. The expression of the same fusion transcript in different (albeit related) cells may have different consequences. Thus, different fusion transcripts may have different effects in the same cells. There is some support for this theory provided by recent developed alveolar rhabdomyosarcoma and synovial sarcoma transgenic mouse models. (*C*) In certain cases, the same fusion transcript can be encountered in more than one mesenchymal neoplasm as seen with the *EWSR1/ATF1* gene fusion that can be associated with clear cell sarcoma and angiomatoid fibrous histiocytoma (the related *EWSR1/CREB1* fusion can act in similar fashion). Presumably, different tumors arise from different precursors, although alternative genetic events also could play a role.

transformed and show some features of myxoid liposarcoma when fused in sarcoma (FUS-CHOP) is expressed, but expression of other fusion genes was not successful in inducing transformation [123].

A transgenic mouse model of myxoid liposarcoma using translocated in sarcoma (TLS-CHOP) produced adipocytic tumors that lacked important histologic features of myxoid liposarcoma; although the chimeric gene was expressed in virtually all cells in the animal, no other neoplastic growths were encountered [124]. Attempts to create other models have failed [125], perhaps because of improper cell targeting or because other genes are necessary to help promote tumorigenesis.

Alveolar rhabdomyosarcomas have been shown to occur at low frequency in a transgenic mouse model using a conditional PAX3/FOXO1A knock-in allele. A low rate of tumor occurrence was remarkably increased by crosses with animals carrying mutations in other loci, perhaps indicating that fusion genes per se are not always sufficient for malignant transformation. It is likely that multiple collaborators are essential for oncogenesis, rather than assuming that a single genetic alternation causes cancer; alternatively, the cellular compartment also may be critical (discussed previously). A *Drosophila* genetic model for PAX7-FOXO1A–associated alveolar rhabdomyosarcoma again underscores the importance of the mutation occurring in a specific myocyte precursor compartment [126]. Many of the translocation-associated sarcomas are found in younger patients and this could be the result of a presumably increased stem or mesenchymal precursor cell compartment associated with growing individuals. Finally, the presumed importance of cell of origin is underscored as exemplified by clear cell sarcoma and angiomatoid fibrous histiocytoma (Fig. 5C). Both can be associated with an EWSR1-ATF1 gene fusion, but the biologic potential and gene expression profiles of these two tumors are remarkably different, perhaps indicating that the initiating cell where the fusion event occurs determines the biology of the subsequent tumor [127]. In the synovial sarcoma mouse model (discussed previously), expression of the SYT-SSX2 fusion transcript-induced myopathy without tumorigenesis in more differentiation myoid precursor cells.

ES serves as a model of the association between fusion genes and cancer development. ES was the first solid tumor noted to have a recurrent translocation identified where the significance of this finding was determined at the molecular level. The first described fusion involved the of *EWSR1* (22q12) and *FLI1*(11q24) genes (see Fig. 4) [116]. *FLI1* is a member of the ETS family of transcription factors and EWSR1 encodes a nuclear protein with unknown function. The fusion protein is comprised of the N-terminal portion of the EWSR1 protein linked to the DNA-binding domain of FLI1. The chimeric protein has transforming activity in cell cultures assays [128] and seems to be the principal event leading to the development of ES. The chimeric protein transforms cells mainly through transcriptional dysregulation. The presence of the fusion transcript invokes an extensive program of altered gene expression that leads to tumorigenesis. Knocking down

EWS/FLI in A673 cells using small hairpin RNA (shRNA) inhibits their transformed phenotype [128]. NKX2.2 is an oncogene from the homeobox family gene that is highly expressed in ES cells. Silencing NKX2.2 in A673 cells causes loss of tumorigenicity in mice, suggesting that NKX2.2 is a key downstream mediator of *EWSR1/FLI1* transformation. Forced expression of NKX2.2 is not sufficient to rescue *EWSR1/FLI1* silencing in A673 cells; therefore, NKX2.2 is essential but not sufficient for cancer development [129]. The ES as a model of cancer development from a known translocation demonstrates a complex pathway involving multiple mediators rather than a single discrete mutation that transforms the cells. The discovery of these key mediators may provide additional therapeutic targets. Fusion genes also are classical potential targets for anticancer therapy. This therapy could be accomplished through direct inhibition of the fusion transcript or perhaps by inhibition of a more amenable critical downstream mediator. Understanding of resultant cellular effects is only partially elucidated and the underlying mechanisms of derangement are yet to be defined. It is now appreciated that although EWSR1/FLI1 is the most common translocation in ES, it is only one of nine types currently described (see Table 4). Other members of the ETS family can substitute for *FLI1,* and the homolog *FUS* can substitute for *EWSR1* on rare occasion. All of these non-*FLI1* variants are extremely rare (less than 1%) other than the *EWSR1-ERG* variant. Within the *EWSR1-FLI1* group, various breakpoints in the introns of these two genes can lead to many fusion transcript structures; however, there are two that predominate, type 1 and type 2 (Fig. 6). In addition, *EWSR1* and *FUS* are involved in translocations in multiple other sarcoma subtypes where they interact with various fusion partners (Fig. 7). In general, *EWSR1* seems to provide an activation domain whereas the fusion partner provides the DNA-binding domain and thus determines what spectrum of genes is dysregulated in each specific tumor type.

Complex genetic alternations. This group of sarcomas includes leiomyosarcoma, osteosarcoma, MFH, angiosarcoma, pleomorphic rhabdomyosarcoma, chondrosarcoma, and MPNST. These diverse tumors are characterized by the presence of highly complex unbalanced karyotypes lacking specific genetic translocations (Fig. 8A). Disruption of normal p53 function is assumed to play a key role in these nonspecific aberrations. In contrast, p53 inactivation is rarely found in sarcomas with discrete genetic alternations. Two pathways are implicated in the generation of complex genetic alternations in sarcomas: telomere dysfunction and impaired joining of nonhomologous ends (NHEJ).

Artandi and colleagues [130] showed an increased rate of epithelial carcinomas in mice lacking the RNA component of telomerase. Telomeres comprise the nucleoprotein complexes that cap the ends of eukaryotic chromosomes and are maintained by the reverse transcriptase telomerase, which adds hexanucleotide repeats to existing telomeres. Lack of telomerase

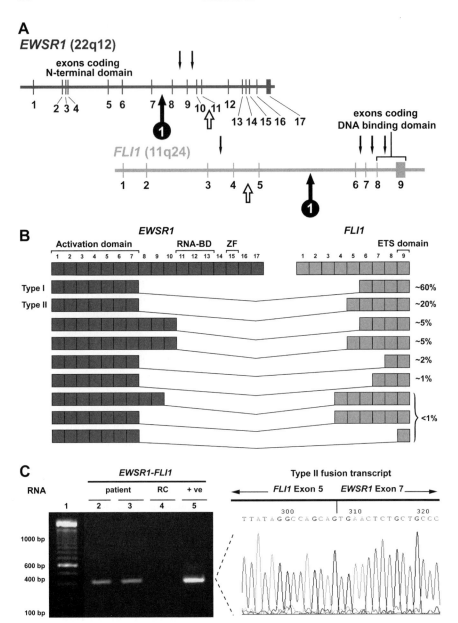

Fig. 6. The genetics of ES. (*A*) The gene structures of *EWSR1* and *FLI1* with the most common breakpoints marked below the genes with arrows and other breakpoints above. (*B*) Exon structures with domains mapped showing that fusion transcripts retain the transcriptional activation domain of *EWSR1* and the ETS DNA-binding domain of *FLI1*, thereby producing an aberrant transcription factor. (*C*) These fusion transcripts can be detected by reverse transcription polymerase chain reaction in the diagnostic setting. It is important to confirm the identity of the amplicons by direct DNA sequencing.

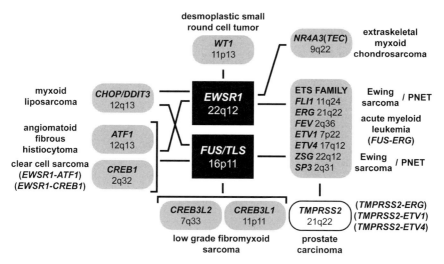

Fig. 7. Gene fusions in sarcoma involving *EWSR1* and *FUS*. *EWSR1* is the most commonly used gene fusion partner in sarcoma combining with multiple genes to produce multiple sarcomas. *FUS* sometimes can substitute for *EWSR1* and vice versa. It is unclear if the prevalence of *EWSR1* results from unique biologic potential, increased propensity for re-arrangement, or perhaps both possibilities. *FUS-ERG* translocations also are documented in acute myeloid leukemia, and fusion genes in prostate carcinoma also can use the ETS family of genes as fusion partners.

activity leads to progressive telomere shortening and ultimately chromosomal instability (end-to-end fusions) as a function of age and successive cell divisions. In the presence of a functional p53/Rb pathway, these cells typically undergo apoptosis as a protective function against severe genetic instability. Abrogation of these pathways is important for tumor cell survival (Fig. 8B). This chromosomal complexity may provide the genetic fodder for selection of a more aggressive tumor phenotype. Ultimately, telomere maintenance usually is recovered at some point as continuous genetic instability becomes counterproductive. This reactivation promotes tumor survival, or immortality, as it sometimes is termed. More recently, a telomerase-independent mechanism has been described in tumors and is termed, alternative lengthening of telomeres (ALT). Although not well understood at the mechanistic level, this pathway seems to be common in sarcoma [131]. Either telomerase itself or ALT apparently are used as a method of telomere maintenance in sarcoma and associated with tumor progression in multiple studies.

p53 mutation may be a common early event in sarcomas with complex nondiscrete gene alternations. Inactivation of p53 may disable cellular defense mechanisms against tumorigenicity that is triggered by telomeric dysfunction and NHEJ.

In telomerase-deficient *p53* mutant mice, the development of epithelial cancers has been promoted by a process of fusion-bridge breakage (BFB).

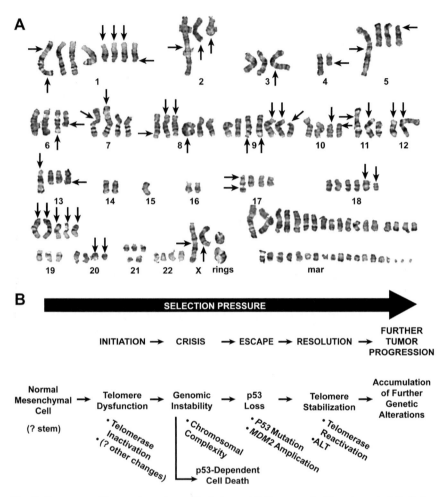

Fig. 8. Sarcomas with complex cytogenetic features. (*A*) Sarcomas lacking characteristic fusion events often show complex karyotypes with chromosomal aneuploidy and nonspecific fusion effects as seen in this high-grade sarcoma. (*B*) A model for tumorigenesis involves telomere dysfunction, resulting in genomic instability, which is rescued with p53 loss of function and telomere stabilization under constant selection pressure. (*Karyotype courtesy of* Dr. Andre Oliveira, Mayo Clinic, Rochester, MN.)

Such BFB events lead to the formation of complex nonreciprocal translocations, a classical cytogenetic feature of human carcinomas. Glisselsson and colleagues [132] have shown a high frequency of BFB events in human sarcoma specimens lacking simple tumor-specific aberrations. In contrast, elevated BFB events have not been observed in any of the cases carrying a fusion gene mutation. ALT is associated with chromosomal instability in osteosarcomas [133], again supporting the role of telomere dysfunction in the development of nondiscrete complex genetic alternations.

In a study examining the impact of haploinsufficiency of a NHEJ component (DNA ligase IV [lig4]) on murine tumorigenesis, lig4 heterozygosity was found to promote the development of STSs possessing clonal amplifications, deletions, and translocations. These genomic alterations were associated with frequent MDM2 amplification. Taken together, these findings support the contention that loss of a single lig4 allele results in NHEJ activity being sufficiently reduced to allow creation of chromosomal aberrations that drive sarcoma tumorigenesis [134].

Summary

Sarcomas are a markedly heterogeneous group of tumors that may have many etiologies. The incidence of different histologic subtypes differs significantly between children and adults. There is an increase in the incidence of sarcoma in the United States that may be the result of improved registry systems, diagnostic tools, and pathologic definitions rather than reflecting a true increase of the disease. Various environmental etiologies, however, also may contribute to a true increased sarcoma incidence in the United States population (eg, use of radiotherapy in cancer patients, immune suppression due to AIDS/solid organ transplants, and exposure to pesticides/herbicides). Genetic alternations, germline or somatic, also may play a key role in the development of sarcoma. As a result of rapidly evolving high throughput of genomic and proteomic technologies, increased knowledge of the oncogenic mechanisms underlying human sarcomagenesis is being generated. Of particular interest are fusion genes, which are sarcoma subtype specific and therefore may be useful as molecular targets for diagnosis and treatment. Understanding of the complex cellular and molecular mechanisms that are involved in sarcomagenesis, however, is still rudimentary at best. We can only hope that future enhanced insight into the molecular basis of sarcoma inception, proliferation, and dissemination ultimately leads to markedly more effective targeted therapies for patients burdened by this all too often devastating malignant disease.

References

[1] Association of Directors of anatomic and Surgical Pathology. Perspectives in pathology: recommendations for the reporting of soft tissue sarcomas. Hum Pathol 1999;30:3–7.

[2] Toro JR, Travis LB, Wu HJ, et al. Incidence patterns of soft tissue sarcomas, regardless of primary site, in the Surveillance, Epidemiology and End Results program, 1978–2001: an analysis of 26,758 cases. Int J Cancer 2006;119:2922–30.

[3] Coindre JM, Terrier P, Guillou L, et al. Predictive value of grade metastasis development in the main histologic types of adult soft tissue sarcomas: a study of 1240 patients from the French Federation of Cancer Centers Sarcoma Group. Cancer 2001;91:1914–8.

[4] Brennan M, Alektiar KM, Maki RG. Soft tissue sarcoma. In: DeVita VT, Hellmann S, Rosenberg SA, editors. Cancer: principles and practice of oncology. 6th edition. Philadelphia: Lippincott Williams & Wilkins; 2001. p. 1844–91.

[5] Greenlee RT, Hill-Harmon MB, Murray T, et al. Cancer statistics, 2001. CA Cancer J Clin 2001;51:15–36.

[6] Zahm SH, Fraumeni JF Jr. The epidemiology of soft tissue sarcoma. Semin Oncol 1997;24: 504–14.

[7] Cameron J. Current surgical therapy. 8th edition. Philadelphia: Mosby; 2004.

[8] Jemal A, Siegel R, Ward E, et al. Cancer statistics, 2006. CA Cancer J Clin 2006;56:106–30.

[9] Jemal A, Siegel R, Ward E, et al. Cancer statistics, 2007. CA Cancer J Clin 2007;57:43–66.

[10] Arndt CAS, Crist WM. Common musculoskeletal tumors of childhood and adolescence. N Engl J Med 1999;341:342–52.

[11] Carola AS. Soft tissue sarcoma. In: Brehman RE, Kliegman RM, Jenson HB, editors. Nelson: textbook of pediatrics. 17th edition. Philadelphia: Elsevier Science; 2004. p. 1714–7.

[12] Gurney JG, Swensen AR, Bultery M. Malignant bone tumors. Cancer incidence and survival among children and adolescents: United States SEER program 1975–1995. Bethesda (MD): National cancer institute, SEER program; 1999. p. 99–110.

[13] Frischi L, Coates M, McCredie M. Incidence of cancer among New South Wales adolescents: which classification scheme describes adolescents better? Int J Cancer 1995;60: 355–60.

[14] Surveillance, Epidemiology, and End Results (SEER) Program. Available at: www.seer.cancer.gov. Accessed September 15, 2007.

[15] Pisters PW, O'Sullivan B, Maki RG, et al. Soft tissue sarcomas. In: Kufe DW, Bast RC, Hait WN, editors. Cancer medicine. 7th edition. Hamilton, Ontario: BC Decker; 2006. p. 1694–720.

[16] Martland HS. Occupational poisoning in manufacture of luminous watch dials. JAMA 1929;92:466–73.

[17] Brady MS, Gaynor JJ, Brennan MF. Radiation-associated sarcoma of bone and soft tissue. Arch Surg 1992;127:1379–85.

[18] Cha C, Antonescu CR, Quan ML, et al. Long-term results with resection of radiation-induced soft tissue sarcomas. Ann Surg 2004;239:903–10.

[19] Stinchcombe TE, Walters R, Khandani AH, et al. Radiation-induced sarcoma after high-dose thoracic radiation therapy in non–small-cell lung cancer. J Clin Oncol 2007;25:1621–3.

[20] Davidson T, Westbury G, Harmer CL. Radiation-induced soft-tissue sarcoma. Br J Surg 1986;73:308–9.

[21] Huvos AG, Woodard HQ, Cahan WG, et al. Postradiation osteogenic sarcoma of bone and soft tissues. A clinicopathologic study of 66 patients. Cancer 1985;55:1244–55.

[22] Pierce SM, Recht A, Lingos TI, et al. Long-term radiation complications following conservative surgery (CS) and radiation therapy (RT) in patients with early stage breast cancer. Int J Radiat Oncol Biol Phys 1992;23:915–23.

[23] Wiklund TA, Blomqvist CP, Raty J, et al. Postirradiation sarcoma. Analysis of a nationwide cancer registry material. Cancer 1991;68:524–31.

[24] Karlsson P, Holmberg E, Samuelsson A, et al. Soft tissue sarcoma after treatment for breast cancer—a Swedish population-based study. Eur J Cancer 1998;34:2068–75.

[25] Tucker MA, D'Angio GJ, Boice JD Jr, et al. Bone sarcomas linked to radiotherapy and chemotherapy in children. N Engl J Med 1987;317:588–93.

[26] Cahan WG, Woodward HG, Higinbotham ND, et al. Sarcoma arising in irradiated bone: report of eleven cases. Cancer 1948;1:3–29.

[27] Arlen M, Higinbotham NL, Huvos HG, et al. Radiationinduced sarcoma of bone. Cancer 1971;28:1087–99.

[28] Falk H, Herbert J, Crowley S, et al. Epidemiology of hepatic angiosarcoma in the United States: 1964–1974. Environ Health Perspect 1981;41:107–13.

[29] Waxweiler RJ, Stringer W, Wagoner JK, et al. Neoplastic risk among workers exposed to vinyl chloride. Ann N Y Acad Sci 1976;271:40–8.

[30] Spirtas R, Kaminski R. Angiosarcoma of the liver in vinyl chloride/polyvinyl chloride workers—1977 update of the NIOSH register. J Occup Med 1978;10:427–9.

[31] Da Silva HJ, Da Motta LC, Tavares MH. Thorium dioxide effects in man-epidemiological, clinical and pathological studies (experience in Portugal). Environ Res 1974;8:131–59.

[32] Faber M. Twenty-eight years of continuous follow-up of patients injected with thorotrast for cerebral angiography. Environ Res 1979;18:37–43.

[33] Roth F. [Arsen Lebertumoren (Hemangioendotheliom)]. Z Krebsforsch 1957;61:468–503 [in German].

[34] Roth F. Delayed sequelae of chronic arsenism in vintners on the Moselle. Deutsche Medizinische Wochenschrift 1957;82:211–7 [German].

[35] Lander JJ, Stanley RJ, Sumner HW, et al. Angiosarcoma of the liver associated with Fowler's solution (potassium arsenite). Gastroenterology 1975;68:1582–6.

[36] Regelson W, Kim U, Ospina J, et al. Hemangioendothelial sarcoma of liver from chronic arsenic intoxication by Fowler's solution. Cancer 1968;21:514–22.

[37] Rennke H, Prat GA, Etcheverry RB, et al. Hemangioendothelioma maligno del higado y arsenicismo cronico. Rev Med Chil 1971;99:664–98.

[38] Sussman EB, Nydick I, Gray GF. Hemangioendothelial sarcoma of the liver and hemochromatosis. Arch Pathol 1974;97:39–42.

[39] Pimentel JC, Menezes AP. Liver disease in vineyard sprayers. Gastroenterology 1977;72: 275–83.

[40] Berk PD, Martin JF, Young RS, et al. Vinyl-chloride-associated liver disease. Ann Intern Med 1976;84:717–31, (1976).

[41] Falk H, Telles NC, Ishak KG, et al. Epidemiology of Thorotrast-induced hepatic angiosarcoma in the United States. Environ Res 1979;18:65–73.

[42] Falk H, Herbert JT, Edmonds L, et al. Review of 4 cases of childhood hepatic angiosarcoma-elevated environmental arsenic exposure in one case. Cancer 1981;47:382–91.

[43] Falk H, Thomas LB, Popper H, et al. Hepatic angiosarcoma associated with androgenic-anabolic steroids. Lancet 1979;2:1120–3.

[44] Zambon P, Ricci P, Bovo E, et al. Sarcoma risk and dioxin emissions from incinerators and industrial plants: a population-based case-control study (Italy). Environ Health 2007;16:6–19.

[45] Tuomisto JT, Pekkanen J, Kiviranta H, et al. Soft-tissue sarcoma and dioxin: a case-control study. Int J Cancer 2004;108:893–900.

[46] Kang H, Enzinger FM, Breslin P, et al. Soft tissue sarcoma and military service in Vietnam: a case- control study. J Natl Cancer Inst 1987;79:693–9.

[47] Rhodes MC, Bucher JR, Peckham JC, et al. Carcinogenesis studies of benzophenone in rats and mice. Food Chem Toxicol 2007;45:843–51.

[48] Hong HL, Ton TV, Devereux TR, et al. Chemical-specific alterations in ras, p53, and beta-catenin genes in hemangiosarcomas from B6C3F1 mice exposed to o-nitrotoluene or riddelliine for 2 years. Toxicol Appl Pharmacol 2003;191:227–34.

[49] Stewart FW, Treves N. Lymphangiosarcoma in post mastectomy lymphedema: a report of six cases of elephantiasis chirurgica. Cancer 1948;1:64–81.

[50] Woodward AH, Ivins JC, Soule EH. Lymphangiosarcoma arising in chronic lymphedematous extremities. Cancer 1972;30:562–72.

[51] Brand KG, Buoen LC, Brand I. Multiphasic incidence of foreign body-induced sarcomas. Cancer Res 1976;36:3681–3.

[52] Mutlu AD, Cavallin LE, Vincent L, et al. In vivo-restricted and reversible malignancy induced by human herpesvirus-8 KSHV: a cell and animal model of virally induced Kaposi's sarcoma. Cancer Cell 2007;11:245–58.

[53] Cattani P, Capuano M, Graffeo R, et al. Kaposi's sarcoma associated with previous human herpesvirus 8 infection in kidney transplant recipients. J Clin Microbiol 2001;39:506–10.

[54] Sarid R, Pizov G, Rubinger D, et al. Detection of human herpesvirus-8 DNA in kidney allografts prior to the development of Kaposi's sarcoma. Clin Infect Dis 2001;33:1502–5.

[55] Eltom MA, Jemal A, Mbulaiteye SM, et al. Trends in Kaposi's sarcoma and non-Hodgkin's lymphoma incidence in the United States from 1973 through 1998. J Natl Cancer Inst 2002; 94:1204–10.

[56] Penn I. Sarcomas in organ allograft recipients. Transplantation 1995;60:1485–91.

[57] Deyrup AT, Lee VK, Hill CE, et al. Epstein-Barr virus-associated smooth muscle tumors are distinctive mesenchymal tumors reflecting multiple infection events: a clinicopathologic and molecular analysis of 29 tumors from 19 patients. Am J Surg Pathol 2006;30:75–82.

[58] Nur S, Rosenblum WD, Katta UD, et al. Epstein-Barr virus-associated multifocal leiomyosarcomas arising in a cardiac transplant recipient: autopsy case report and review of the literature. J Heart Lung Transplant 2007;26(9):944–52.

[59] McClain KL, Leach CT, Jenson HB, et al. Association of Epstein–Barr virus with leiomyosarcomas in children with AIDS. N Engl J Med 1995;332:12–8.

[60] Rubin BP, Heinrich MC, Corless CL. Gastrointestinal stromal tumour. Lancet 2007;369: 1731–41.

[61] Heinrich MC, Corless CL, Demetri GD, et al. Kinase mutations and imatinib response in patients with metastatic gastrointestinal stromal tumor. J Clin Oncol 2003;21:4342–9.

[62] Hirota S, Isozaki K, Moriyama Y, et al. Gain-of-function mutations of c-kit in human gastrointestinal stromal tumors. Science 1998;279:577–80.

[63] Takazawa Y, Sakurai S, Sakuma Y, et al. Gastrointestinal stromal tumors of neurofi bromatosis type I (von Recklinghausen's disease). Am J Surg Pathol 2005;29:755–63.

[64] Yantiss RK, Rosenberg AE, Sarran L, et al. Multiple gastrointestinal stromal tumors in type I neurofibromatosis: a pathologic and molecular study. Mod Pathol 2005;18:475–84.

[65] Beghini A, Tibiletti MG, Roversi G, et al. Germline mutation in the juxtamembrane domain of the kit gene in a family with gastrointestinal stromal tumors and urticaria pigmentosa. Cancer 2001;92:657–62.

[66] Chompret A, Kannengiesser C, Barrois M, et al. PDGFRA germline mutation in a family with multiple cases of gastrointestinal stromal tumor. Gastroenterology 2004;126:318–21.

[67] Blume-Jensen P, Claesson-Welsh L, Siegbahn A, et al. Activation of the human c-kit product by ligand-induced dimerization mediates circular actin reorganization and chemotaxis. EMBO J 1991;10:4121–8.

[68] Li FP, Fraumeni JF Jr. Soft-tissue sarcomas, breast cancer, and other neoplasms. A familial syndrome? Ann Intern Med 1969;71:747–52.

[69] Li FP, Fraumeni JF Jr, Mulvihill JJ, et al. A cancer family syndrome in twenty-four kindreds. Cancer Res 1988;48:5358–62.

[70] Das P, Kotilingam D, Korchin B, et al. High prevalence of p53 exon 4 mutations in soft tissue sarcoma. Cancer 2007;109(11):2323–33.

[71] Hieken TJ, Das Gupta TK. Mutant p53 expression: a marker of diminished survival in well-differentiated soft tissue sarcoma. Clin Cancer Res 1996;2:1391–5.

[72] Vogelstein B, Lane D, Levine AJ. Surfing the p53 network. Nature 2000;408:307–10.

[73] Oren M. Decision making by p53: life, death and cancer. Cell Death Differ 2003;10:431–42.

[74] Vogelstein B, Kinzler KW. P53 function and dysfunction. Cell 1992;70:523–6.

[75] Levine AJ. P53, the cellular gate keeper for growth and division. Cell 1997;88:323–31.

[76] Lozano G. The oncogenic roles of p53 mutants in mouse models. Curr Opin Genet Dev 2007;17:66–70.

[77] Cordon-Cardo C, Latres E, Drobnjak M, et al. Molecular abnormalities of *mdm2* and *p53* genes in adult soft tissue sarcomas. Cancer Res 1994;54:794–9.

[78] Sherr CJ. Cancer cell cycles. Science 1996;274:1672–7.

[79] Singer S, Socci ND, Ambrosini G, et al. Gene expression profiling of liposarcoma identifies distinct biological types/subtypes and potential therapeutic targets in well-differentiated and dedifferentiated liposarcoma. Cancer Res 2007;67:6626–36.

[80] Shimada S, Ishizawa T, Ishizawa K, et al. The value of MDM2 and CDK4 amplification levels using real-time polymerase chain reaction for the differential diagnosis of liposarcomas and their histologic mimickers. Hum Pathol 2006;37:1123–9.

[81] Gisselsson D, Palsson E, Hoglund M, et al. Differentially amplified chromosome 12 sequences in low and high grade osteosarcoma. Genes Chromosomes Cancer 2002;33:133–40.

[82] Pollack IF, Mulvihill JJ. Neurofibromatosis 1 and 2. Brain Pathol 1997;7:823–36.

[83] Guha A. Ras activation in astrocytomas and neurofibromas. Can J Neurol Sci 1998;25: 267–81.

[84] Wong FL, Boice JD Jr, Abramson DH, et al. Cancer incidence after retinoblastoma. Radiation dose and sarcoma risk. JAMA 1997;278:1262–7.

[85] Moll AC, Imhof SM, Bouter LM, et al. Second primary tumors in hereditary retinoblastoma: a register-based follow-up study, 1945–1994. Int J Cancer 1996;67:515–9.

[86] Draper GJ, Sanders BM, Kingston JE. Second primary neoplasms in patients with retinoblastoma. Br J Cancer 1986;53:661–71.

[87] Derkinderen DJ, Koten JW, Nagelkerke ND, et al. Non-ocular cancer in patients with hereditary retinoblastoma and their relatives. Int J Cancer 1988;41:499–504.

[88] Hansen MF, Koufos A, Gallie BL, et al. Osteosarcoma and retinoblastoma: a shared chromosomal mechanism revealing recessive predisposition. Proc Natl Acad Sci U S A 1985;82: 6216–20.

[89] Weinberg RA. The retinoblastoma protein and cell cycle control. Cell 1995;81:323–30.

[90] Thannhauser SJ. Werner's syndrome (progeria of the adult) and Rothmund's syndrome: two types of closely related heredofamilial atrophic dermatosis with juvenile cataracts and endocrine features. A critical study with five new cases. Ann Intern Med 1945;23:559–625.

[91] Goto M, Miller RW, Ishikawa Y, et al. Excess of rare cancers in Werner syndrome (adult progeria). Cancer Epidemiol Biomarkers Prev 1996;5:239–46.

[92] Faragher RG, Kill IR, Hunter JA, et al. The gene responsible for Werner syndrome may be a cell division "counting" gene. Proc Natl Acad Sci U S A 1993;90:12030–4.

[93] Salk D, Au K, Hoehn H, et al. Cytogenetics of Werner's syndrome cultured skin fibroblasts: variegated translocation mosaicism. Cytogenet Cell Genet 1981;30:92–107.

[94] Martin GM, Oshima J. Lessons from human progeroid syndromes. Nature 2000;408: 263–6.

[95] Hickson ID. RecQ helicases: caretakers of the genome. Nat Rev Cancer 2003;3:169–78.

[96] Lebel M, Leder P. A deletion within the murine Werner syndrome helicase induces sensitivity to inhibitors of topoisomerase and loss of cellular proliferative capacity. Proc Natl Acad Sci U S A 1998;95:13097–102.

[97] Lebel M, Cardiff RD, Leder P. Tumorigenic effect of nonfunctional p53 or p21 in mice mutant in the Werner syndrome helicase. Cancer Res 2001;61:1816–9.

[98] Ellis NA, Groden J, Ye TZ, et al. The Bloom's syndrome gene product is homologous to RecQ helicases. Cell 1995;83:655–66.

[99] German J, Ellis NA. Bloom syndrome. In: Vogelstein B, Kinzler KW, editors. The genetic basis of human cancer. Columbus, OH: McGraw-Hill Companies; 1997. p. 733–51 (Chapter 30).

[100] Roa BB, Savino CV, Richards CS. Ashkenazi Jewish population frequency of the Bloom syndrome gene 2281 delta 6ins7 mutation. Genet Test 1999;3:219–21.

[101] Chaganti RSK, Schonberg S, German J. A manifold increase in sister chromatid exchanges in Bloom's syndrome lymphocytes. Proc Natl Acad Sci U S A 1974;71:4508–12.

[102] Wu L, Hickson ID. The Bloom's syndrome helicase suppresses crossing over during homologous recombination. Nature 2003;426:870–4.

[103] Luo G, Santoro IM, McDaniel LD, et al. Cancer predisposition caused by elevated mitotic recombination in Bloom mice. Nat Genet 2000;26:424–9.

[104] Kansara M, Thomas DM. Molecular pathogenesis of osteosarcoma. DNA Cell Biol 2007; 26:1–18.

[105] Nishijo K, Nakayama T, Aoyama T, et al. Mutation analysis of the RECQL4 gene in sporadic osteosarcomas. Int J Cancer 2004;111(3):367–72.

[106] Wang LL, Gannavarapu A, Kozinetz CA, et al. Association between osteosarcoma and deleterious mutations in the RECQL4 gene in Rothmund-Thomson syndrome. J Natl Cancer Inst 2003;95:669–74.

[107] Launonen V, Vierimaa O, Kiuru M, et al. Inherited susceptibility to uterine leiomyomas and renal cell cancer. Proc Natl Acad Sci U S A 2001;98:3387–92.

[108] Tomlinson IP, Alam NA, Rowan AJ, et al. Multiple Leiomyoma Consortium. Germline mutations in FH predispose to dominantly inherited uterine fibroids, skin leiomyomata and papillary renal cell cancer. Nat Genet 2002;30:406–10.

[109] Kiuru M, Launonen V, Hietala M, et al. Familial cutaneous leiomyomatosis is a two-hit condition associated with renal cell cancer of characteristic histopathology. Am J Pathol 2001;159:825–9.

[110] Lehtonen HJ, Kiuru M, Ylisaukko-Oja SK, et al. Increased risk of cancer in patients with fumarate hydratase germline mutation. J Med Genet 2006;43:523–6.

[111] Pollard PJ, Wortham N, Barclay E, et al. Evidence of increased microvessel density and activation of the hypoxia pathway in tumours from the hereditary leiomyomatosis and renal cell cancer syndrome. J Pathol 2005;205:41–9.

[112] Pollard PJ, Briere JJ, Alam NA, et al. Accumulation of Krebs cycle intermediates and overexpression of HIF1{alpha} in tumours which result from germline FH and SDH mutations. Hum Mol Genet 2005;14:2231–9.

[113] Pollard PJ, Spencer-Dene B, Shukla D, et al. Targeted inactivation of fh1 causes proliferative renal cyst development and activation of the hypoxia pathway. Cancer Cell 2007;11:303–5.

[114] Xia SJ, Barr FG. Chromosome translocations in sarcomas and the emergence of oncogenic transcription factors. Eur J Cancer 2005;41:2513–27.

[115] Scheidler S, Fredericks WJ, Rauscher FJ III, et al. The hybrid PAX3–FKHR fusion protein of alveolar rhabdomyosarcoma transforms fibroblasts in culture. Proc Natl Acad Sci U S A 1996;93:9805–9.

[116] May WA, Gishizky ML, Lessnick SL, et al. Ewing sarcoma 11;22 translocation produces a chimeric transcription factor that requires the DNA-binding domain encoded by FLI1 for transformation. Proc Natl Acad Sci U S A 1993;90:5752–6.

[117] Nagai M, Tanaka S, Tsuda M, et al. Analysis of transforming activity of human synovial sarcoma-associated chimeric protein SYT-SSX1 bound to chromatin remodeling factor hBRM/ hSNF2 alpha. Proc Natl Acad Sci U S A 2001;98:3843–8.

[118] Schwarzbach MH, Koesters R, Germann A, et al. Comparable transforming capacities and differential gene expression patterns of variant FUS/CHOP fusion transcripts derived from soft tissue liposarcomas. Oncogene 2004;23:6798–805.

[119] Arvand A, Welford SM, Teitell MA, et al. The COOH-terminal domain of FLI-1 is necessary for full tumourigenesis and transcriptional modulation by EWS/FLI-1. Cancer Res 2001;61:5311–7.

[120] Garraway LA, Sellers WR. Lineage dependency and lineage-survival oncogenes in human cancer. Nat Rev Cancer 2006;6:593–602.

[121] Haldar M, Hancock JD, Coffin CM, et al. A conditional mouse model of synovial sarcoma: insights into a myogenic origin. Cancer Cell 2007;11:375–88.

[122] Davis SR, Meltzer PS. Modeling synovial sarcoma: timing is everything. Cancer Cell 2007;11:305–7.

[123] Riggi N, Cironi L, Provero P, et al. Expression of the FUS-CHOP fusion protein in primary mesenchymal progenitor cells gives rise to a model of myxoid liposarcoma. Cancer Res 2006;66:7016–23.

[124] Perez-Losada J, Pintado B, Gutierrez-Adan A, et al. The chimeric FUS/TLS-CHOP fusion protein specifically induces liposarcomas in transgenic mice. Oncogene 2000;19:2413–22.

[125] Anderson MJ, Shelton GD, Cavenee WK, et al. Embryonic expression of the tumor-associated PAX3-FKHR fusion protein interferes with the developmental functions of Pax3. Proc Natl Acad Sci U S A 2001;98:1589–94.

[126] Galindo RL, Allport JA, Olson EN. A Drosophila model of the rhabdomyosarcoma initiator PAX7-FKHR. Proc Natl Acad Sci U S A 2006;103:13439–44.

[127] Antonescu CR, Dal Cin P, Nafa K, et al. EWSR1-CREB1 is the predominant gene fusion in angiomatoid fibrous histiocytoma. Genes Chromosomes Cancer 2007;46:1051–60.

[128] Davis S, Meltzer PS. Ewing's sarcoma: general insights from a rare model. Cancer cell 2006; 9:331–2.

[129] Smith R, Owen LA, Trem DJ, et al. Expression profiling of EWS/FLI identifies NKX2.2 as a critical target gene in Ewing's sarcoma. Cancer cell 2006;9:405–16.

[130] Artandi SE, Chang S, Lee SL, et al. Telomere dysfunction promotes non-reciprocal translocations and epithelial cancers in mice. Nature 2000;10:641–5.

[131] Henson JD, Hannay JA, McCarthy SW, et al. A robust assay for alternative lengthening of telomeres in tumors shows the significance of alternative lengthening of telomeres in sarcomas and astrocytomas. Clin Cancer Res 2005;11:217–25.

[132] Gisselsson D, Pettersson L, Höglund M, et al. Chromosomal breakage-fusion-bridge events cause genetic intratumor heterogeneity. Proc Natl Acad Sci U S A 2000;97:5357–62.

[133] Scheel C, Schaefer KL, Jauch A, et al. Alternative lengthening of telomeres is associated with chromosomal instability in osteosarcomas. Oncogene 2001;20:3835–44.

[134] Sharpless NE, Ferguson DO, O'Hagan RC, et al. Impaired nonhomologous end-joining provokes soft tissue sarcomas harboring chromosomal translocations, amplifications, and deletions. Mol Cell 2001;8:1187–96.

ELSEVIER
SAUNDERS

SURGICAL
CLINICS OF
NORTH AMERICA

Surg Clin N Am 88 (2008) 483–520

Classification and Pathology

Julie M. Wu, MD*, Elizabeth Montgomery, MD

*The Johns Hopkins University, 401 N. Broadway, Weinberg 2242,
Baltimore, MD 21231, USA*

Soft tissue tumors are a heterogeneous group of benign and malignant processes. Some are assumed to be reactive, and others are clearly neoplastic. Because of their rarity, they frequently pose diagnostic problems for surgical pathologists. Accurate diagnosis of these tumors is enhanced by knowledge of the clinical features of the given lesions and, at times, by application of immunohistochemical and molecular techniques. In this article the lesions are described essentially in accordance with the World Health Organization classification [1,2]. A description of all classified soft tissue entities is beyond the scope of this article. Both detailed [3] and abbreviated [4] textbooks are available.

Grading and staging

Grading soft tissue tumors applies only to sarcomas. Histologic grade is an important (if not the most important) prognostic parameter in soft tissue neoplasia [5–7]. Many sarcomas can be assigned a grade definitionally, based on their subtype. In practice, the overall rarity of soft tissue tumors does not allow separate grading criteria for each subtype. Therefore, during the past several decades general grading schemes have been devised and studied that correlate with prognosis, recurrence, and metastasis-free and overall survival. For example, in one early study, overall survival rates for grades 1, 2, and 3 tumors were 97%, 67%, and 38%, respectively [7]. The National Cancer Institute (NCI) regards tumor necrosis as the most important prognostic indicator in separating grades 2 and 3. The key in the NCI histopathologic grading system is the use of necrosis greater or less than 15% to separate grades 2 and 3. Necrosis also is predictive of survival after the first recurrence

---
* Corresponding author.
E-mail address: juliemwu@gmail.com (J.M. Wu).

0039-6109/08/$ - see front matter. Published by Elsevier Inc.
doi:10.1016/j.suc.2008.03.007

[5]. Many authors have found that this scheme accurately predicts prognosis in soft tissue tumors. The NCI system is presented in Box 1.

Perhaps the ultimate goal in staging soft tissue tumors is to identify patients (such as those who have grade 2 tumors) who may benefit from surgery alone versus a combination of surgery with adjuvant therapy. A large number of proliferation markers have been explored for this purpose. At present, however, histologic grading remains the foundation of clinical decision making for most sarcomas, although genetic markers are promising in well-studied pediatric sarcomas and in sarcomas with established translocations such as synovial sarcoma and alveolar rhabdomyosarcoma.

The staging of any cancer is a portrait of its anatomic location and the extent of disease at the time of initial diagnosis, and a detailed discussion is beyond the scope of this article. Readers are referred to other articles in this issue.

Classification of soft tissue tumors

Soft tissue tumors are classified according to the adult tissue types that the lesional cells resemble. This classification does not necessarily indicate that the tumor arose from such cells. In the future, classification may be established on molecular grounds, but presently morphologic features remain the basis of classification. Table 1 presents known translocations and their associated gene products.

Fibrous tissue tumors: fibroma

Collagenous fibromas tend to occur in adults over a wide age range (16–81 years) with a wide anatomic distribution (arm, shoulder, girdle, posterior neck and upper back, feet and ankles, leg, hand, abdominal wall, and hip) [8]. These tumors are painless and slow growing and often are present for years, ranging in size 1 to 20 cm (median, 3 cm). Collagenous fibromas are predominantly subcutaneous, lobulated, and typically infiltrative into fat. On microscopic examination the lesions are composed of bland stellate and spindle-shaped fibroblasts set in a densely collagenized or myxocollagenous matrix. Mitotic activity is absent or minimal. Collagenous fibromas are recognized readily as benign without recurrences or metastasis despite incomplete excision in some cases.

Fibroma of tendon sheath was first well characterized by Chung and Enzinger [9]. It tends to occur between the third and fifth decades and is more common in men. Most affect the tendons and tendon sheaths of the fingers, hand, and wrist and usually present as insidiously growing masses. They are associated with mild tenderness and pain in about one third of patients. Fibroma of tendon sheath typically is well circumscribed and lobulated and measures approximately 2 cm. On gross examination the tumors are found

Box 1. National Cancer Institute histopathologic grading of soft tissue tumors

Histologic parameters
- Tumor type
- Necrosis
- Mitoses

Grade
- I: Well differentiated
- II: < 15% necrosis (none or minimal)
- III: > 15% necrosis (moderate or marked)

National Cancer Institute three-grade system
Grade I
- Well-differentiated liposarcoma
- Myxoid liposarcoma
- Dermatofibrosarcoma protuberans

Grade I–III
- Leiomyosarcoma[a]
- Chondrosarcoma
- Malignant peripheral nerve sheath tumor[c]
- Hemangiopericytoma[b]
- Fibrosarcoma[a]
- Myxoid chodrosarcoma[d]

Grade II–III
- Round cell liposarcoma
- Malignant fibrous histiocytoma
- Clear cell sarcoma
- Angiosarcoma
- Epithelioid sarcoma
- Malignant granular cell tumor
- Fibrosarcoma
- Synovial sarcoma
- Rhabdomyosarcoma
- Pleomorphic liposarcoma

Grade III
- Ewing's sarcoma
- Osteosarcoma
- Alveolar soft part sarcoma
- Ewing's sarcoma and peripheral primitive neuroectodermal tumor
- Malignant triton tumor
- Mesenchymal chondrosarcoma

---

[a] Grade I, absent necrosis, low mitotic activity (< 6 mitoses per 10 high-power field).

[b] Grade I, <1 mitosis per 10 high-power field.

[c] Grade I, appearance of neurofibroma but with mitoses (< 6 mitoses per 10 high-power field).

[d] Grade I, uniformly hypocellular, myxoid, devoid of mitoses.

Data from Guillou L, Coindre JM, Bonichon F, et al. Comparative study of the National Cancer Institute and French Federation of Cancer Centers Sarcoma Group grading systems in a population of 410 adult patients with soft tissue sarcoma. J Clin Oncol 1997;(15):350–62.

Table 1
Specific cytogenetically established chromosomal translocations and the corresponding gene changes in mesenchymal tumors

Tumor type	Translocation	Gene changes
Alveolar rhabdomyosarcoma	t(2;13)(q35;q14)	*PAX3-FKHR*
	t(1;13)(p36;q14)	*PAX7-FKHR*
Alveolar soft part sarcoma	t(X;17)(p11.2;q25)	*ASPL-TFE3*
Clear cell sarcoma (malignant melanoma of soft parts)	t(12;22)(q13;q12)	*ATF1-EWS*
Congenital fibrosarcoma and mesoblastic nephroma	t(12;15)(p13;q25)	*ETV6-NTRK3*
Dermatofibrosarcoma protuberans (giant cell fibroblastoma)	t(17;22)(q22;q13)	*COL1A1-PDGFB*
Desmoplastic small round cell tumor	t(11;22)(p13;q12)	*WT1-EWS*
Endometrial stromal sarcoma	t(7;17)(p15;q21)	*JAZF1-JJAZ1*
Ewing's sarcoma and peripheral primitive neuroectodermal tumors	t(11;22)(q24;q12)	*EWS-FLI1*
	t(21;22)(q22;q12)	*EWS-ERG*
	t(7;22)(p22;q12)	*EWS-ETV1*
	t(17;22)(q12;q12)	*EWS-E1AF*
	t(2;22)(q33;q12)	*FEV-EWS*
	t(2;19)(p23;p13.1)	*ALK-TPM4*
Inflammatory myofibroblastic tumor	t(1;2)(q22-23;p23)	*TPM3-ALK*
	t(9;22)(q22;q12)	*EWS-CHN(TEC)*
Myxoid chondrosarcoma, extraskeletal	t(9;17)(q22;q11)	*RBP56-CHN(TEC)*
	t(9;15)(q22;q21)	*TEC/TCF12*
Myxoid liposarcoma	t(12;16)(q13;p11)	*TLS(FUS)-CHOP*
	t(12;22)(q13;q12)	*EWS-CHOP*
Synovial sarcoma	t(X;18)(p11;q11)	*SYT-SSX1*
		SYT-SSX2
Low-grade fibromyxoid sarcoma	t(7;16)(q33;p11)	*FUS-BBF2H7*

Data from Sandberg AA. Translocations in malignant tumors. Am J Pathol 2001;159:1979.

attached to tendons and tendon sheaths and have a firm consistency. Microscopically, fibroma of tendon sheath is lobulated and consists of spindle-shaped fibroblasts associated with dense collagenation, admixed with zones of myxoid degeneration with stellate fibroblasts. Fibroma of tendon sheath may recur locally if incompletely excised but is benign.

Elastofibroma is a slowly growing fibroelastic proliferation typically occurring on the backs of female patients. Although in the past these lesions were assumed to be reactive [10], recent studies suggest that they have a variety of chromosomal alterations and could be neoplasms instead [11]. Bilaterality is also known [12]. On microscopic examination the mass consists of intertwining eosinophilic collagen and thickened, serrated, deeply eosinophilic elastic fibers that have a degenerated beaded appearance or are fragmented into globules or flowerlike arrangements. Elastofibromas are benign.

Calcifying aponeurotic fibroma primarily affects the hands and feet of children between birth and age16 years [13]. The tumor usually presents as a slow-growing, poorly circumscribed mass. There is a tendency for local recurrence. Microscopically the nodules are characterized by infiltrative fibrous growth of plump, oval fibroblasts arranged in cords. There is rich cellularity and dense collagen. Frequently, the nodules may be attached to an aponeurosis or tendon. Typically bandlike or serpiginous central calcification is surrounded by chondroid matrix. Variable numbers of giant cells also may be seen.

Fibroblastic/myofibroblastic proliferations

Pseudosarcomatous proliferative lesions of soft tissue are fascia-based fibroblastic and myofibroblastic lesions that have the potential to be overdiagnosed as sarcoma. They usually are subtyped according to the location, depth of involvement, age at presentation, and histologic features. They are assumed to be reactive, and they recur only rarely after surgical excision. There are reports of cytogenetic alterations, however [14,15].

Nodular fasciitis, first described in the 1950s [16], is the most frequently encountered pseudosarcomatous lesion, presenting mostly in the third to fourth decades as a rapidly growing mass of the upper extremities and usually attaining a size of 2 to 3 cm. Because of its rapid growth, increased cellularity, and high mitotic index, it sometimes is mistaken for a sarcoma [17–21]. The second most common site is the head and the neck region, which is the most frequent site in infants and children. No gender predilection has been observed.

Nodular fasciitis classically involves subcutaneous tissue, but intramuscular and fascial forms also occur. The nodule consists primarily of plump myofibroblasts that appear similar to those seen in tissue culture or granulation tissue (Fig. 1). The cells are bland in appearance, with pale nuclei and small nucleoli. The mitotic rate is fairly high, but atypical mitoses are absent. Intermixed with the fibroblasts are lymphocytes and extravasated erythrocytes with variable numbers of macrophages and giant cells (Fig. 2). The intervening matrix is myxoid, imparting a feathery appearance, whereas cellular forms exhibit dense cellularity with less matrix.

Proliferative fasciitis and myositis are less common than nodular fasciitis [22], mainly occurring in adults and with no gender predilection. This proliferation often presents as a palpable, mobile, rapidly growing subcutaneous nodule in the extremities, especially the forearm and the thigh.

Grossly proliferative fasciitis appears as poorly circumscribed, elongated mass mainly involving the interlobular fibrous tissue septa of the subcutis. Histologically, in addition to stellate cells, there are ganglion-like cells with basophilic cytoplasm, one or two nucleoli, and occasional cytoplasmic inclusions. There is variable myxoid stroma that becomes more collagenized as lesions persist. The large ganglion-like cells are mistaken readily as malignant.

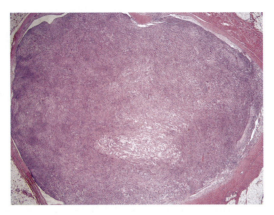

Fig. 1. Nodular fasciitis, low power. The subcutaneous nodule has well-delineated margins, comprised of loose myofibroblastic cells with central myxoid degeneration (hematoxylin-eosin, original magnification ×2).

Proliferative myositis is the deep or intramuscular counterpart of proliferative fasciitis affecting the muscles of the trunk and the limb girdles.

Fibromatoses

The fibromatoses are classified as superficial or deep [1,2]. This discussion focuses on deep fibromatoses, also called "aggressive fibromatoses" and "desmoid tumors." In children, most desmoid tumors are extra-abdominal with a female predominance, whereas in young adults desmoid tumors almost always occur in the abdominal wall (of women). As patients approach

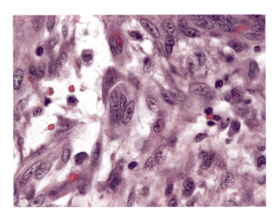

Fig. 2. Nodular fasciitis, high-power. A higher-power examination reveals plump myofibroblasts with spindle cytoplasm and vesicular nuclei. There is a background of extravasated erythrocytes and lymphocytes (hematoxylin-eosin, original magnification ×40).

their sixth decade, the sex ratio approaches 1:1, and most tumors continue to affect the abdominal wall. As patients age still further, the sex ratio remains 1:1, but the sites of disease vary. It is important for the treating surgeon to be aware of these trends, because the "juvenile" type is particularly prone to recurrence (70% in one series, versus 45% for extra-abdominal, and 10% for abdominal presentations) [23]. These tumors usually are large, and local control can prove difficult, but despite their capacity for local aggression, deep fibromatoses do not metastasize. They are managed clinically in the same fashion as low-grade sarcomas, however.

Hormonal effects and pregnancy are believed to influence the growth of this tumor. Some tumors express hormone receptors (estrogen and progesterone), and therefore tamoxifen and other hormonal modulators are among the adjuvant therapies for this tumor [24,25].

Extra-abdominal desmoid is a relatively common lesion that has deceptively bland histomorphology but a tendency to recur locally and to infiltrate the surrounding tissue. These tumors arise primarily in the connective tissue of muscle and the overlying fascia; the most common location is the shoulder girdle followed by chest wall, back, thigh, and head and neck [24–39]. Fibromatosis of the head and neck is seen more commonly in children, in which case the lesions tend to be more cellular and may grow more aggressively, even encroaching on the trachea with destruction of adjacent bone and a fatal outcome. Although these tumors do not metastasize, multicentricity has been described [40,41].

Clinically the lesions present as deep-seated, firm, nonencapsulated, slowly growing, locally invasive, painless masses. They are seen most commonly in young women, although children and even infants may be affected.

Microscopically, the lesion is poorly defined with infiltrative margins consisting of spindled fibroblasts separated by abundant collagen. The vessels, although thin-walled, are conspicuous at scanning magnification (Fig. 3). The nuclei of the proliferating lesion typically are tinctorially lighter than those of the endothelial cells, and the smooth muscle cytoplasm in vessel walls is pinker than the surrounding myofibroblastic cytoplasm of the tumor cells. Mitotic figures are infrequent.

Abdominal fibromatosis is far less prone to recurrences than desmoid tumors in other sites. It usually occurs in the abdominal wall of women of childbearing age during or after pregnancy. It typically manifests as a slow-growing, progressive mass that becomes more prominent on abdominal muscle contraction. The gross and microscopic features are identical to those of extra-abdominal fibromatosis.

Intra-abdominal fibromatosis includes several entities that have similar morphologic findings but distinct clinical presentations [34,39]. Pelvic fibromatosis typically involves the lower portion of the pelvis, where it presents as a slowly growing mass in young females but has no relationship to gestation. Mesenteric fibromatosis, probably the commonest among the group,

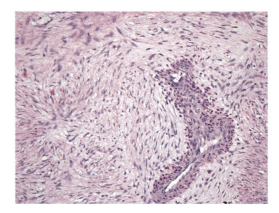

Fig. 3. Fibromatosis (hematoxylin-eosin, original magnification ×10). A thin-walled vessel stands out in a background of lightly colored spindled fibroblasts.

usually presents as a slowly growing mass that involves small bowel mesentery or retroperitoneum. The recurrence rate of mesenteric fibromatosis seems to be substantially higher in patients who have Gardner's syndrome than in patients who do not have this syndrome [34,39,42].

Fibrosarcomas

Once regarded as the most common type of sarcoma [43], adult fibrosarcoma now is rarely diagnosed. With current criteria and modern ancillary studies, many lesions classified as fibrosarcomas in the past are readily recognized as malignant peripheral nerve sheath tumors (MPNST), synovial sarcomas, or pseudosarcomas, and fibrosarcoma has become essentially a diagnosis of exclusion.

Adult fibrosarcoma probably accounts for 1% to 5% of adult sarcomas [44]. Classical fibrosarcoma is most common in middle-aged and older adults with no gender predilection. Fibrosarcoma usually involves deep soft tissues of the extremities, trunk, and head and neck. Hypoglycemia has been reported and has been related to the elaboration of insulin-like growth factor by the tumor cells, a phenomenon also observed in association with solitary fibrous tumors of the pleura [45,46]. Fibrosarcoma can arise in dermatofibrosarcoma protuberans (DFSP) (Fig. 4).

This neoplasm is composed of spindle-shaped cells, characteristically arranged in sweeping fascicles that are angled in a herringbone pattern. Storiform areas can be seen. The cells have tapered, darkly staining nuclei with variably prominent nucleoli and scant cytoplasm. Mitotic activity almost always is present but is variable. Higher-grade tumors have more densely staining nuclei and can display focal round cell change and multinucleated cells, but sarcomas with significant pleomorphism currently are classified as

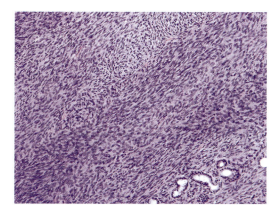

Fig. 4. Fibrosarcoma (hematoxylin-eosin, original magnification ×10). There is a classic herringbone pattern with interwoven, angled fascicles. This particular case arose in a pre-existing dermatofibrosarcoma protuberans; the cutaneous adnexal structures allude to a superficial location.

malignant fibrous histiocytoma (MFH). The stroma has variable collagen, from a delicate intercellular network to paucicellular areas with diffuse or keloidlike sclerosis.

There are no recent series of fibrosarcomas classified using modern techniques. In the older literature, behavior relates to grade and to general factors of tumor size and depth from the skin. The probability of local recurrence relates to the completeness of excision [47–49]. Fibrosarcomas metastasize to lungs and bone, especially the axial skeleton, and rarely to lymph nodes, in about 10% to 65% of patients. Five-year survival is on the order of 50%.

Low-grade fibromyxoid sarcoma is a tumor affecting young and middle-aged adults. It is composed of bland, fibroblast-like cells with a swirling, vaguely storiform pattern in a fibrous and focally myxoid stroma, occasionally with plexiform vasculature. These tumors have little mitotic activity and minimal nuclear pleomorphism. Seemingly innocuous, these lesions recur and frequently metastasize (eg, to lung). This tumor is not equivalent to low-grade examples of myxofibrosarcoma, because the latter occur in older patients, are more pleomorphic and less fibrous, and seldom metastasize when superficial. The differential diagnosis of low-grade fibromyxoid sarcoma is predominantly with fibromatosis.

Hyalinizing spindle cell tumor with giant rosettes is an entity closely resembling low-grade fibromyxoid sarcoma that affects the proximal extremities in young to middle-aged adults [50]. Although grossly circumscribed, the tumors have infiltrative borders microscopically and are composed of bland spindled cells situated in a hyalinized to myxoid stroma, often with "cracking" artifact in the collagen. Scattered large, rosette-like structures that often merge with areas of dense hyalinization are characteristic. These rosettes consist of a central collagen core surrounded by a rim of rounded cells that are morphologically and immunophenotypically different from the cells of the spindled stroma. This lesion, in fact, is related to fibromyxoid sarcoma [51,52]. The tumors share an identical characteristic translocation [53] with its own fusion gene product [54,55]; t(7;16)(q33;p11) fuses the *FUS* gene to *BBF2H7*.

Fibrohistiocytic tumors

DFSP is a nodular, subcutaneous tumor that arises in early or middle adulthood, predominantly in truncal sites. The clinical progression is characterized by the onset of a plaquelike lesion that, after an indefinite time interval, proceeds to a phase of more rapid growth with one or multiple (satellite) nodules.

Although grossly circumscribed, the tumor is diffusely infiltrative on histologic sections; the tumor extends along the fibrous septa, interweaves among adnexal structures, and partitions the subcutaneous fat into a characteristic lacelike appearance (Fig. 5). The center of the tumor is comprised of a uniform population of spindled cells organized in a storiform pattern. Because of its infiltrative nature, recurrences are common (up to 50%) [56,57], and wide local excision is advised. Metastases have been reported in 4 of 96 patients with a 15-year follow-up, with three of the four showing lung metastasis and the other showing lymphatic spread [58]. Local resection is recommended for metastatic lesions.

Nearly all DFSPs express CD34 [54,55,59,60], which has been used to distinguish DFSP from its primary mimicker, benign fibrous histiocytoma. Although some fibrous histiocytomas also may express CD34, the expression usually is focal. DFSP is characterized by a supernumerary ring chromosome comprised of sequences from chromosomes 17 and 22 [61,62],

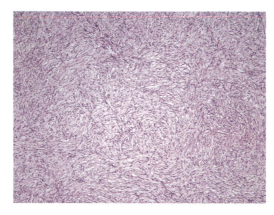

Fig. 5. Dermatofibrosarcoma protuberans (hematoxylin-eosin, original magnification ×4). The tumor is comprised of dark, spindled cells arranged in a storiform architecture. Compared with fibromatosis, vessels are comparatively obscure.

resulting in the fusion of platelet-derived growth factor β-chain (*PDGFβ*) to the collagen type 1 gene (*COL1A1*) [63]. The resultant overproduction of PDGFβ has been thought to stimulate cell proliferation [64].

MFH comprises a collection of tumors whose description has been evolving. It was the most common sarcoma diagnosis rendered in the 1980s and early 1990s, but the use of newer techniques has reduced the number of cases so diagnosed in more recent years. It has been suggested that MFH is not an entity but a collection of poorly differentiated neoplasms better classified with comprehensive examination [65]. Certainly this classification may contain neoplasms that could be better characterized, but the term remains a reasonable descriptive one, and the phenotype can be recognized reproducibly. Masqueraders now are unmasked readily with modern immunohistochemistry. Many observers prefer to diagnose such tumors as "undifferentiated pleomorphic sarcoma," but this discussion retains the old terminology.

Storiform pleomorphic MFH is the most common variant of MFH. It is a tumor of older adults and usually affects the limbs and limb girdles, followed by the retroperitoneum, trunk, or head and neck. Pediatric cases are uncommon but behave similarly [66]. These neoplasms typically attain a large size with zones of hemorrhage and necrosis. Deep tumors usually are circumscribed, whereas superficial ones sometimes can track along connective tissue septa and often require a wider excision than palpation would suggest [67]. Overall survival is usually on the order of 50%. The key prognosticators are tumor grade and tumor size [68–71].

Histologically there is at least a focal storiform pattern, and the tumor consists of a variable proportion of atypical pleomorphic spindle cells and pleomorphic multinucleated cells with ample eosinophilic cytoplasm (Fig. 6). The stroma has variable amounts of collagen. There is no specific immunohistochemical profile for MFH. Cytogenetic/molecular studies yield complex karyotypes [72], and there is no specific genetic alteration.

The differential diagnosis of pleomorphic spindle cell tumors includes spindled carcinomas, lymphomas, and melanomas, as well as pleomorphic sarcomas. Among sarcomas, pleomorphic liposarcoma, leiomyosarcoma, rhabdomyosarcoma, and dedifferentiated sarcomas, especially liposarcoma, require consideration. For these, even focal specific differentiation suffices for diagnosis of various subtypes of pleomorphic sarcomas.

Pleomorphic sarcomas of various histologic types are remarkably similar clinically. The prognosis of pleomorphic sarcomas generally is poor, and about 40% of patients who have high-grade MFH die of the disease within 5 years of diagnosis. Dedifferentiated liposarcomas have a slightly better prognosis, with 28% mortality at 5 years [73]. On the other end of the spectrum, pleomorphic rhabdomyosarcomas have a worse prognosis, with 70% mortality. Thus, in clinical practice it is important to identify pleomorphic rhabdomyosarcomas and dedifferentiated liposarcomas, but the specific distinction of pleomorphic liposarcoma, pleomorphic leiomyosarcoma, or

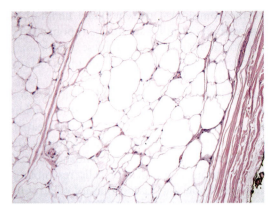

Fig. 7. Lipoma (hematoxylin-eosin, original magnification ×10). There is striking similarity to mature adipose tissue.

the most common location. Men are affected more frequently than women. In lipomatosis there is a diffuse, nonlobular proliferation of fat in the affected tissues. The subcutaneous fat of the back of the neck and shoulder is involved in nearly every individual [78–81]. Lipomatosis is thought to be secondary to a defect in lipid metabolism, and patients who have diffuse lipomatosis have the clinical appearance of obesity. Mediastinal involvement can cause venous obstruction with stasis and airway obstruction [78–81]. The lipomas in these patients have the same gross and histologic features as conventional lipoma. The adipocytes have a normal appearance, except for slightly smaller size.

Lipoblastoma is a benign tumor arising exclusively in infants, typically during the first 3 years of life [82–85]. Lipoblastoma is more common in boys and typically involves the subcutaneous tissues of the extremities. Local recurrence has been reported in 9% to 22% of patients. These tumors have alterations (rearrangements) of chromosome 8q [86]. Microscopically, lipoblastoma is lobular, composed of primitive stellate/spindle-shaped cells, multivacuolated adipocytes, and univacuolated adipocytes. Sometimes these tumors mature to conventional lipomas.

Angiolipoma occurs as a subcutaneous nodule in young adults, most commonly in the forearm. These tumors present more commonly as multiple lesions rather than solitary occurrences [87]. Angiolipomas are characteristically painful on palpation. Histologically, the tumor is comprised of lobules of mature fat separated by vascular channels containing fibrin thrombi. Unlike classical lipomas, angiolipomas typically do not have karyotypic abnormalities.

Spindle-cell lipoma and pleomorphic lipoma often are recognized as fatty tumors by the surgeon but cause difficulty for the pathologist [88]. Both tend to present in the shoulder girdle of elderly men. Spindle cell lipoma is composed of an admixture of mature adipocytes and spindle cells embedded in myxoid matrix that contains brightly eosinophilic collagen fibers. Cytogenetic studies have shown abnormalities involving 13q and 16q [89,90]. Pleomorphic lipoma can be considered a pleomorphic variant of spindle cell lipoma [89–92]. Microscopically, these tumors resemble spindle cell lipomas with the additional presence of hyperchromatic multinucleated giant cells that frequently demonstrate a concentric or "floretlike" arrangement of the nuclei.

Distinguishing pleomorphic lipoma from well-differentiated sclerosing liposarcoma can be problematic, especially because lipoblast-like cells can be seen in pleomorphic lipoma. A subcutaneous location suggests pleomorphic lipoma, whereas a deeper or retroperitoneal location suggests sclerosing liposarcoma.

Other lipoma subtypes include chondroid lipomas, angiomyolipomas, myolipomas, and hibernomas [93–97].

Adipose tissue tumors: liposarcoma

The World Health Organization recognizes the following subtypes of liposarcoma [1–3]: well-differentiated liposarcoma/dedifferentiated liposarcoma, myxoid liposarcoma/round cell liposarcoma, and pleomorphic liposarcoma.

Well-differentiated liposarcoma is the most common subtype of liposarcoma. These tumors nearly always occur in adults and have no gender predilection [98–104]. They arise most commonly in the deep soft tissues of the proximal extremities and the retroperitoneum. Occasionally retroperitoneal liposarcomas may present as groin masses because of local extension into the peritoneal-lined scrotal sac and therefore may simulate groin hernia [105,106].

In the absence of dedifferentiation, distant metastases almost never occur. Extremity tumors often recur many years after the original surgical procedure, but local recurrence in the extremities typically is not associated with destructive growth. Therefore well-differentiated liposarcoma is managed by wide local excision without major functional compromise, if technically possible. Retroperitoneal tumors are treated by debulking that almost always results in residual gross or microscopic tumor. Treated in this way, well-differentiated liposarcoma of the extremity demonstrates a recurrence rate of approximately 40% to 50%, whereas the groin and retroperitoneal tumors nearly always recur (80%–90%). The extremity tumors do not result in patient death, but the retroperitoneal and groin tumors have poor long-term prognosis because of uncontrolled local growth within the abdominal cavity [98,100,101,107].

Well-differentiated liposarcomas demonstrate ring chromosomes and long marker chromosomes derived from the q13-15 region of chromosome 12. These findings are present regardless of anatomic location [108,109].

Well-differentiated liposarcomas usually are large: tumors in excess of 20 cm are common. They typically demonstrate a multinodular growth within and between skeletal muscles. The tumors are soft and pale yellow on cut section. Three microscopic variants of well-differentiated liposarcoma occur. None of the histologic variants of low-grade liposarcoma is clinically or prognostically relevant.

The term "atypical lipoma" has been applied to well-differentiated liposarcomas that occur in the subcutis [98,101,110]. Tumors in this location have an excellent prognosis and an extremely low rate of dedifferentiation.

Well-differentiated liposarcoma and dedifferentiated liposarcoma are related; the latter arises from the former. Similarly, myxoid and round cell liposarcoma are two biologic and clinical ends of a spectrum. Both have a single cytogenetic abnormality.

Dedifferentiated liposarcoma is a spindle cell nonlipogenic sarcoma occurring in association with a well-differentiated low-grade liposarcoma [73,101,102,107,111,112]. Dedifferentiation portends a capacity for distant metastasis (15%–30%), more aggressive local growth, increased risk of local recurrence, and higher mortality. It is cytogenetically related to low-grade liposarcoma and exhibits ring chromosome transformation. It is treated by radical surgical excision. Adjuvant therapy also may be considered.

Up to half of all liposarcomas are of myxoid/round cell type, which represent histologic spectrums of the same entity [113–119]. Tumors with pure myxoid liposarcoma morphology have a better prognosis than those with round cell features [113,114,117]. These tumors typically affect adults and are most common in the fifth decade. Men are affected more often than women. The deep soft tissue of the thigh is the single most common location for these neoplasms.

Patients typically complain of a painless soft tissue mass. Myxoid/round cell liposarcoma is treated by wide surgical excision with or without radiation therapy. Approximately 30% of patients develop distant metastases. Like most other sarcomas, these metastases often involve the lungs, but myxoid/round cell liposarcoma also often metastasizes to nonpulmonary sites including the retroperitoneum, soft tissue, and skeleton [116]. Histologic grading seems to be of value in identifying patients at risk for metastases. Specifically, as the cellularity of the tumor increases, and the degree of tumor composed of round cell liposarcoma or cellular myxoid liposarcoma increases, so does the risk of metastasis.

Most myxoid/round cell liposarcomas demonstrate a specific chromosomal translocation t(12;16)(q13;p11) that results in the rearrangement of the *CHOP* and *FUS* genes [115,118–121]. A minority demonstrates variants of this translocation that typically also involve the12q13 breakpoint.

Myxoid liposarcoma is composed of univacuolar and multivacuolar lipoblasts embedded in a richly myxoid ground substance. Characteristically, there is an acute angle (plexiform) branching capillary vasculature (Fig. 8). Round cell liposarcoma is characterized by a relative increase in

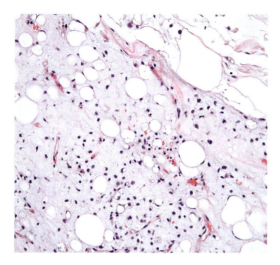

Fig. 8. Liposarcoma, myxoid (hematoxylin-eosin, original magnification ×10). There are darkly stained but relatively uniform oval cells in a background of a myxoid and lipomatous stroma. Note the delicate, arcuate vessels.

the cellularity of the tumor so that individual tumor cells lie in direct continuity with each other without intervening matrix. One of the difficulties in precise classification of myxoid/round cell liposarcoma is that there are no universally acceptable criteria for minimum levels of cellularity and nuclear atypia that define round cell foci within these tumors. Prognostic cutoff points proposed by some authors range from cellular areas of 5% to 25% [107,114,117].

Pleomorphic liposarcoma is the rarest subtype of liposarcoma. It typically occurs in adults older than 50 years. Both men and women are affected. Most tumors arise in the deep soft tissues of the thigh, trunk, or retroperitoneum where they produce symptoms related to a painless mass. There are no specific cytogenetic abnormalities within this subgroup of liposarcoma, and they display complex karyotypes [72]. Pleomorphic liposarcomas have a very high incidence of metastases and tumor-related mortality.

Clusters of markedly pleomorphic multivacuolated lipoblasts are present. Mitotic figures, including atypical forms, are found readily (Fig. 9).

Skeletal muscle tumors

When soft tissue tumors are considered in total, benign lesions outnumber malignant ones by a ratio of more than 100:1. Skeletal muscle tumors are the exception: rhabdomyosarcomas are 50-fold more common than rhabdomyomas. Most rhabdomyosarcomas are found in children.

Rhabdomyosarcoma is the most common pediatric soft tissue sarcoma, comprising 80% to 90% of reported cases. Reported areas of involvement

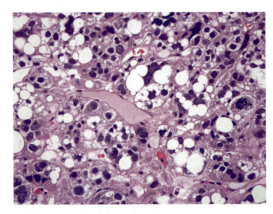

Fig. 9. Liposarcoma, pleomorphic (hematoxylin-eosin, original magnification ×40). There is striking nuclear pleomorphism and hyperchromatism in these lipoblasts. Mitotic figures are present.

include urinary bladder, prostate, common bile duct, and vagina. The term reflects the tendency of the tumors to recapitulate skeletal myoblasts rather than to arise from them.

Embryonal rhabdomyosarcomas most frequently occur as head and neck and genitourinary lesions in young children, whereas alveolar rhabdomyosarcomas most frequently occur as extremity and parameningeal lesions in adolescents. Clinical symptomatology reflects the affected organ system. Orbital tumors present with proptosis and diplopia. Cervicovaginal tumors cause vaginal bleeding, and large masses extruding from the introitus may be evident. Extremity tumors typically present as painless masses.

Rhabdomyosarcomas generally are fleshy, nondescript pale gray-yellow masses with areas of necrosis and hemorrhage. They insidiously invade adjacent tissues, so that microscopic areas of marginal involvement may be apparent even with grossly resected lesions.

The primary distinguishing characteristic of rhabdomyosarcomas is their capacity for myogenesis at the microscopic level. Rhabdomyoblasts display brightly eosinophilic cytoplasm and when more differentiated acquire microscopically visible cytoplasmic cross striations that result from the submicroscopic alignment of myofilaments in register. More commonly, at the less differentiated end of the spectrum, ancillary methods of demonstrating myogenesis often are necessary for diagnostic confirmation.

The most common subtype is embryonal rhabdomyosarcoma, which is typified by alternating areas of cellular condensation and hypocellularity, with cells floating in mucoid ground substance (Fig. 10). Over the past century, the prognosis for embryonal rhabdomyosarcomas has improved dramatically.

Botryoid rhabdomyosarcoma, named for its resemblance to a cluster of grapes, has a distinctive gross appearance. This tumor arises exclusively along mucosa-lined surfaces, such as the bladder, vagina, or conjunctiva.

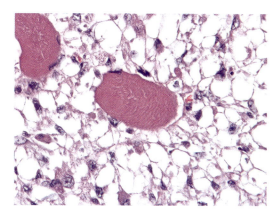

Fig. 10. Rhabdomyosarcoma, embryonal (hematoxylin-eosin, original magnification ×20). There are scattered enlarged cells with prominent nucleoli in a background of mucoid material. The cytoplasm shows skeletal muscle differentiation; note the brightly eosinophilic cytoplasm.

It displays a characteristic histologic feature, a cambium layer, which is a subepithelial condensation of tumor cells named for its resemblance to the more rapidly growing layer of a tree just beneath the bark. This variant is genetically identical to other embryonal rhabdomyosarcomas but has a proven superior prognosis [122].

Spindle cell rhabdomyosarcoma is another subtype that is associated with a better prognosis. Spindle cell variants, however, arise almost exclusively in the paratesticular region, a site with an independently better prognosis, so it could be argued that this improved prognosis is site dependent. Grossly, spindle cell rhabdomyosarcoma has a fibrous, whorled appearance. Microscopically, these tumors are more differentiated than the usual rhabdomyosarcomas and exhibit a heavy content of muscle proteins by immunohistochemistry [123].

Alveolar rhabdomyosarcoma is a highly aggressive sarcoma. Microscopically, alveolar rhabdomyosarcomas form nests of discohesive cells separated by a prominent framework of fibrovascular septa, thus displaying some resemblance to lung alveoli (Fig. 11) [124].

Alveolar rhabdomyosarcoma displays a characteristic fusion between the *PAX3* gene on chromosome 2 and the *FKHR* gene of chromosome 13 forming the t(2;13)(q35;q14) translocation [125–130]. This translocation fuses two DNA-binding transcription factors and seems to cause the abnormal cell proliferation [131,132]. Another *PAX* gene, *PAX7*, located on chromosome 1, may also fuse with the *FKHR* gene and produce alveolar rhabdomyosarcomas containing a similar aberrant fusion gene, the t(1;13)(p36;q14) translocation. Although similar in molecular composition and in tumorigenesis, t(1;13)(p36;q14) lesions are associated with less aggressive tumors and occur in younger children [127].

Unfortunately the improvements in outcome for embryonal rhabdomyosarcoma have not been matched in alveolar rhabdomyosarcoma, although

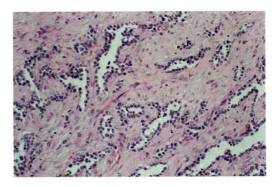

Fig. 11. Rhabdomyosarcoma, alveolar (hematoxylin-eosin, original magnification ×10). The pseudoglandular formations are lined by small, blue, poorly differentiated tumor cells. There is a suggestion of discohesion toward the center of the spaces.

the more aggressive therapy used to treat the latter tumors may ameliorate some of the differences in outcome [133].

Pleomorphic rhabdomyosarcoma accounts for 5% to 7% of all pleomorphic adult soft tissue sarcomas. Two series report a wide age range (27 or 28–84 years) with a mean of 61 or 56 years [134,135]. No pediatric cases were identified in either series.

Pleomorphic rhabdomyosarcoma usually arises in the large skeletal muscles of the extremities, most commonly in the thigh. Men seem to be affected more frequently than women. Patients usually present with a painless but rapidly growing soft tissue mass. Metastases to the lungs often are present at time of diagnosis.

Microscopically these tumors are pleomorphic sarcomas composed of undifferentiated round to spindle-shaped cells and an admixture of polygonal cells with densely eosinophilic cytoplasm in spindle, tadpole, and racquet-like contours (Fig. 12). Cross striations are vanishingly rare in all cases. Diagnosis requires the presence of pleomorphic rhabdomyoblasts on routine hematoxylin and eosin stains coupled with immunohistochemical evidence of at least one skeletal muscle–specific marker [136]. Preliminary cytogenetic study has yielded complex karyotypes [72,137].

The prognosis for these tumors is poor, but prognostic factors have yet to be developed. In two series with follow-up, about 75% of patients died of disease [135,136].

Peripheral nerve sheath tumors

Schwannomas are nerve sheath tumors arising most commonly in the head and neck area [138], although they can be found emanating from nerves anywhere in the body. Most schwannomas are sporadic (90%), although some are associated with neurofibromatosis type 2 (3%) [139].

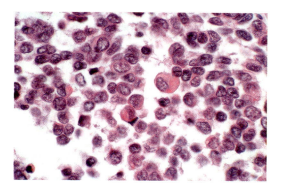

Fig. 12. Rhabdomyosarcoma, pleomorphic (hematoxylin-eosin, original magnification ×40). The cells display a wide range of morphology and some contain eosinophilic cytoplasm intimating muscle differentiation.

Because they are encapsulated by epineurium, schwannomas appear as a circumscribed mass attached to the originating nerve.

Microscopic findings correspond to the gross description: schwannomas are comprised of alternating areas of cellularity. Antoni A areas are comprised of packed spindled cells with club-shaped nuclei forming Verocay bodies, collections of palisading spindled cells surrounding a central area of pink fibrillary processes. Antoni B areas are less cellular, comprised of similar spindled cells floating in a myxoid matrix that is comprised of loose collagen bands and inflammatory cells.

Schwannomas are regarded as benign tumors that rarely, if ever, recur even after incomplete resection [140].

Neurofibromas occur sporadically as solitary lesions or syndromically as diffuse lesions seen in neurofibromatosis type 1. Sporadic neurofibromas arise as superficial, painless nodules in young adults (age 20–30 years).

Neurofibromas that arise in large nerves cause a circumferential expansion that surrounds the normal nerve; these tumors are still encapsulated by epineurium. More commonly, neurofibromas arise from smaller nerves and appear circumscribed but have no capsule.

Histologically, neurofibromas are comprised of spindled tumor cells with wavy nuclei interspersed with delicate collagen strands in a background of myxoid stroma. Neurofibromas usually are not encapsulated. Diagnosis of malignant transformation is problematic, because neurofibromas, atypical neurofibromas, and MPNST exist in a morphologic continuum. Criteria for malignancy are based on nuclear atypia, presence of mitotic activity, and/or marked increase in cellularity [141].

In neurofibromatosis, tumors emerge during childhood or adolescence in three forms: solitary neurofibromas are indistinguishable from sporadic lesions; plexiform neurofibromas are pathognomonic of neurofibromatosis and involve an entire extremity with associated skin hyperpigmentation and bone hypertrophy; diffuse neurofibromas are seen in 10% of patients who have neurofibromatosis [3] and present as an ill-defined plaque-like thickening of the subcutis, most commonly in the head and neck region.

MPNST accounts for approximately 5% to 10% of all soft tissue sarcomas [3]. Approximately 50% of MPNST cases have been reported in patients who have neurofibromatosis [142,143], whereas 3% to 5% of patients who have neurofibromatosis type 1 develop MPNST [144]. The average age of presentation is 32 years regardless of neurofibromatosis 1 status [145]. Most MPNSTs arise in the proximal major truncal nerves and present as an enlarging mass with or without pain.

The tumors typically present as a fusiform enlargement of, or as a sessile mass associated with, a large nerve. On microscopy, the cells of MPNSTs resemble those of schwannomas and neurofibromas in having spindle-shaped outlines and comma-shaped nuclei, although cells may become rounded or oval. A fascicular architecture with alternating cellularity is typical of the lesion. More specific but less common features include neuroid-type whorls, hyalinized nodules, nuclear palisading, and subintimal proliferation of tumor cells encroaching on blood vessels. Heterotopic elements also are more prevalent in MPNSTs than in other types of sarcomas [146,147]. The role of immunohistochemistry in the diagnosis MPNSTs is one of exclusion. Most MPNSTs display focal staining with S100, which is helpful in differentiating the lesions from cellular schwannomas, which often display diffuse and strong positivity. MPNSTs are not characterized by a single translocation but instead are associated with a number of chromosomal alterations.

Both local recurrence and distant metastasis are common [143,148,149]. The most common site of metastasis is lung, followed by bone and pleura [3]. Lymph node metastasis is rare, whereas direct spread along nerve sheath is common. Therefore a frozen section is reasonable to assess adequacy of excision.

Miscellaneous tumor types

Clear cell sarcoma (malignant melanoma of soft parts) affects the distal extremities, particularly the feet and ankles, of young adults [150–153].

The tumor consists of a packeted and fascicular arrangement of uniform round to spindle-shaped cells with clear to eosinophilic cytoplasm and often containing abundant glycogen (Fig. 13). The individual cells have uniform and prominent nucleoli. Melanin can be seen occasionally. Most cases are reactive with S100 protein and melanoma markers, both HMB-45 [150–153] and newer ones.

Based on the staining pattern, some observers have speculated that these tumors are simply melanomas of connective tissue. This proposal probably is incorrect for several reasons. (1) The histologic features of clear cell sarcoma are very monotonous, whereas skin melanomas feature more

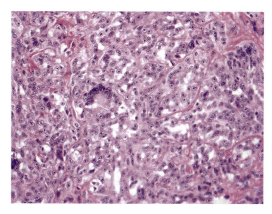

Fig. 13. Clear cell sarcoma (hematoxylin-eosin, original magnification ×20). There are packets of cells arranged in a loosely cohesive pattern. Although there are some multinucleated forms, most cells are monotonous with single, cherry-red nucleoli.

prominent cytologic pleomorphism. (2) Their clinical behavior also is markedly different: an excellent prognosis would be expected for a 1-cm clear cell sarcoma, whereas a nodular skin melanoma of this size would be rapidly lethal. In fact, most patients who have clear cell carcinoma tumors smaller than 2.5 cm fare well on follow-up [151]. (3) Clear cell sarcoma has a characteristic 12;22 translocation, whereas skin melanomas have complex karyotypes [154–161]. The gene product afforded by this translocation, the *EWS-ATF1* fusion transcript, can be detected by reverse transcriptase polymeric chain reaction (RT-PCR), and thus diagnosis of clear cell sarcoma can be made by molecular means, although diagnosis usually is not difficult by light microscopy [161].

Alveolar soft part sarcoma (ASPS) principally affects adolescents and young adults with a slight female predominance [162–167]. The tumor arises primarily in the deep soft tissues of the lower extremity, particularly the anterior thigh and the buttock [163], followed by the chest and abdominal wall. In children, ASPS has a proclivity for the head and neck region, especially the periorbital soft tissue and tongue. ASPS clinically presents as a slow-growing, painless mass which may be apparent for months to years before the patient seeks medical attention. Unfortunately, metastatic disease to the lung or brain sometimes heralds the presence of an occult sarcoma.

ASPS has a poor long-term survival. In a clinicopathologic study covering more than 60 years, Lieberman and colleagues [163] documented a 5-year survival rate of 60%, a 10-year survival rate of 38%, and a 20-year survival rate of only15% for patients presenting without metastatic disease. Death usually results from metastases to vital organs. The principal metastatic sites are the lung, followed by the brain and bone [163]. Children who have ASPS fare better than adults; earlier detection may be a factor in their improved survival rate [166,168].

At low magnification, ASPS displays a distinctive nested or organoid arrangement of large, polygonal cells with eosinophilic cytoplasm (Fig. 14). The nests are separated by thin-walled vascular channels. The neoplastic cells have distinct cell borders with eccentrically placed nuclei and prominent nucleoli. Periodic acid-Schiff stain detects intracytoplasmic glycogen and highlights elongated and rhomboid-shaped crystalline structures within the cytoplasm (Fig. 15). Tumors have the *ASPL-TFE3* fusion gene characterized by der(17)t(X;17)(p11.2;q25). The protein product can be detected immunohistochemically [169] as well as by molecular techniques.

Epithelioid sarcoma is the most common primary sarcoma of the hand and wrist [3]. The clinical and histologic features of epithelioid sarcoma can mimic those of a nonneoplastic process, so the sarcoma may be misdiagnosed until recurrence or metastasis reveals its true nature. Genetic evaluation of epithelioid sarcoma has yet to yield a consistent event.

Epithelioid sarcoma is most prevalent in patients between 10 and 39 years of age [170] and has a male predominance [171]. The flexor surface of the hand, fingers, and forearm are the most commonly involved sites, followed by the knee and lower leg, proximal lower and upper extremity, ankle, and the feet and toes. A history of trauma is elicited in about 20% to 25% of cases [170,171].

Epithelioid sarcoma arising in the dermis most often presents as a slow-growing, painless, usually solitary nodule or plaque. Epithelioid sarcoma situated in the subcutaneous or fascial tissue frequently presents as a fixed, relatively hard nodule. Tumors of the hand and penis clinically can mimic superficial fibromatoses. Dermal and subcutaneous lesions characteristically develop a cleft of the overlying skin that eventually ulcerates [172]. These innocuous clinical presentations commonly lead the clinician to the erroneous diagnosis of a benign lesion. The neoplasm spreads proximally up the extremity producing numerous cutaneous nodules and ulcerative lesions.

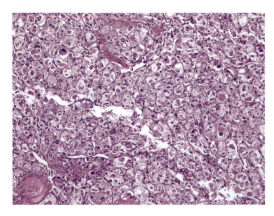

Fig. 14. Alveolar soft part sarcoma (hematoxylin-eosin, original magnification ×10). The tumor is arranged in organoid clusters containing cells with eosinophilic cytoplasm. There is prominent discohesion, rendering a pseudoalveolar appearance.

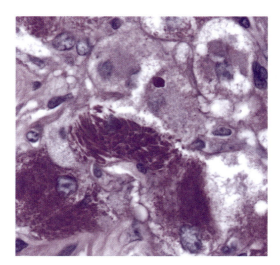

Fig. 15. Alveolar soft part sarcoma, periodic acid-Schiff (PAS) stain (hematoxylin-eosin, original magnification ×40). The PAS stain shows striking intracytoplasmic eosinophilic crystals. The crystalline deposition is attributed to the *ASPL-TFE* fusion.

Documented recurrence rates range from about 35% to more than 75% [170,173,174]. Multiple recurrences are characteristic. Metastases were reported in 45% of patients [170]. Lung and regional lymph nodes are the most common metastatic sites, followed by skin, soft tissue, and the central nervous system. Although the reported 5-year survival rate for epithelioid sarcoma is at least 60% in most studies [171,173–176], the overall survival of patients who have epithelioid sarcoma probably is quite low. Because lymph node involvement is more common in epithelioid sarcoma than in other types of sarcoma, regional lymph node dissection has a role.

Epithelioid sarcoma is characterized by a predominantly nodular growth pattern of epithelioid and plump spindle cells. The center of the nodule commonly undergoes degenerative change. At the periphery of the nodules, the epithelioid cells occasionally grow in a cordlike fashion, and the spindled cells form vague fascicles as these elements mingle with dense, eosinophilic collagen. When the tumor spreads along fascial planes and aponeurotic connective tissue, the confluent nodules align themselves along the length of the tissue plane, resulting in a band of tumor cells surrounding hypocellular or necrotic zones (garlandlike configuration).

Synovial sarcoma is a rare but distinctive soft tissue neoplasm showing epithelial differentiation. The term "synovial sarcoma" has become well established but is a misnomer: this tumor has no demonstrable relationship with synovium.

Between 5% and 10% of all soft tissue sarcomas are synovial sarcoma. Approximately 800 new cases per year are diagnosed in the United States [177]. Synovial sarcomas are mainly tumors of young adults with a male

predominance. Synovial sarcoma typically presents as an otherwise asymptomatic deep-seated, slow-growing mass. About 90% occur on the extremities, with a third around the knee. Fewer than 5% of cases originate within
a joint or bursa [178,179]. A distinct region of involvement is the head and
neck, most commonly the paravertebral region with pharyngeal
presentation.

Some tumors, especially in the lower limb, have radiologically detectable
scattered calcifications. This identification is diagnostically useful, because
such calcifications are rare in other types of sarcoma although they can be
found in benign processes (eg, calcifying fibrous pseudotumor).

Biphasic synovial sarcoma has an epithelial and a spindle-cell component
(Fig. 16). The epithelial cells have round vesicular nuclei, abundant cytoplasm, and distinct cell borders. Classically, they form glands with lumina
or prominent papillary structures with spindle cells rather than connective
tissue in the papillary core. The nuclei of the spindle cells typically are uniform, relatively small, ovoid, and pale staining with inconspicuous nucleoli.
Cytoplasm is scant, and the cell membranes are indistinct, so that nuclei
overlap. Mitotic figures can be scarce despite the cellularity.

Monophasic synovial sarcoma is comprised predominantly of only the
spindle cell component and therefore closely resembles other spindle cell sarcomas (Fig. 17). Its distinctive features have become appreciated and fully
accepted only in the last 2 decades. Many display, at least focally, a prominent hemangiopericytoma-like vascular architecture with open, branching
thin-walled vessels of variable caliber. An obvious epithelial component
sometimes can be found by extensive sampling, but this identification is
not necessary to make the diagnosis.

About one third of synovial sarcomas have focal calcification, with or
without ossification. Calcification is extensive in some tumors, and the

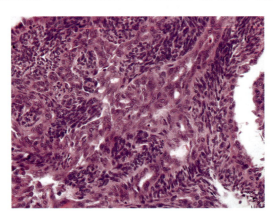

Fig. 16. Synovial sarcoma, biphasic (hematoxylin-eosin, original magnification ×10). There is
a dimorphic population: the epithelial component has plump, cohesive clusters with vesicular
nuclei; the spindle cell component has fascicular bundles with hyperchromatic and elongated
nuclei. The two elements are closely juxtaposed.

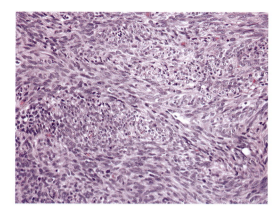

Fig. 17. Synovial sarcoma, monophasic (hematoxylin-eosin, original magnification ×10). In contrast to the biphasic variant, there is a monotonous population of spindle cells. Compare the loose fascicular architecture and the tightly woven fascicles of fibrosarcoma (see Fig. 4).

improved prognosis in such cases merits their separation as a subtype. This phenomenon is more common in synovial sarcoma of the lower extremities and is seen rarely in examples arising in the head and neck. The 32 calcifying synovial sarcoma described by Varela-Duran and Enzinger [180] were all biphasic, but calcifying monophasic synovial sarcoma exists.

A specific translocation involving chromosomes X and 18 has been described in synovial sarcoma [181]. This balanced reciprocal translocation, t(x;18)(p11.2;q11.2), is found in most reported synovial sarcomas. The resultant fusion gene product, SYT-SSX chimeric RNA [182], can be detected by RT-PCR in frozen and paraffin-embedded material [183,184]. These techniques are of diagnostic use, because this translocation has not been demonstrated convincingly in any other tumor types [184].

Bone tumors

Ewing's sarcoma and peripheral primitive neuroectodermal tumor (PNET) are biologically related tumors with histologic and ultrastructural commonalities [185–190]. Soft tissue examples of these neoplasms now are recognized as the second most common pediatric soft tissue sarcoma, following rhabdomyosarcoma. They also are the second most common bone tumors in young adults.

Ewing family tumors are primarily bone lesions; only a relatively small percentage arises in soft tissue. The most commonly affected areas are the diaphysis or metaphyseal-diaphyseal portions of long bone. Patients present with pain and an associated mass. Ewing family tumors are best considered as systemic phenomena, because systemic symptoms accompany the initial presentation. Fever, anemia, leukocytosis, and an elevated erythrocyte sedimentation rate may occur. As with all sarcomas, metastases at presentation (typically to lungs) are indicators of poor prognosis.

The distinction between Ewing's sarcoma and PNET lies in the presence of Homer Wright rosettes, which are present in PNET and are absent in Ewing's sarcoma. These microscopic structures comprise wreaths of dark, oval nuclei that circumscribe wispy, lightly pink, neurofibrillary cores. The presence of well-defined rosettes suffices to categorize a lesion histologically as PNET.

In contrast, Ewing's sarcoma is the quintessential "small round blue cell" tumor (Fig. 18). These tumors are composed of highly compressed cellular masses in diffuse sheets. The tumor cell nuclei typically possess round, even contours and smooth chromatin with inconspicuous nucleoli, being similar to but larger than lymphoid cells. One prominent distinction is their cytoplasm, which often is clear or bubbly because of an abundance of glycogen demonstrable by periodic acid-Schiff stains. Another prominent feature is the presence of interspersed amorphous clusters of cells with more condensed nuclei and lightly eosinophilic cytoplasm creating a pattern of alternating "light" cells and "dark" cells. Although these lesions grow rapidly, the mitotic index often is paradoxically low in typical Ewing's sarcoma.

The Ewing family of tumors is characterized genetically by a gene fusion between the *FLI1* gene on chromosome 11 and the *EWS* gene on chromosome 22. Karyotypically this fusion is expressed by the reciprocal translocation, t(11;22)(q24;q12). A variety of fusions may occur, all of which fuse the two translated protein molecules. The resultant protein is a fusion of a DNA transcription factor (*EWS*) joined to a RNA binding factor (*FLI1*) causing abnormal DNA regulation and leading to tumorigenesis. The genetic aberrations of the Ewing family tumors can be exploited for diagnosis.

Osteosarcomas are the most common primary malignancy of bone, comprising 35% of all bone tumors [191]. The most frequently diagnosed bone

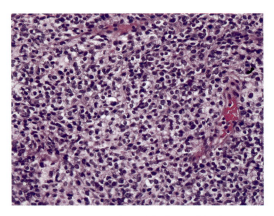

Fig. 18. Ewing's sarcoma (hematoxylin-eosin, original magnification ×20). Primitive blue cells display no distinguishable architectural attributes. Note the absence of rosette formation, distinguishing this tumor from peripheral primitive neuroectodermal tumor.

tumor in patients under the age of 20 years is osteosarcoma, followed by Ewing's sarcoma. Osteosarcomas classically arise as fast-growing metaphyseal lesions in the area of the knee and affect patients who have no known bone conditions. One third of osteosarcomas, however, occur in patients over the age of 40 years, in whom radiation exposure and pre-existing Paget disease should be considered. The most commonly affected site is the axial skeleton, followed by the proximal tibia and distal femur [192]. There is a gender predilection toward males in younger patients, but this trend diminishes with age. Regardless of age, patients present with deep, unremitting pain that develops over a period of weeks of months.

Osteosarcomas have a spectrum of gross appearance, ranging from well circumscribed to infiltrate, and display areas of dense yellow-white sclerosis to gray-tan pumice-like granularity. The histologic appearance is similarly wide ranging. There is a pleomorphic composition of cells which appear small and round, clear, multinucleated, spindled, epithelioid, plasmacytoid, or fusiform. Hence, the diagnosis of osteosarcoma hinges on the presence of osteoid, which is comprised of pink, dense, curvilinear extracellular material found in the center of the lesion. As can be expected from their heterogeneous appearance, osteosarcomas have no consistent genetic abnormalities.

Prognosis is best predicted by response to preoperative chemotherapy. Lesions with more than 90% tumor necrosis correspond to an 80% to 90% long-term survival rate, but lesions with less than 90% tumor necrosis correspond to a survival rate of less than 15% [193]. Current treatment is surgery combined with pre- and postoperative chemotherapy. With this multidisciplinary approach, long-term survival has increased to 70% [194], but patients who have h recurrent disease or metastatic lesions (typically to lungs) at diagnosis have a lower survival rate of 20%.

References

[1] Fletcher C, Unni K, Mertens FE. World Health Organization classification of tumours. Pathology and genetics of tumours of soft tissue and bone. Lyon (France): IACR Press; 2002.
[2] Weiss S. Histological typing of soft tissue tumours. Berlin: Springer-Verlag; 1994.
[3] Weiss S, Goldblum J. Enzinger and Weiss's soft tissue tumors. 4th edition. St. Louis (MO): Mosby; 2001.
[4] Montgomery E, Aaron AE. Clinical pathology of soft tissue tumors. New York: Marcel Dekker; 2001.
[5] Costa J, Wesley RA, Glatstein E, et al. The grading of soft tissue sarcomas. Results of a clinicohistopathologic correlation in a series of 163 cases. Cancer 1984;53:530–41.
[6] Markhede G, Angervall L, Stener B. A multivariate analysis of the prognosis after surgical treatment of malignant soft-tissue tumors. Cancer 1982;49:1721–33.
[7] Myhre-Jensen O, Kaae S, Madsen EH, et al. Histopathological grading in soft-tissue tumours. Relation to survival in 261 surgically treated patients. Acta Pathol Microbiol Immunol Scand [A] 1983;91:145–50.
[8] Miettinen M, Fetsch JF. Collagenous fibroma (desmoplastic fibroblastoma): a clinicopathologic analysis of 63 cases of a distinctive soft tissue lesion with stellate- shaped fibroblasts. Hum Pathol 1998;29:676–82.

[57] Mentzel T, Beham A, Katenkamp D, et al. Fibrosarcomatous ("high-grade") dermatofi-brosarcoma protuberans: clinicopathologic and immunohistochemical study of a series of 41 cases with emphasis on prognostic significance. Am J Surg Pathol 1998;22:576–87.

[58] Petoin DS, Verola O, Banzet P, et al. [Darier-Ferrand dermatofibrosarcoma. Study of 96 cases over 15 years]. Chirurgie 1985;111:132–8 [in French].

[59] Goldblum JR, Tuthill RJ. CD34 and factor-XIIIa immunoreactivity in dermatofibrosar-coma protuberans and dermatofibroma. Am J Dermatopathol 1997;19:147–53.

[60] Weiss SW, Nickoloff BJ. CD-34 is expressed by a distinctive cell population in peripheral nerve, nerve sheath tumors, and related lesions. Am J Surg Pathol 1993;17:1039–45.

[61] Minoletti F, Miozzo M, Pedeutour F, et al. Involvement of chromosomes 17 and 22 in der-matofibrosarcoma protuberans. Genes Chromosomes Cancer 1995;13:62–5.

[62] Mandahl N, Heim S, Willen H, et al. Supernumerary ring chromosome as the sole cytoge-netic abnormality in a dermatofibrosarcoma protuberans. Cancer Genet Cytogenet 1990; 49:273–5.

[63] O'Brien KP, Seroussi E, Dal Cin P, et al. Various regions within the alpha-helical domain of the COL1A1 gene are fused to the second exon of the PDGFB gene in dermatofibrosarco-mas and giant-cell fibroblastomas. Genes Chromosomes Cancer 1998;23:187–93.

[64] Simon MP, Pedeutour F, Sirvent N, et al. Deregulation of the platelet-derived growth fac-tor B-chain gene via fusion with collagen gene COL1A1 in dermatofibrosarcoma protuber-ans and giant-cell fibroblastoma. Nat Genet 1997;15:95–8.

[65] Fletcher CD. Pleomorphic malignant fibrous histiocytoma: fact or fiction? A critical reap-praisal based on 159 tumors diagnosed as pleomorphic sarcoma. Am J Surg Pathol 1992;16: 213–28.

[66] Cole CH, Magee JF, Gianoulis M, et al. Malignant fibrous histiocytoma in childhood. Can-cer 1993;71:4077–83.

[67] Fanburg-Smith JC, Spiro IJ, Katapuram SV, et al. Infiltrative subcutaneous malignant fibrous histiocytoma: a comparative study with deep malignant fibrous histiocytoma and an observation of biologic behavior. Ann Diagn Pathol 1999;3:1–10.

[68] Montgomery E, Fisher C. Myofibroblastic differentiation in malignant fibrous histiocy-toma (pleomorphic myofibrosarcoma): a clinicopathologic study. Histopathology 2001; 38:499–509.

[69] Pezzi CM, Rawlings MS Jr, Esgro JJ, et al. Prognostic factors in 227 patients with malig-nant fibrous histiocytoma. Cancer 1992;69:2098–103.

[70] Le Doussal V, Coindre JM, Leroux A, et al. Prognostic factors for patients with localized primary malignant fibrous histiocytoma: a multicenter study of 216 patients with multivar-iate analysis. Cancer 1996;77:1823–30.

[71] Weiss SW, Enzinger FM. Malignant fibrous histiocytoma: an analysis of 200 cases. Cancer 1978;41:2250–66.

[72] Mertens F, Fletcher CD, Dal Cin P, et al. Cytogenetic analysis of 46 pleomorphic soft tissue sarcomas and correlation with morphologic and clinical features: a report of the CHAMP Study Group. Chromosomes and Morphology. Genes Chromosomes Cancer 1998;22:16–25.

[73] Henricks WH, Chu YC, Goldblum JR, et al. Dedifferentiated liposarcoma: a clinicopatho-logical analysis of 155 cases with a proposal for an expanded definition of dedifferentiation. Am J Surg Pathol 1997;21:271–81.

[74] Guccion JG, Enzinger FM. Malignant giant cell tumor of soft parts. An analysis of 32 cases. Cancer 1972;29:1518–29.

[75] Merino MJ, LiVolsi VA. Inflammatory malignant fibrous histiocytoma. Am J Clin Pathol 1980;73:276–81.

[76] Kyriakos M, Kempson RL. Inflammatory fibrous histiocytoma. An aggressive and lethal lesion. Cancer 1976;37:1584–606.

[77] Coindre JM, Hostein I, Maire G, et al. Inflammatory malignant fibrous histiocytomas and dedifferentiated liposarcomas: histological review, genomic profile, and MDM2 and CDK4 status favour a single entity. J Pathol 2004;203:822–30.

[78] Gamez J, Playan A, Andreu AL, et al. Familial multiple symmetric lipomatosis associated with the A8344G mutation of mitochondrial DNA. Neurology 1998;51:258–60.

[79] Ronan SJ, Broderick T. Minimally invasive approach to familial multiple lipomatosis. Plast Reconstr Surg 2000;106:878–80.

[80] Tsao H, Sober AJ. Multiple lipomatosis in a patient with familial atypical mole syndrome. Br J Dermatol 1998;139:1118–9.

[81] Stoll C, Alembik Y, Truttmann M. Multiple familial lipomatosis with polyneuropathy, an inherited dominant condition. Ann Genet 1996;39:193–6.

[82] Chung EB, Enzinger FM. Benign lipoblastomatosis. An analysis of 35 cases. Cancer 1973; 32:482–92.

[83] Hicks J, Dilley A, Patel D, et al. Lipoblastoma and lipoblastomatosis in infancy and childhood: histopathologic, ultrastructural, and cytogenetic features. Ultrastruct Pathol 2001; 25:321–33.

[84] Mentzel T, Calonje E, Fletcher CD. Lipoblastoma and lipoblastomatosis: a clinicopathological study of 14 cases. Histopathology 1993;23:527–33.

[85] Collins MH, Chatten J. Lipoblastoma/lipoblastomatosis: a clinicopathologic study of 25 tumors. Am J Surg Pathol 1997;21:1131–7.

[86] Dal Cin P, Sciot R, De Wever I, et al. New discriminative chromosomal marker in adipose tissue tumors. The chromosome 8q11-q13 region in lipoblastoma. Cancer Genet Cytogenet 1994;78:232–5.

[87] Howard WR, Helwig EB. Angiolipoma. Arch Dermatol 1960;82:924–31.

[88] Enzinger FM, Harvey DA. Spindle cell lipoma. Cancer 1975;36:1852–9.

[89] Dal Cin P, Sciot R, Polito P, et al. Lesions of 13q may occur independently of deletion of 16q in spindle cell/pleomorphic lipomas. Histopathology 1997;31:222–5.

[90] Mandahl N, Mertens F, Willen H, et al. A new cytogenetic subgroup in lipomas: loss of chromosome 16 material in spindle cell and pleomorphic lipomas. J Cancer Res Clin Oncol 1994;120:707–11.

[91] Shmookler BM, Enzinger FM. Pleomorphic lipoma: a benign tumor simulating liposarcoma. A clinicopathologic analysis of 48 cases. Cancer 1981;47:126–33.

[92] Azzopardi JG, Iocco J, Salm R. Pleomorphic lipoma: a tumour simulating liposarcoma. Histopathology 1983;7:511–23.

[93] Meis JM, Enzinger FM. Chondroid lipoma. A unique tumor simulating liposarcoma and myxoid chondrosarcoma. Am J Surg Pathol 1993;17:1103–12.

[94] Tsutsumi M, Yamauchi A, Tsukamoto S, et al. A case of angiomyolipoma presenting as a huge retroperitoneal mass. Int J Urol 2001;8:470–1.

[95] Meis JM, Enzinger FM. Myolipoma of soft tissue. Am J Surg Pathol 1991;15:121–5.

[96] Furlong MA, Fanburg-Smith JC, Miettinen M. The morphologic spectrum of hibernoma: a clinicopathologic study of 170 cases. Am J Surg Pathol 2001;25:809–14.

[97] Gisselsson D, Hoglund M, Mertens F, et al. Hibernomas are characterized by homozygous deletions in the multiple endocrine neoplasia type I region. Metaphase fluorescence in situ hybridization reveals complex rearrangements not detected by conventional cytogenetics. Am J Pathol 1999;155:61–6.

[98] Evans HL, Soule EH, Winkelmann RK. Atypical lipoma, atypical intramuscular lipoma, and well differentiated retroperitoneal liposarcoma: a reappraisal of 30 cases formerly classified as well differentiated liposarcoma. Cancer 1979;43:574–84.

[99] Elgar F, Goldblum JR. Well-differentiated liposarcoma of the retroperitoneum: a clinicopathologic analysis of 20 cases, with particular attention to the extent of low-grade dedifferentiation. Mod Pathol 1997;10:113–20.

[100] Lucas DR, Nascimento AG, Sanjay BK, et al. Well-differentiated liposarcoma. The Mayo Clinic experience with 58 cases. Am J Clin Pathol 1994;102:677–83.

[101] Evans HL. Liposarcoma: a study of 55 cases with a reassessment of its classification. Am J Surg Pathol 1979;3:507–23.

[102] Weiss SW, Rao VK. Well-differentiated liposarcoma (atypical lipoma) of deep soft tissue of the extremities, retroperitoneum, and miscellaneous sites. A follow-up study of 92 cases with analysis of the incidence of "dedifferentiation". Am J Surg Pathol 1992;16: 1051–8.

[103] Enzinger F, Winslow D. Liposarcoma: a study of 103 cases. Virchows Arch Pathol Anat Physiol Klin Med 1962;335:367–88.

[104] Shmookler BM, Enzinger FM. Liposarcoma occurring in children. An analysis of 17 cases and review of the literature. Cancer 1983;52:567–74.

[105] Montgomery E, Fisher C. Paratesticular liposarcoma; a clinicopathologic study. Am J Surg Pathol 2003;27:40–7.

[106] Montgomery E, Fisher C. Paratesticular liposarcoma: a clinicopathologic study. Am J Surg Pathol 2003;27:40–7.

[107] Evans H. Liposarcomas and atypical lipomatous tumors: a study of 66 cases followed for a minimum of 10 years. Surg Pathol 1988;1:41–54.

[108] Rosai J, Akerman M, Dal Cin P, et al. Combined morphologic and karyotypic study of 59 atypical lipomatous tumors. Evaluation of their relationship and differential diagnosis with other adipose tissue tumors (a report of the CHAMP Study Group). Am J Surg Pathol 1996;20:1182–9.

[109] Fletcher CD, Akerman M, Dal Cin P, et al. Correlation between clinicopathological features and karyotype in lipomatous tumors. A report of 178 cases from the Chromosomes and Morphology (CHAMP) Collaborative Study Group. Am J Pathol 1996;148: 623–30.

[110] Azumi N, Curtis J, Kempson RL, et al. Atypical and malignant neoplasms showing lipomatous differentiation. A study of 111 cases. Am J Surg Pathol 1987;11:161–83.

[111] Yoshikawa H, Ueda T, Mori S, et al. Dedifferentiated liposarcoma of the subcutis. Am J Surg Pathol 1996;20:1525–30.

[112] McCormick D, Mentzel T, Beham A, et al. Dedifferentiated liposarcoma. Clinicopathologic analysis of 32 cases suggesting a better prognostic subgroup among pleomorphic sarcomas [see comments]. Am J Surg Pathol 1994;18:1213–23.

[113] Oliveira AM, Nascimento AG, Okuno SH, et al. p27(kip1) protein expression correlates with survival in myxoid and round-cell liposarcoma. J Clin Oncol 2000;18:2888–93.

[114] Kilpatrick SE, Doyon J, Choong PF, et al. The clinicopathologic spectrum of myxoid and round cell liposarcoma. A study of 95 cases. Cancer 1996;77:1450–8.

[115] Tallini G, Akerman M, Dal Cin P, et al. Combined morphologic and karyotypic study of 28 myxoid liposarcomas. Implications for a revised morphologic typing, (a report from the CHAMP Group). Am J Surg Pathol 1996;20:1047–55.

[116] Spillane AJ, Fisher C, Thomas JM. Myxoid liposarcoma—the frequency and the natural history of nonpulmonary soft tissue metastases. Ann Surg Oncol 1999;6:389–94.

[117] Smith TA, Easley KA, Goldblum JR. Myxoid/round cell liposarcoma of the extremities. A clinicopathologic study of 29 cases with particular attention to extent of round cell liposarcoma. Am J Surg Pathol 1996;20:171–80.

[118] Antonescu CR, Elahi A, Healey JH, et al. Monoclonality of multifocal myxoid liposarcoma: confirmation by analysis of TLS-CHOP or EWS-CHOP rearrangements. Clin Cancer Res 2000;6:2788–93.

[119] Antonescu CR, Tschernyavsky SJ, Decuseara R, et al. Prognostic impact of P53 status, TLS-CHOP fusion transcript structure, and histological grade in myxoid liposarcoma: a molecular and clinicopathologic study of 82 cases. Clin Cancer Res 2001;7:3977–87.

[120] Sreekantaiah C, Karakousis CP, Leong SP, et al. Trisomy 8 as a nonrandom secondary change in myxoid liposarcoma. Cancer Genet Cytogenet 1991;51:195–205.

[121] Paulien S, Turc-Carel C, Dal Cin P, et al. Myxoid liposarcoma with t(12;16) (q13;p11) contains site-specific differences in methylation patterns surrounding a zinc-finger gene mapped to the breakpoint region on chromosome 12. Cancer Res 1990;50:7902–7.

[122] Newton WA Jr, Soule EH, Hamoudi AB, et al. Histopathology of childhood sarcomas, Intergroup Rhabdomyosarcoma Studies I and II: clinicopathologic correlation. J Clin Oncol 1988;6:67–75.

[123] Cavazzana AO, Schmidt D, Ninfo V, et al. Spindle cell rhabdomyosarcoma. A prognostically favorable variant of rhabdomyosarcoma. Am J Surg Pathol 1992;16:229–35.

[124] Enzinger FM, Shiraki M. Alveolar rhabdomyosarcoma. An analysis of 110 cases. Cancer 1969;24:18–31.

[125] Parham DM. Pathologic classification of rhabdomyosarcomas and correlations with molecular studies. Mod Pathol 2001;14:506–14.

[126] Chen B, Dias P, Jenkins JJ 3rd, et al. Methylation alterations of the MyoD1 upstream region are predictive of subclassification of human rhabdomyosarcomas. Am J Pathol 1998;152:1071–9.

[127] Sorensen PH, Lynch JC, Qualman SJ, et al. PAX3-FKHR and PAX7-FKHR gene fusions are prognostic indicators in alveolar rhabdomyosarcoma: a report from the children's oncology group. J Clin Oncol 2002;20:2672–9.

[128] Douglass EC, Rowe ST, Valentine M, et al. Variant translocations of chromosome 13 in alveolar rhabdomyosarcoma. Genes Chromosomes Cancer 1991;3:480–2.

[129] Barr FG, Qualman SJ, Macris MH, et al. Genetic heterogeneity in the alveolar rhabdomyosarcoma subset without typical gene fusions. Cancer Res 2002;62:4704–10.

[130] Douglass EC, Shapiro DN, Valentine M, et al. Alveolar rhabdomyosarcoma with the t(2;13): cytogenetic findings and clinicopathologic correlations. Med Pediatr Oncol 1993;21:83–7.

[131] Shapiro DN, Sublett JE, Li B, et al. Fusion of PAX3 to a member of the forkhead family of transcription factors in human alveolar rhabdomyosarcoma. Cancer Res 1993;53:5108–12.

[132] Shapiro DN, Valentine MB, Sublett JE, et al. Chromosomal sublocalization of the 2;13 translocation breakpoint in alveolar rhabdomyosarcoma. Genes Chromosomes Cancer 1992;4:241–9.

[133] Crist W, Gehan EA, Ragab AH, et al. The Third Intergroup Rhabdomyosarcoma Study. J Clin Oncol 1995;13:610–30.

[134] Schurch W, Begin LR, Seemayer TA, et al. Pleomorphic soft tissue myogenic sarcomas of adulthood. A reappraisal in the mid-1990s. Am J Surg Pathol 1996;20:131–47.

[135] Gaffney EF, Dervan PA, Fletcher CD. Pleomorphic rhabdomyosarcoma in adulthood. Analysis of 11 cases with definition of diagnostic criteria. Am J Surg Pathol 1993;17:601–9.

[136] Furlong MA, Mentzel T, Fanburg-Smith JC. Pleomorphic rhabdomyosarcoma in adults: a clinicopathologic study of 38 cases with emphasis on morphologic variants and recent skeletal muscle-specific markers. Mod Pathol 2001;14:595–603.

[137] Sonobe H, Takeuchi T, Taguchi T, et al. A new human pleomorphic rhabdomyosarcoma cell-line, HS-RMS-1, exhibiting MyoD1 and myogenin. Int J Oncol 2000;17:119–25.

[138] Das Gupta TK, Brasfield RD, Strong EW, et al. Benign solitary schwannomas (neurilemomas). Cancer 1969;24:355–66.

[139] Antinheimo J, Sankila R, Carpen O, et al. Population-based analysis of sporadic and type 2 neurofibromatosis-associated meningiomas and schwannomas. Neurology 2000;54:71–6.

[140] Stout A. The peripheral manifestations of specific nerve sheath tumor (neurilemoma). Am J Cancer 1935;24:751–96.

[141] Scheithauer B, Woodruff JM, Erlandson RA. Tumors of the peripheral nervous system. Washington, DC: American Registry of Pathology; 1999.

[142] Ducatman BS, Scheithauer BW, Piepgras DG, et al. Malignant peripheral nerve sheath tumors. A clinicopathologic study of 120 cases. Cancer 1986;57:2006–21.

[143] Kourea HP, Bilsky MH, Leung DH, et al. Subdiaphragmatic and intrathoracic paraspinal malignant peripheral nerve sheath tumors: a clinicopathologic study of 25 patients and 26 tumors. Cancer 1998;82:2191–203.

[144] Sorensen SA, Mulvihill JJ, Nielsen A. Long-term follow-up of von Recklinghausen neurofibromatosis. Survival and malignant neoplasms. N Engl J Med 1986;314:1010–5.

[145] Guccion JG, Enzinger FM. Malignant schwannoma associated with von Recklinghausen's neurofibromatosis. Virchows Arch A Pathol Anat Histol 1979;383:43–57.

[146] Daimaru Y, Hashimoto H, Enjoji M. Malignant peripheral nerve-sheath tumors (malignant schwannomas). An immunohistochemical study of 29 cases. Am J Surg Pathol 1985;9:434–44.

[147] deCou JM, Rao BN, Parham DM, et al. Malignant peripheral nerve sheath tumors: the St. Jude Children's Research Hospital experience. Ann Surg Oncol 1995;2:524–9.

[148] Hruban RH, Shiu MH, Senie RT, et al. Malignant peripheral nerve sheath tumors of the buttock and lower extremity. A study of 43 cases. Cancer 1990;66:1253–65.

[149] Wong WW, Hirose T, Scheithauer BW, et al. Malignant peripheral nerve sheath tumor: analysis of treatment outcome. Int J Radiat Oncol Biol Phys 1998;42:351–60.

[150] Lucas DR, Nascimento AG, Sim FH. Clear cell sarcoma of soft tissues. Mayo Clinic experience with 35 cases. Am J Surg Pathol 1992;16:1197–204.

[151] Montgomery E, Meis J, Ramos A, et al. Clear cell sarcoma of tendons and aponeuroses. A clinicopathologic study of 58 cases with analysis of prognostic factors. Int J Surg Pathol 1993;1:89–100.

[152] Enzinger F. Clear cell sarcoma of tendons and aponeuroses: an analysis of 21 cases. Cancer 1965;18:1163–74.

[153] Chung EB, Enzinger FM. Malignant melanoma of soft parts. A reassessment of clear cell sarcoma. Am J Surg Pathol 1983;7:405–13.

[154] Reeves BR, Fletcher CD, Gusterson BA. Translocation t(12;22)(q13;q13) is a nonrandom rearrangement in clear cell sarcoma. Cancer Genet Cytogenet 1992;64:101–3.

[155] Bridge JA, Sreekantaiah C, Neff JR, et al. Cytogenetic findings in clear cell sarcoma of tendons and aponeuroses. Malignant melanoma of soft parts. Cancer Genet Cytogenet 1991;52:101–6.

[156] Fujimura Y, Ohno T, Siddique H, et al. The EWS-ATF-1 gene involved in malignant melanoma of soft parts with t(12;22) chromosome translocation, encodes a constitutive transcriptional activator. Oncogene 1996;12:159–67.

[157] Langezaal SM, Graadt van Roggen JF, Cleton-Jansen AM, et al. Malignant melanoma is genetically distinct from clear cell sarcoma of tendons and aponeurosis (malignant melanoma of soft parts). Br J Cancer 2001;84:535–8.

[158] Mrozek K, Karakousis CP, Perez-Mesa C, et al. Translocation t(12;22)(q13;q12.2-12.3) in a clear cell sarcoma of tendons and aponeuroses. Genes Chromosomes Cancer 1993;6:249–52.

[159] Nedoszytko B, Mrozek K, Roszkiewicz A, et al. Clear cell sarcoma of tendons and aponeuroses with t(12;22) (q13;q12) diagnosed initially as malignant melanoma. Cancer Genet Cytogenet 1996;91:37–9.

[160] Zucman J, Delattre O, Desmaze C, et al. EWS and ATF-1 gene fusion induced by t(12;22) translocation in malignant melanoma of soft parts. Nat Genet 1993;4:341–5.

[161] Antonescu CR, Tschernyavsky SJ, Woodruff JM, et al. Molecular diagnosis of clear cell sarcoma: detection of EWS-ATF1 and MITF-M transcripts and histopathological and ultrastructural analysis of 12 cases. J Mol Diagn 2002;4:44–52.

[162] van Ruth S, van Coevorden F, Peterse JL, et al. Alveolar soft part sarcoma. a report of 15 cases. Eur J Cancer 2002;38:1324–8.

[163] Lieberman PH, Brennan MF, Kimmel M, et al. Alveolar soft-part sarcoma. A clinico-pathologic study of half a century. Cancer 1989;63:1–13.

[164] Evans HL. Alveolar soft-part sarcoma. A study of 13 typical examples and one with a histologically atypical component. Cancer 1985;55:912–7.

[165] Portera CA Jr, Ho V, Patel SR, et al. Alveolar soft part sarcoma: clinical course and patterns of metastasis in 70 patients treated at a single institution. Cancer 2001;91:585–91.

[166] Matsuno Y, Mukai K, Itabashi M, et al. Alveolar soft part sarcoma. A clinicopathologic and immunohistochemical study of 12 cases. Acta Pathol Jpn 1990;40:199–205.

[167] Auerbach HE, Brooks JJ. Alveolar soft part sarcoma. A clinicopathologic and immunohistochemical study. Cancer 1987;60:66–73.

[168] Pappo AS, Parham DM, Cain A, et al. Alveolar soft part sarcoma in children and adolescents: clinical features and outcome of 11 patients. Med Pediatr Oncol 1996;26:81–4.

[169] Argani P, Lal P, Hutchinson B, et al. Aberrant nuclear immunoreactivity for TFE3 in neoplasms with TFE3 gene fusions. Am J Surg Pathol 2003;27:750–61.

[170] Chase DR, Enzinger FM. Epithelioid sarcoma. Diagnosis, prognostic indicators, and treatment. Am J Surg Pathol 1985;9:241–63.

[171] Prat J, Woodruff JM, Marcove RC. Epithelioid sarcoma: an analysis of 22 cases indicating the prognostic significance of vascular invasion and regional lymph node metastasis. Cancer 1978;41:1472–87.

[172] Dabska M, Koszarowski T. Clinical and pathologic study of aponeurotic (epithelioid) sarcoma. Pathol Annu 1982;17(Pt 1):129–53.

[173] Halling AC, Wollan PC, Pritchard DJ, et al. Epithelioid sarcoma: a clinicopathologic review of 55 cases. Mayo Clin Proc 1996;71:636–42.

[174] Ross HM, Lewis JJ, Woodruff JM, et al. Epithelioid sarcoma: clinical behavior and prognostic factors of survival. Ann Surg Oncol 1997;4:491–5.

[175] Bos GD, Pritchard DJ, Reiman HM, et al. Epithelioid sarcoma. An analysis of fifty-one cases. J Bone Joint Surg Am 1988;70:862–70.

[176] Evans HL, Baer SC. Epithelioid sarcoma: a clinicopathologic and prognostic study of 26 cases. Semin Diagn Pathol 1993;10:286–91.

[177] Kransdorf MJ. Malignant soft-tissue tumors in a large referral population: distribution of diagnoses by age, sex, and location. AJR Am J Roentgenol 1995;164:129–34.

[178] Dardick I, O'Brien PK, Jeans MT, et al. Synovial sarcoma arising in an anatomical bursa. Virchows Arch A Pathol Anat Histol 1982;397:93–101.

[179] McKinney CD, Mills SE, Fechner RE. Intraarticular synovial sarcoma. Am J Surg Pathol 1992;16:1017–20.

[180] Varela-Duran J, Enzinger FM. Calcifying synovial sarcoma. Cancer 1982;50:345–52.

[181] Smith S, Reeves BR, Wong L, et al. A consistent chromosome translocation in synovial sarcoma [letter]. Cancer Genet Cytogenet 1987;26:179–80.

[182] Clark J, Rocques PJ, Crew AJ, et al. Identification of novel genes, SYT and SSX, involved in the t(X;18)(p11.2;q11.2) translocation found in human synovial sarcoma. Nat Genet 1994;7:502–8.

[183] Coindre JM, Hostein I, Benhattar J, et al. Malignant peripheral nerve sheath tumors are t(X;18)-negative sarcomas. Molecular analysis of 25 cases occurring in neurofibromatosis type 1 patients, using two different RT-PCR-based methods of detection. Mod Pathol 2002;15:589–92.

[184] van de Rijn M, Barr FG, Collins MH, et al. Absence of SYT-SSX fusion products in soft tissue tumors other than synovial sarcoma. Am J Clin Pathol 1999;112:43–9.

[185] Douglass EC, Rowe ST, Valentine M, et al. A second nonrandom translocation, der(16)t(1;16)(q21;q13), in Ewing sarcoma and peripheral neuroectodermal tumor. Cytogenet Cell Genet 1990;53:87–90.

[186] Downing JR, Head DR, Parham DM, et al. Detection of the (11;22)(q24;q12) translocation of Ewing's sarcoma and peripheral neuroectodermal tumor by reverse transcription polymerase chain reaction. Am J Pathol 1993;143:1294–300.

[187] Sorensen PH, Lessnick SL, Lopez-Terrada D, et al. A second Ewing's sarcoma translocation, t(21;22), fuses the EWS gene to another ETS-family transcription factor, ERG. Nat Genet 1994;6:146–51.

[188] Weidner N, Tjoe J. Immunohistochemical profile of monoclonal antibody O13: antibody that recognizes glycoprotein p30/32MIC2 and is useful in diagnosing Ewing's sarcoma and peripheral neuroepithelioma. Am J Surg Pathol 1994;18:486–94.

[189] Yunis EJ. Ewing's sarcoma and related small round cell neoplasms in children. Am J Surg Pathol 1986;10(Suppl 1):54–62.

[190] Delattre O, Zucman J, Melot T, et al. The Ewing family of tumors—a subgroup of small-round-cell tumors defined by specific chimeric transcripts. N Engl J Med 1994;331:294–9.

[191] Dorfman HD, Czerniak B. Bone cancers. Cancer 1995;75:203–10.
[192] Huvos AG. Osteogenic sarcoma of bones and soft tissues in older persons. A clinicopath-ologic analysis of 117 patients older than 60 years. Cancer 1986;57:1442–9.
[193] Raymond AK, Chawla SP, Carrasco CH, et al. Osteosarcoma chemotherapy effect: a prog-nostic factor. Semin Diagn Pathol 1987;4:212–36.
[194] Nagarajan R, Clohisy D, Weigel B. New paradigms for therapy for osteosarcoma. Curr Oncol Rep 2005;7:410–4.

ELSEVIER
SAUNDERS

SURGICAL
CLINICS OF
NORTH AMERICA

Surg Clin N Am 88 (2008) 521–537

Advanced Modalities
for the Imaging of Sarcoma

Dalia Fadul, MD, Laura M. Fayad, MD*

*The Russell H. Morgan Department of Radiology and Radiological Science,
Johns Hopkins University, 601 North Caroline Street, Baltimore, MD 21287, USA*

There is a diversity of modalities available for the imaging of soft tissue and skeletal sarcomas. However, conventional radiography remains the first line imaging modality in the diagnostic work-up, as it provides superior spatial resolution for the evaluation of bone trabecular detail [1]. In the assessment of skeletal sarcomas, radiography is used for initial detection and characterization of the lesion. In the assessment of soft tissue sarcomas, radiography is less valuable for detection, given its poor contrast resolution compared with cross-sectional modalities, though it is often employed for the assessment of tumor calcification patterns that aid the characterization of these masses.

Cross-sectional imaging techniques have become essential for the comprehensive analysis of sarcomas, for the primary purpose of treatment planning and when additional characterization is needed beyond radiography. Magnetic resonance imaging (MRI) is most advantageous for the determination of the extent of newly discovered masses and for the assessment of tumors following treatment. MRI may allow further characterization of a mass, based on such features as the enhancement pattern, location, and signal strength. Computed tomography (CT) may be used for initial staging when MRI is contra-indicated, but is most valuable for the characterization of skeletal masses and soft tissue mineralization patterns. A final technique that has emerged is that of positron emission tomography (PET) imaging, which affords the advantage of whole body imaging rather than locoregional staging. This article focuses on the advanced imaging modalities of CT, MRI, and PET in the evaluation of sarcomas.

* Corresponding author.
  E-mail address: lfayad1@jhmi.edu (L.M. Fayad).

Computed tomography

CT is a noninvasive diagnostic technique that uses a rotational radiographic source to generate cross-sectional images [2]. It essentially maps the density of electrons in tissue to create an image. An important benefit of using CT is its ability to provide rapid image acquisition, which reduces the need for sedation. This feature is especially useful in the pediatric population and in critically ill patients [3,4]. CT is less expensive than MRI and provides excellent osseous cortical detail and definition of lesion matrix mineralization patterns. It can also be used to image those patients with contraindications to MRI. CT represents a cost-effective modality for a wide range of clinical problems and is widely available [1,2].

CT offers better spatial resolution than MRI, though it still remains inferior to radiography in this respect. However, it can provide a clear anatomic depiction of complex areas not well evaluated by radiography, such as the axial skeleton and small joints. With recent technologic advances and the introduction of thin-section multi-detector scanners (16-, 64-detector, and beyond), CT offers the capability of producing imaging datasets with isotropic resolution that result in improved image quality. Such datasets in turn allow the reconstruction of multiplanar reformatted images and three-dimensional (3D) CT images with optimal spatial resolution. In addition, faster gantry rotation speed allows more volume coverage at improved temporal resolution, decreasing motion artifact. Finally, more efficient X-ray tube usage minimizes beam-hardening artifact with metallic hardware, allowing for a better postoperative evaluation than MRI, in the presence of metal [2].

CT angiography is another facet of CT that is evolving. Technologic advances in this area include improved isotropic datasets and temporal resolution, allowing enhanced visualization of the vascularity of sarcomas. Specifically, CT angiography can delineate tumor size, extent, source, and degree of vascularity, which aids in establishing the grade of malignancy [5], though the contrast resolution afforded by CT is inferior to that of MRI. Intravenous contrast is necessary when evaluating soft tissue sarcomas, though not so for skeletal sarcomas, which are evaluated by their characteristic patterns of bone destruction rather than their contrast enhancement patterns.

Disadvantages of using CT include the exposure to radiation and its poor contrast resolution when compared with MRI. In addition, if the use of intravenous contrast is necessary, there is a risk of allergic reaction or contrast nephropathy [1,2].

With regard to the evaluation of the primary mass, CT is most frequently indicated for the characterization of the mass. Other indications include the assessment of surrounding bone destruction and fracture risk, the identification of potential tumor recurrence in the presence of hardware and, finally, the detection of metastatic disease. For example, metastatic disease to the lungs is common with osteosarcoma and early detection improves survival rates. Therefore, as part of the diagnostic work-up, lung evaluation is required, and CT represents the most sensitive technique for detecting lung metastases [3,4,6].

Skeletal sarcomas

When evaluating skeletal tumors, CT is useful for characterizing the pattern of bone destruction, tumor margins, and matrix, to guide the diagnosis between benign and malignant lesions as well as to determine the histology of the lesion. Analysis of any matrix mineralization patterns can be helpful in offering a more specific diagnosis. Sarcomas may produce chondroid, osteoid, or fibrous matrix. Chondroid matrix tends to produce small punctuate or swirled areas of calcification, sometimes described as "arcs and whorls," "popcorn" calcification, or "speckled," as can be seen with chondrosarcoma (Fig. 1). Osseous matrix tends to appear dense and confluent, sometimes described as "cloud-like," and is characteristically seen in osteosarcomas (Fig. 2) [4,7], while fibrous matrix is not calcified, occasionally with a "ground glass" quality.

To distinguish between a benign and a malignant process, CT evaluation includes the assessment of tumor margins and the pattern of cortical and periosteal bone destruction. Well-defined margins indicate a more benign process, whereas ill-defined or irregular margins are indicative of a destructive or malignant process. Regarding the periosteum, benign periosteal reaction is described as solid or continuous, while malignant periosteal reaction can have a number of appearances, described as interrupted, spiculated

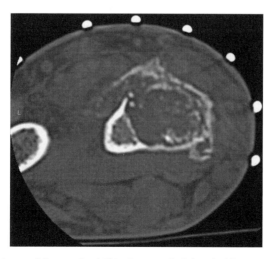

Fig. 1. Axial CT image of the proximal tibia shows typical chondroid-type matrix with stippled and curvilinear calcifications, and cortical destruction in a chondrosarcoma of the proximal tibia.

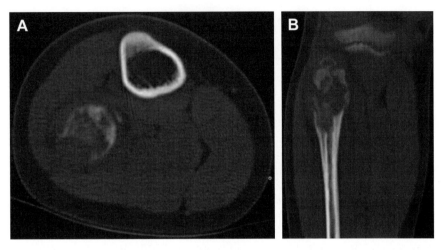

Fig. 2. Axial (*A*) and coronal volume rendered 3D (*B*) CT images of the proximal fibula. Typical "cloud-like" osseous matrix is shown, with cortical destruction in a proven case of osteosarcoma of the proximal fibula.

(hair-on-end or sunburst), lamellated (onion skinning), or triangular (Codman's triangle) [4,8,9]. As an example, Ewing's sarcoma can demonstrate all of the aforementioned types of periosteal reaction, though the lamellated and hair-on-end appearances are classic descriptors. The Codman's triangle and sunburst periosteal reaction are classically associated with osteosarcoma or chondrosarcoma [4,9].

Soft tissue sarcomas

Soft tissue sarcomas may contain components of varying densities, which can be demonstrated by CT. Most importantly, a solid lesion such as a sarcoma can be accurately differentiated from a simple cyst by the presence of enhancement within the lesion following contrast administration. Often, however, especially when large, sarcomas will have necrotic areas, which will appear cystic on CT (Fig. 3). Other densities may be observed within a mass that may allude to its histology. For example, lesions that contain fat (lipomatous lesions) are well characterized by CT and liposarcomas are fat-containing lesions that will also demonstrate soft tissue density, including thickened, irregular septa and nodular components [10] in addition to fat density, to differentiate them from their benign counterparts (lipomas). Another density characteristic that may be used to distinguish the histology of a lesion is high-density material, which may reflect proteinaceous or hemorrhagic content within the mass.

When evaluating soft tissue sarcomas, CT provides the capability for detecting mineralization (calcification or ossification) within a mass that may guide the diagnosis toward soft tissue chondrosarcomas or osteosarcomas.

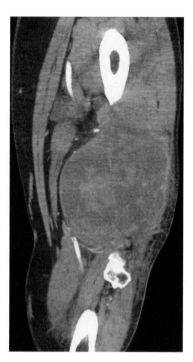

Fig. 3. Coronal CT image of a high-grade sarcoma shows a very large heterogeneous soft tissue mass of the thigh with solid and cystic components, causing displacement of the surrounding vessels without evidence of cortical involvement.

However, known as the great mimicker, myositis ossificans circumscripta refers to localized bone and cartilage formation in the soft tissues and is usually post-traumatic. Often mistaken for a sarcoma, CT is essential for characterizing its benign nature through the presence of a peripheral zonal pattern of calcification (Fig. 4) [11]. While the mineralization pattern is typically peripheral, it is not contiguous with the underlying bone and does not cause periosteal reaction, characteristics that are nicely confirmed by CT.

Magnetic resonance imaging

MRI is a noninvasive technique that uses the proton within hydrogen atoms in the body to create an image based on an applied magnetic field [12]. Advantages of MRI over other imaging techniques include its high contrast resolution, superior to other cross-sectional imaging modalities, resulting in the visualization of exquisite soft tissue detail. In addition, it is more sensitive than CT for the detection of bone marrow abnormalities. MRI also requires no radiation exposure, but like CT, offers multiplanar imaging capability [4,12].

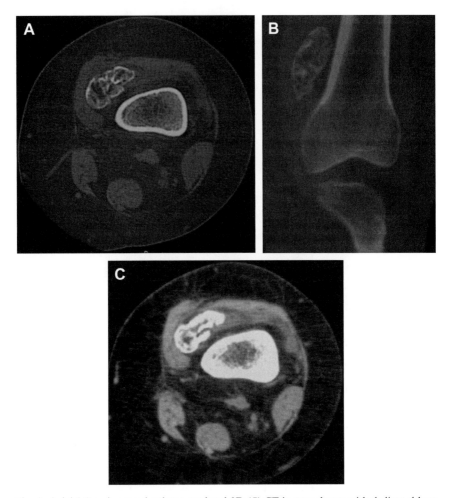

Fig. 4. Axial (*A*) and coronal volume rendered 3D (*B*) CT images shown with dedicated bone windows, and axial (*C*) CT image with dedicated soft tissue window of the distal thigh, show a peripherally calcified, well-defined soft tissue lesion with lobular borders and no evidence of underlying bone involvement in a case of myositis ossificans circumscripta. There is associated surrounding soft tissue edema.

Disadvantages of MRI include a long imaging acquisition time, much longer than CT, which may require the use of sedation, a challenge in the pediatric patient. Additionally, there are numerous contraindications to the performance of MRI based on the fact that the strong magnetic field can move implanted metal structures in the body. Absolute contraindications include the presence of a cardiac pacemaker, implanted cardiac defibrillator, aneurysm clips, carotid artery vascular clamp, neurostimulator, insulin or infusion pump, implanted drug infusion device, bone growth or fusion stimulator, and cochler or otologic or ear implant. Patients suffering from claustrophobia may also be unable to tolerate the procedure, a problem also occasionally encountered with CT, although to a much lesser degree. More open configurations for the magnet have been invented to circumvent this problem, but the quality of the images produced by such magnets is poorer [12].

MRI is the modality of choice for the locoregional staging of musculoskeletal masses. The particular sequences that are useful for tumor evaluation differ from other indications for MRI, such as for the identification of the internal derangement of joints. When evaluating tumors, whether soft tissue or osseous in nature, pure spin echo T1-weighted and fluid-sensitive sequences are indicated to detect the mass, characterize it, and determine its extent. T1-weighted images provide high signal-to-noise images for good anatomic detail of the affected structures and, in the setting of osseous tumors, are especially necessary for the identification of the tumor extent within the bone marrow. Also, most musculoskeletal tumors demonstrate increased fluid signal, so that fluid sensitive sequences (fat-saturated T2-weighted and short tau inversion recovery sequences) are also fundamental. Sarcomas may be homogeneous or heterogeneous. However, malignancies, by virtue of their very nature and potential for autonomous growth, are generally larger and more likely to outgrow their vascular supply with subsequent infarction, necrosis, and heterogeneous signal intensity on MR imaging. Consequently, the larger a mass is, the greater its heterogeneity, the greater is the concern for malignancy [12–15]. In addition to spin echo sequences, gradient echo sequences may be indicated to evaluate for the presence of calcification or hemosiderin [15].

Intravenous contrast administration is not absolutely indicated for the evaluation of de novo skeletal sarcomas, as routine noncontrast images are adequate for defining the presence of a mass. Contrast is, however, required for the assessment of de novo soft tissue masses and for the posttreatment evaluation of all sarcomas. For de novo soft tissue masses, contrast is used for characterization and is especially useful to distinguish simple cystic lesions (for example, ganglions) from solid tumors; it may also be used to guide the selection of a biopsy site (to a non-necrotic portion of the mass). Enhancement following contrast administration reflects tissue vascularity and tissue perfusion, and, in general, the rate of enhancement in malignant lesions is greater than that seen in benign lesions [16,17]. However, it should be noted that MRI with contrast has relatively low specificity for characterizing lesions for malignancy, estimated to be between 25% and 48% [17–19].

On the other hand, an important use of contrast lies in the assessment of tumors that have been treated, whereby contrast helps determines if viable tumor remains [12,14]. Following the treatment of sarcomas, MRI is used to monitor preoperative neoadjuvant therapy to predict the percentage of tumor necrosis, the most important factor differentiating treatment responders from nonresponders and one of the most reliable predictors of outcome. For this purpose, MRI may provide an estimate of the percentage of tissue necrosis that has occurred, but a change in the size of the lesion, the most commonly used feature, is not an accurate measure of response. Other measures of treatment response include the use of dynamic contrast-enhanced techniques, but these are often cumbersome and provide information on only a portion of the lesion. Following surgery, MRI is the modality of choice for the distinction between residual or recurrent tumor and post-operative fibrosis or inflammation. For this purpose, there is some overlap in the features of benign postsurgical inflammation and the presence of subtle residual or recurrent disease. In fact, only when there is an absence of T2 signal can the MRI absolutely rule out the presence of tumor in the surgical bed [17,18], as increased T2 signal and contrast enhancement can be observed in tumor, as well as immature scar tissue and nonmalignant reactive tissue. It should be noted that a recent drawback for using contrast (gadolinium) has emerged in the form of nephrogenic systemic fibrosis, occurring in patients with pre-existing renal disease [20].

Advanced techniques, such as diffusion weighted imaging and MR spectroscopy, are under investigation and may become a fundamental part of the routine evaluation of sarcomas. These sequences do not require the use of intravenous contrast administration and may prove to add specificity to conventional MRI for the characterization of disease processes. Preliminary research has shown that diffusion-weighted imaging has the potential to differentiate between benign and malignant soft tissue masses. With MR spectroscopy, the metabolic make-up of a mass may be ascertained, with the focus on detecting metabolites that are characteristically elevated in malignancy. Recent studies indicate that the metabolite choline is elevated in malignant musculoskeletal lesions [21–23].

Skeletal sarcomas

When evaluating skeletal sarcomas, MRI is not particularly useful for characterization of the mass (which is typically done by radiography). However, it is the modality of choice for determining the extent of bone marrow involvement of a lesion, for the purpose of treatment planning, including the detection of any skip lesions. Tumors appear as a marrow replacement process on T1-weighted images and can have either well-defined or ill-defined margins. T2-weighted images are useful for defining the extent of masses into the adjacent soft tissues, but are not specific for this purpose [4]. Contrast is generally not required for de novo lesions, although occasionally, intravenous contrast may add specificity to the characterization of a mass by MRI. Contrast is used primarily in the setting of prior treatment for differentiating posttreatment residual or recurrent disease from fibrosis, and as a preliminary estimate of postneoadjuvant therapy response [12–14,16–18].

Many sarcomas have a nonspecific appearance by MRI. However, there are a handful of lesions with specific MRI characteristics. For instance, telangectatic osteosarcoma can have a distinctive appearance on MRI, demonstrating fluid-fluid levels, internal septations, enhancement and peripheral heterogeniety (Fig. 5). However, such features must be considered in the setting of other findings that would suggest malignancy, because fluid-fluid levels may also be identified in benign processes, such as bone cysts, giant cell tumors, and any lesion with a fracture [14,16,17].

Low-grade cartilage lesions often have a distinctive appearance by MRI as well. Encondromas are typically ovoid in configuration, occurring adjacent to a physeal scar, containing increased T2 signal with a lobulated appearance, and occasional signal voids that signify calcifications. When a suspected enchondroma demonstrates more aggressive features of increased endosteal scalloping or cortical destruction, chondrosarcoma is likely. Osteochondromas can be diagnosed, as they are on other modalities, by the contiguity of their cortex and medullary canal with the host bone. MRI is particularly useful in assessing the thickness of the cartilage cap of osteochondromas to identify chondrosarcoma transformation [24]. With regard to contrast enhancement of chondrosarcomas, low-grade lesions show a lobulated pattern with enhanced septations after intravenous injection of contrast, while high-grade tumors do not have septations and show more diffuse, heterogeneous enhancement [16,19].

Soft tissue sarcomas

Soft tissue sarcomas originate in the mesenchymal tissues of muscles, connective tissue, vessels, joints, and fat. As such, MRI represents an ideal modality to evaluate them, given its superior contrast resolution compared with other modalities, particularly CT. When evaluating soft tissue

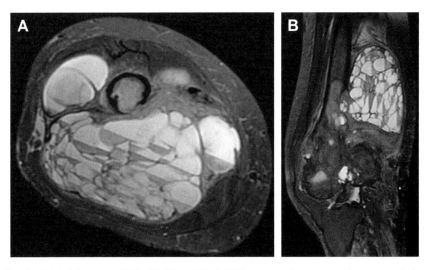

Fig. 5. Axial (A) and sagittal (B) T2-weighted MRI images show a very large mass lesion extending from the distal femoral diaphysis associated with multiple fluid-fluid levels, internal septations, and heterogeneity characteristic of a telangiectatic osteorsarcoma. Note the intramedullary component of the mass with extensive soft tissue component posteriorly.

sarcomas, MRI exquisitely defines the extent of the lesion with respect to compartmental involvement in the muscles, fascia, bones, and joints, as well as any involvement of the neurovascular bundles (Fig. 6). In addition, for posttreatment evaluation, MRI is the modality of choice for detecting residual or recurrent disease.

However, with respect to the characterization of disease, MRI allows for the accurate characterization of only a small number of soft tissue lesions and is frequently deficient in its ability to distinguish whether a mass is benign or malignant. As such, many soft tissue masses encountered in clinical practice will require a biopsy for characterization and diagnosis. There are several lesions, however that can be well characterized by MRI. Lipomas, for example, contain fat signal almost exclusively as seen on all pulse sequences and may occasionally demonstrate thin internal septations (Fig. 7). Cysts are well-circumscribed lesions of decreased signal on T1-weighted images and increased signal on T2-weighted images, with the hallmark that they do not demonstrate any internal enhancement with contrast administration. Vascular malformations have a characteristic infiltrating appearance, are of increased signal on T2 weighted images, and may contain flow voids if they possess an arterial component. There are also some lesions with a few, though not entirely, specific MRI characteristics, which include nerve sheath tumors, myxoid masses, giant cell tumors of the tendon sheath, and some fibrous tumors, such as elastofibroma and desmoid tumors [13].

As a general rule, contrast enhancement characteristics may help distinguish benign and malignant soft tissue lesions, even though there is much overlap in the enhancement patterns of benign tumors and sarcomas. Malignant masses tend to demonstrate greater heterogeneity, liquefaction, and rapid early enhancement than benign lesions [13,18,19], but overall, with MRI a correct diagnosis of a soft tissue mass is made in only approximately 25% to 40% of cases [25]. That being said, the characteristics that a lesion demonstrates on the various MR sequences will help direct the final decision as to whether it is benign or malignant. For example, liposarcoma is a common soft tissue sarcoma and, depending on the subtypes, will often demonstrate internal lipomatous tissue with intervening solid components and variable enhancement patterns (Fig. 8), features that will direct the management toward an invasive biopsy, differentiating it from a simple lipoma.

Positron emission tomography

PET is a noninvasive diagnostic technique that involves the acquisition of physiologic images by the detection of radiation emitted from positrons administered to the patient [26,27]. It is considered the gold standard in metabolic imaging and provides information about both the anatomic extent as well as the behavior of tumors, which, in turn, will guide therapeutic choices. The most widely used tracer for PET is fluorine-18 fluorodeoxyglucose (FDG). FDG is a glucose analog that accumulates in cells in proportion to the rate of glucose metabolism. FDG provides a means of quantifying glucose metabolism as the radiotracer becomes trapped in a cell in proportion to the rate of glycolysis [28]. The standard uptake value (SUV) is a quantification measure of FDG uptake (metabolic activity) in a region of interest. Because increased metabolism is a recognized feature of malignant cells when compared with normal cells, PET is a useful tool for the assessment of malignancies. In addition, although there is much overlap, high-grade malignancies tend to have increased rates of glycolysis and FDG uptake (and therefore higher SUV values) than low-grade and benign lesions [26,28].

Studies suggest that PET is a reliable test for determining the biologic activity of a tumor and for predicting tumor necrosis after neoadjuvant therapy. For the evaluation of sarcomas, PET is showing promise for staging of the tumors, especially distant metastases and monitoring the effect of treatment. It has also shown some potential for targeting high-yield portions of a mass for biopsy [29–33]. Fig. 9 is an example of a mass with distant metastases in the lung.

Nevertheless, although promising, there are limitations to the use of PET. Clearly, PET imaging does not allow the prediction of the histology of a mass [27]. Also, when compared with CT and MRI, PET has poor spatial resolution and should, in fact, be interpreted in conjunction with a cross-sectional study. In this way, common pathologies, such as insufficiency fractures that may be found in oncology patients and have been shown to demonstrate increased FDG uptake, are not misinterpreted as metastastic disease on a PET study. PET/CT has become more widely available in recent years and helped to alleviate the challenges of interpreting PET examinations by themselves. PET/CT has high sensitivity for the initial staging of tumors as well as for the assessment of recurrence; the literature shows an overall 66% sensitivity and 96% specificity of FDG-PET for diagnosing recurrent sarcomas. While combined PET/CT has higher accuracy than either modality by itself, PET overall remains more accurate than CT [34].

Skeletal sarcomas

There has been limited work on the characterization of skeletal sarcomas by PET, although the grading of sarcomas using PET has been recently studied. For example, in general, the higher the grade of the cartilage lesion, the greater its SUV value [35]. However, this poses a diagnostic dilemma for low-grade chondrosarcomas, which can have values less than the cut-off typically observed with malignancy: 2.5. Additionally, SUV values may be above 2.5 with benign inflammatory lesions, such as osteomyelitis or eosinophilic granuloma, as well as any lesion with high giant cell or fibrous content [35,36], such as giant cell tumors, aneurysmal bone cysts, osteoblastomas, Paget's disease, and fibrous dysplasia [26,36]. In such cases, PET will be deficient in distinguishing benign and malignant disease.

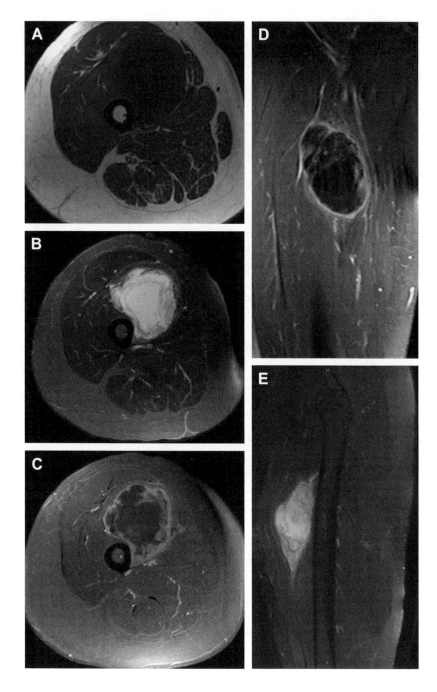

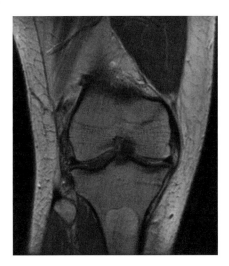

Fig. 7. Coronal T1-weighted MRI image shows a well-corticated, slightly expansile lesion of increased signal in the proximal tibial metaphysis. Notice the T1 signal is similar to fatty tissue, and this lesion represents an intraosseous lipoma.

Regarding osteosarcomas, although FDG-PET may provide important information regarding the biologic features of the mass, it has a limited role in primary staging. First-line diagnostic tools remain radiography and MRI. But in the pediatric population, FDG PET may be especially useful to detect intraosseus skip metastases in cases of equivocal MRI findings because of physiologic marrow distribution [34].

PET is most valuable for detecting metastatic disease because it represents a whole-body imaging technique, whereas CT and MRI are limited to the body area scanned. In addition, the response to preoperative neoadjuvant therapy is the most important prognostic factor in sarcomas because the degree of drug-induced tumor necrosis is highly correlated with disease-free survival after therapy [26]. As a functional imaging tool, PET studies have shown that biochemical changes in tumors in response to treatment tend to occur sooner than morphologic changes, and as such, may be better detected with PET than with anatomic cross-sectional imaging [33,34].

Fig. 6. Axial precontrast T1-weighted (A) and axial T2-weighted (B) MRI images of the thigh show slightly heterogeneous noncontrast intermediate T1 and increased T2 signal in a soft tissue mass adjacent to the osseous cortex of the femur. This lesion is displacing adjacent structures. Axial T1-weighted postcontrast (C) and coronal T1-weighted postcontrast (D) MRI images show heterogeneous contrast enhancement, mostly at the periphery of the lesion with central necrosis, more commonly indicating a malignant than benign state and negating the possibility of a cyst. Sagittal T2-weighted (E) MRI image shows an ovoid, hyperintense but heterogeneous soft tissue mass paralleling the long axis of the body, commonly seen with synovial sarcoma.

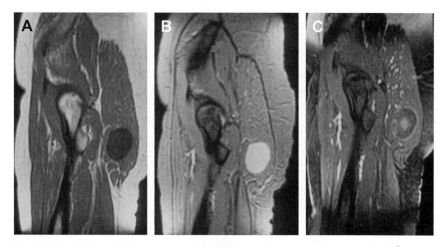

Fig. 8. Sagittal T1-weighted precontrast (*A*) MRI image shows a well-circumscribed, low signal intensity lesion within the soft tissues of the posterior thigh. Sagittal T2-weighted MRI image (*B*) shows that the lesion is increased T2 signal. Sagittal T1-weighted postcontrast MRI image (*C*) shows the lesion demonstrates heterogeneous enhancement internally, negating the possibility that it is a cyst, even though the precontrast features suggest the possibility of a cystic nature. This mass was proven to be a myxoid liposarcoma.

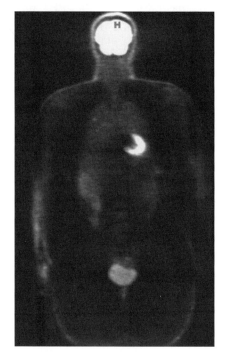

Fig. 9. Coronal PET image shows focal radiotracer uptake in a right upper lobe pulmonary nodule, representing a single distant focus of metastatic disease in a patient with newly diagnosed osteosarcoma.

Soft tissue tumors

An important feature of sarcomas, especially soft tissue sarcomas, is that they are often inhomogeneous, with different portions of the tumor having different degrees of aggressiveness and malignancy grades [26]. Biopsy is a key step in the diagnosis of these masses, but improperly performed biopsies are a frequent cause of misdiagnosis, amputation, and local recurrence [26,29]. As such, selecting a high-yield biopsy site is paramount. PET may allow the determination of the most metabolically active region of the lesion to be visualized, thus providing information on tumor biology, which is not done by any other imaging modality [27]. Targeting the area with the highest metabolic activity within the tumor helps determine the accurate histologic tumor grade and predicts outcome [30].

Summary

The advanced imaging techniques of CT, MRI, and PET available for the evaluation of soft tissue and skeletal sarcomas have been discussed in this article. There are benefits and disadvantages to the use of each modality and the choice of modality must be tailored to each patient and particular lesion. In general, CT is more suited to characterization of a mass while MRI will better define the extent of disease for treatment planning. PET is a promising tool for determining the metabolic activity of a lesion, and for use as a potential guide to biopsy and management. Often, however, a multi-modality approach to the evaluation of sarcomas is most effective, as complimentary information is gained from each technique.

References

[1] Scott WW, Didie WJ, Fayad LM. Imaging of rheumatologic diseases. Primer on the Rheumatic Diseases 2008;28–41.

[2] Siemens AG. Medical solutions. Computed tomography: its history and technology. Available at: http://www.medical.siemens.com/siemens/en_INT/qq_ctFBAs/files/brochures/CT_History_and_Technology.pdf. September 1, 2007.

[3] Boone JM, Geraghty EM, Seibert JA, et al. Dose reduction in pediatric CT: a rational approach. Radiology 2003;228:352–60.

[4] Fayad LM, Johnson P, Fishman EK. Multi-detector CT of musculoskeletal disease in the pediatric patient; principles, techniques, and clinical applications. Radiographics 2005;25: 603–18.

[5] Lois JF, Fischer HJ, Deutsch LS, et al. Angiography in soft tissue sarcomas. Cardiovasc Intervent Radiol 2007;7(6):309–16.

[6] Fayad LM, Bluemke DA, Weber KL, et al. Characterization of pediatric skeletal tumors and tumor-like condition: specific cross-sectional imaging signs. Skeletal Radiol 2006;35(5): 259–68.

[7] Fishman EK, Kuszyk B. 3D imaging: musculoskeletal applications. Crit Rev Diagn Imaging 2001;42:59–100.

[8] Teo HE, Peh WC. Primary bone tumors of adulthood. Cancer Imaging 2004;4(2):74–83.

[9] Sander TG, Parsons TW. Radiological imaging of musculoskeletal neoplasia. Cancer Control 2001;8(3):221–31.

[10] Kim T, Murakami T, Oi H, et al. CT and MR imaging of abdominal liposarcoma. AJR Am J Roentgenol 1996;166:829–33.

[11] Amendola MA, Glazer GM, Agha FP, et al. Myositis ossificans circumscripta: CT diagnosis. Radiology 1983;139:775–9.

[12] O'Bray R, Carrino JA, Fayad LM. Magnetic resonanc imaging of the musculoskeletal system, in press.

[13] Kaplan PA, Helms CA, Dussault R, et al. Musculoskeletal MRI. Philadelphia: WB Sauders; 2001.

[14] Nomikos GS, Murphey MD, Kransdorf MJ, et al. Primary bone tumors of the lower extremities. Radiol Clin North Am 2002;40:971–90.

[15] Bitar R, Leung G, Perng R, et al. MR pulse sequences: what every radiologist wants to know but is afraid to ask. Radiographics 2006;26(2):513–37.

[16] Kransdorf M, Murphey M. Radiologic evaluation of soft tissue masses. AJR Am J Roentgenol 2000;175:575–87.

[17] van der Woude HJ, Verstraete KL, Hogondoom PC, et al. Musculoskeletal tumors: does fast dynamic constrast-enhanced subtraction MR imaging contribute to the characterization? Radiology 1998;208:821–8.

[18] Berquist TH, Ehman RL, King BF, et al. Value of MR imaging in differentiating benign from malignant soft tissue masses: study of 95 lesions. AJR Am J Roentgenol 1990;155: 1251–5.

[19] Borden EC, Baker LH, Bell RB, et al. Soft tissue sarcomas of adults. Clin Cancer Res 2003;9: 1941–56.

[20] Musculoskeletal tumors, staging and treatment planning. Available at: www.emedicine.com. Accessed February 7, 2007.

[21] Fayad LM, Bluemke DA, McCarthy EF, et al. Musculoskeletal tumors: use of proton MR spectroscopic imaging for characterization. J Magn Reson Imaging 2006;23(1):23–8.

[22] Fayad LM, Barker PB, Bluemke DA, et al. Molecular characterization of musculoskeletal tumors by proton MR spectroscopy. Semin Musculoskelet Radiol 2007;188:1513–20.

[23] Wang CK, Li CW, Hsieh TJ, et al. Characterization of bone and soft tissue tumors with in vivo 1H MR spectroscopy: initial results. Radiology 2004;232:599–605.

[24] Chondrosarcoma. Available at: www.emedicine.com. Accessed August 11, 2005.

[25] Ollivier L, Vanel D, Leclere J. Imaging of chondrosarcomas. Cancer Imaging 2004;4(1): 36–8.

[26] Freudenberg LS, Antoch G, Eising EG, et al. PET/CT and PET using [18F]-FDG in a patient with soft tissue sarcoma. J Nucl Med 2005;2(2):19–23.

[27] Ioannidis JPA, Lau J. F18-FDG PET for the diagnosis and grading of soft-tissue sarcoma: a meta-analysis. J Nucl Med 2003;44(5):717–24.

[28] Delbeke D, Coleman RE, Guiberteau MJ, et al. Procedure guideline for tumor imaging with 18F-FDG PET/CT. J Nucl Med 2006;47(5):885–95.

[29] Nieweg OE, Pruim J, van Ginkel RJ, et al. Fluorine-18-Flurordeoxyglucose PET Imaging of Soft-Tissue Sarcoma. J Nucl Med 1996;37(2):257–61.

[30] Eary JS, Mankoff EA. Tumor metabolic rates in sarcoma using FDG PET. J Nucl Med 1998; 39:250–4.

[31] Jones DN, McCowage GB, Sostman HT, et al. Monitoring of neoadjuvant therapy response of soft tissue and musculoskeletal sarcoma using fluorine-18 FDG PET. J Nucl Med 1996;37: 1438–44.

[32] Dimitrakopoulou-Strauss A, Strauss LG, Schwarzbach M, et al. Dynamic PET ^{18}F-FDG studies in patients with primary and recurrent soft tissue sarcomas: impact on diagnosis and correlation with grading. J Nucl Med 2001;42:713–20.

[33] Studies favor PET-CT for imaging soft-tissue sarcoma. Radiological Society of North America. Available at: http://links.mkt256.com/servlet/MailView?ms=NDc3NTqxS0&r= OTQ1MDc5NTA4S0&j=MzQ1ODAxMjQS1&mt=1. Accessed August 23, 2007.

[34] Brenner W, Bohuslavizki KH, Eary JF. PET imaging of osteosarcoma. J Nucl Med 2003;44: 930–42.

[35] Feldman F, van Heertum R, Saxena C, et al. 18FDG-PET applications for cartilage neoplasms. Skeletal Radiol 2005;34(7):367–74.

[36] Aoki J, Watanabe H, Shinozaki T, et al. FDG PET of primary benign and malignant bone tumors: standardized uptake value in 52 lesions. Radiology 2001;219:774–7.

ELSEVIER
SAUNDERS

SURGICAL
CLINICS OF
NORTH AMERICA

Surg Clin N Am 88 (2008) 539–557

Management of Extremity Soft Tissue Sarcomas

Matthew T. Hueman, MD[a], Katherine Thornton, MD[b],
Joseph M. Herman, MD, MSc[c], Nita Ahuja, MD[d],*

[a]Department of Surgery, The Johns Hopkins University School of Medicine, 600 North Wolfe Street,
Blalock 665, Baltimore, MD 21287, USA
[b]Department of Medical Oncology, The Sidney Kimmel Comprehensive Cancer Center at
Johns Hopkins, 1650 Orleans Street, CRB I Room 1M88, Baltimore, MD 21231, USA
[c]Department of Radiation Oncology, The Sidney Kimmel Comprehensive Cancer Center at
Johns Hopkins, 401 North Broadway, Weinberg 1440–Oncology, Baltimore, MD 21231, USA
[d]Department of Surgery, The Johns Hopkins University School of Medicine, 1650 Orleans
Street, CRB1-342, Baltimore, MD 21231, USA

Soft tissue sarcomas are relatively rare tumors, with approximately 9220 cases anticipated in the United States in 2007 [1]. Although soft tissue sarcomas can arise in virtually any anatomic site, patients with extremity sarcomas represent almost half of all patients [2]. In a series of 3442 patients from Memorial Sloan-Kettering Cancer Center, 33% of all soft tissue sarcomas originated in the lower extremities and 14% in the upper extremities [2].

Given the rarity of presentation at other anatomic sites, much of the treatment of sarcomas at non-extremity sites has been extrapolated from evidence in clinical trials of patients with extremity sarcomas. This extrapolation of treatment is largely defined by the use and timing of adjuvant therapy such as radiotherapy and systemic chemotherapy. An understanding of the management of extremity sarcoma is a keystone to optimal treatment of patients with soft tissue sarcomas at other anatomic sites.

This article provides an understanding of the evaluation, staging, and management of patients with extremity sarcoma. Although there are straightforward guidelines to the management of patients with extremity sarcoma, each patient presents with unique considerations for tumor control, functional outcome, and potential toxicities. As is true for patients diagnosed with sarcoma at other anatomic sites, a multidisciplinary team

---

* Corresponding author.
E-mail address: nahuja@jhmi.edu (N. Ahuja).

approach streamlines care with attention to the complexities and intricacies of choosing and delivering optimal therapy.

Staging

Although soft tissue sarcomas are, in fact, a heterogeneous mixture of histologies and presentations, the sixth edition of the American Joint Committee on Cancer (AJCC) staging system applies to all soft tissue sarcomas with the exception of angiosarcoma, dermatofibrosarcoma, infantile fibrosarcoma, and malignant mesenchymoma. Histologic grade, tumor size, and depth are the primary determinants of AJCC stage (Table 1). The central importance of histologic grade in the staging system is unique to soft tissue sarcoma. The presence or absence of distant or nodal disease completes the staging system. Although the histologic subtype and anatomic site of origin clearly influence outcomes [3–5], these factors are not included in the staging system; histologic subtype does help influence the analysis of histologic grade and is thus indirectly measured.

Table 1
American Joint Committee on Cancer staging for soft tissue sarcomas

Parameter	Finding			
Primary tumor				
TX	Primary tumor cannot be assessed			
T0	No evidence of primary tumor			
T1	Tumor ≤5 cm in greatest dimension			
T1a	Superficial tumor			
T1b	Deep tumor			
T2	Tumor >5 cm in greatest dimension			
T2a	Superficial tumor			
T2b	Deep tumor			
Regional lymph nodes				
NX	Regional lymph nodes cannot be assessed			
N0	No regional lymph node metastases			
N1	Regional lymph node metastases			
Distant metastases				
MX	Distant metastases cannot be assessed			
M0	No distant metastases			
M1	Distant metastases			
Stage grouping				
Stage I	G1-2	T1a, 1b, 2a, 2b	N0	M0
Stage II	G3-4	T1a, T1b, T2a	N0	M0
Stage III	G3-4	T2b	N0	M0
Stage IV	Any G	Any T	N1	M0
	Any G	Any T	Any N	M1

Superficial defined as above and not invading the superficial fascia; deep defined as invading fascia (retroperitoneal and visceral lesions and most head and neck lesions are considered deep).
Abbreviation: G, grade.
Data from Greene F, Page D, Norrow M. AJCC cancer staging manual. 6th edition. New York: Springer; 2002.

Although histologic grade can be measured on a two-, three-, or four-tiered system, the staging system incorporates all of these grades. This approach allows simplification to the more common use in everyday clinical application of a two-tiered system, low (G1, G2) or high (G3, G4) grade. This incorporation of histologic grade into the staging system reflects the finding in comparative multivariate analyses that histologic grade is the most important factor in predicting the risk for distant metastasis and tumor-related death [5,6].

Tumor size is defined by whether the sarcoma is greater than 5 cm measured clinically or radiographically. Tumor size has been shown to be an important predictive factor in determining metastasis-free and overall survival [7]. Tumor size is further subcategorized by the depth, that is, "a" if superficial (lack of involvement of superficial investing muscular fascia of the extremity) or "b" if deep (deep to, or involves, superficial fascia). Sarcomas located deep to the investing muscle fascia have been shown to have a worse prognosis [5,6].

Of all the applicable anatomic sites, the AJCC staging system is best designed for extremity sarcomas. In the sixth edition, the AJCC reclassified tumors that were T2b, G1-2, N0, M0 as stage I instead of stage II. In the current modification, the four different stages are divided by the following descriptions: (1) stage I tumors are low grade (G1-2), small or large, and superficial or deep; (2) stage II tumors are high grade (G3-4), small and superficial, or deep or large and superficial only; (3) stage III tumors are high grade (G3-2), large, and deep; and (4) stage IV tumors involve metastasis to a distant site or regional nodes.

Although tumor grade, size, and depth are important prognostic factors for metastasis-free and overall survival, the most important factor in predicting local recurrence is the presence of positive margins on surgical excision [7]. Although tumor grade, size, depth, and histotype are the strongest factors for metastasis-free and overall survival, data suggest that positive margin status may also affect systemic control and disease-free survival [8,9]. Both of these points argue for re-resection to negative surgical margins whenever possible, because radiotherapy typically can compensate for inadequate resections.

Presentation and natural history

The most common presentation of a soft tissue sarcoma is a painless mass. Surgeons routinely evaluate patients with soft tissue masses of the extremities, and the majority of these masses are benign. For benign masses, a simple excision results in cure. Occasionally, the surgeon encounters a patient with either a preoperatively suspicious mass or an unexpected sarcoma after local excision and pathologic review. Patients with sarcomas have a high rate of local recurrence and mortality; therefore, it is crucial that the treating surgeon understand the appropriate diagnostic, staging, and treatment options.

Ideally, the soft tissue mass is identified as a possible sarcoma before plans for biopsy (or excision), because both the technique for biopsy and the pretreatment confirmation of malignancy are crucial to ensure optimal outcomes. Multidisciplinary evaluation and planning of the treatment of patients with sarcoma should be performed before initiation of any therapy. The natural history of sarcomas may help the surgeon identify suspicious masses upon examination. Extremity sarcomas most commonly occur proximally in the hip and shoulder regions [10]. A rapid rate of growth in combination with areas of differing consistency and fixation may alert the clinician to the possibility of sarcoma, but slow growth does not rule out malignancy. It is not unusual for such proximal extremity sarcomas to grow to a large size before the patient recognizes the need to seek medical attention. The patient may first notice the mass when an unrelated injury occurs to the affected extremity. Distal extremity soft tissue masses are generally identified sooner; therefore, they are usually smaller in size on presentation [11]. When the sarcomas become large enough, involvement of critical nearby neurovascular structures or locally compressed muscles may cause symptoms of radiating pain, numbness, or swelling [12].

The histology of extremity sarcoma is often related to the site of origin. The most common histologic subtypes seen in proximal extremity sarcoma are malignant fibrous histiocytomas, liposarcomas, and leiomyosarcomas [6]. Distal extremity sarcomas tend to be of different histologic subtype in comparison with more common proximal extremity sarcomas and include synovial sarcomas, epithelioid sarcomas, and clear cell sarcomas, which occur more frequently in the hands and feet. The most common histology occurring in the hand is epithelioid sarcoma [13], whereas synovial sarcoma and clear cell sarcoma occur more commonly in the feet. Most epithelioid, synovial, and clear cell sarcomas occur in the distal extremities [13,14]. Each of these histologic subtypes is associated with distinct clinical and biologic behavior.

Lymph node spread by sarcomas is generally rare (<3%) but is more commonly seen in patients with epithelioid sarcomas (up to 15%) and occurs with increased frequency in patients with clear cell sarcomas [15].

Most patients with extremity sarcoma present with clinically localized disease. Approximately 10% of patients have evidence of metastatic disease after staging evaluation [16,17]. The most common site of metastases for extremity sarcomas is the lung. Other sites of metastases include the lymph nodes and bone [15,17].

The most common site of metastasis after primary treatment of an apparently localized extremity sarcoma is the lung. Metachronous lung metastases usually occur within 2 to 3 years after resection. Patients with larger (greater than 5 cm), deeper (deep to superficial fascia), and higher grade tumors, as well as patients with high-risk histologic subtypes, are at increased risk for distant metastasis. The survival for patients with stage IV sarcoma is poor. Local control does not govern overall survival, and most patients with extremity sarcoma die of systemic manifestations of the disease.

Diagnosis and evaluation

The use of pretreatment biopsy is often helpful but not always necessary. Knowledge of the histology and grade of the tumor, recognizing the possibility of sampling error with a minimally invasive biopsy, helps plan multidisciplinary treatment. Pretreatment biopsy is mandatory when the tumor seems to involve critical structures or when neoadjuvant therapy is considered. Additionally, evidence suggestive of metastatic disease may prompt biopsy. With the insight of the grade and histology of the tumor obtained from biopsy, the surgeon can help plan the optimal margins for the best oncologic and functional outcome. Although several options for biopsy exist, one should preferably use the least invasive method sufficient to obtain a definitive histologic subtype and grade. The site of biopsy can also be crucial; the biopsy needle tract can result in local recurrence if this area is not excised during definitive surgical therapy [18]. Most commonly, core needle biopsy is used and provides adequate tissue diagnosis [19].

An essential step once the diagnosis of sarcoma is made is to assess the extent of local disease and the presence or absence of distant disease. For the assessment of local disease burden, physical examination provides an estimation of tumor size and depth and of the proximity of the tumor to critical structures such as bone, tendon, nerves, and blood vessels. A high-quality MRI or CT scan should confirm the clinical suspicion of proximity to vital structures and the local extent and will provide the most reliable information for operative planning. At the same time, this imaging may help guide plans for biopsy. Both CT and MRI provide detailed information of the tumor in relationship to surrounding anatomy. Although MRI is often thought to be superior in evaluation of soft tissue masses, at least one study has shown MRI and CT to be equally efficacious in local staging [20]. This equal ability to provide anatomic detail allows both CT and MRI to delineate tumors from vessels, nerves, bone, and muscle groups, suggesting that the surgeon should use the imaging that he or she and the collaborating radiologist feel most comfortable interpreting. This local staging should guide operative planning and help determine the possibility for limb- and function-preserving wide local excision, which is possible in approximately 95% of patients.

Given the predilection of sarcoma to metastasize to the lung, the systemic disease burden is most appropriately evaluated with radiographic imaging of the chest. Based on current guidelines, a chest radiograph may be sufficient and is the minimum requirement (National Comprehensive Cancer Network practice guidelines, www.nccn.org), however a CT scan is generally preferred. Depending on the histologic subtype, grade, depth, and size, coupled with the clinician's preference, some experts may argue for high-resolution chest CT. Positron emission tomography (PET) has an increasing role in the management of sarcoma, particularly in assessing for evidence of metastatic disease and the response to therapy, but is currently not performed as part of standard staging [21–23]. As a reflection of this increasing role, a large prospective study is currently accruing patients with soft tissue sarcoma who are receiving neoadjuvant chemotherapy to determine the value of the FDG-PET scan (combined with CT) in predicting disease-free survival (www.cancer.gov/clinicaltrials/UMN-2005LS080).

Limb function-preserving surgery for extremity sarcoma

Surgical resection with negative margins is the mainstay of therapy for extremity sarcomas. Historically, successful local control of extremity sarcomas has been obtained with amputation [24]. Although amputation provides local control in the vast majority of patients, functional and psychologic consequences may be significant. Contemporary approaches to surgical management of extremity soft tissue sarcomas have focused on functional resections with wide negative margins with the addition of radiotherapy when appropriate to provide local control. In suitable patients, the use of limited surgery and radiotherapy can provide a function-preserving alternative without sacrificing local control or survival when compared with amputation [25].

Successful conservative resection obtains negative surgical margins while preserving limb function. Microscopic and grossly positive surgical margins are associated with inferior outcomes, including a significantly increased risk of local recurrence [7,26,27]; therefore, careful preoperative planning and a realistic determination of the likelihood of a margin-negative resection with primary surgical management should be undertaken before intervention. As described previously, preoperative MRI and CT can be helpful in planning the surgical approach and determining whether initial surgery is likely to provide adequate resection margins of at least 1 to 2 cm. MRI may be most useful for determining the extent of soft tissue and neurovascular invasion, whereas CT can be useful for determining the extent of local invasion as well as the extent and degree of any bone invasion.

At the time of surgery, care must be taken to excise all sites of known and suspected disease and prior areas of violation. Most often, this region includes the biopsy site and the tumor mass with a wide margin of normal appearing tissue. Soft tissue sarcomas often appear on gross inspection to be contained within a well-defined capsule; however, on histologic evaluation microscopic disease is often appreciated outside of this pseudocapsule. Removal of the tumor mass and pseudocapsule without a margin of normal appearing tissue is associated with a high incidence of positive margins and frequently requires a second operation to obtain negative margins.

Several principles of surgical resection can help the practitioner provide an adequate oncologic resection while maintaining maximal function. The resected tissue should include the unviolated tumor, pseudocapsule, and reactive zone with a wide margin. In addition, any previous biopsy site or scars should be contained within the final specimen. In general, incisions should be placed longitudinally to facilitate resection with minimal violation of normal tissues and to minimize the toxicity of eventual radiotherapy. Drain sites should be placed in proximity to the surgical incision to facilitate the safe inclusion in radiotherapy field.

The concept of a barrier to spread is an important component of surgical resection guidelines [28]. A barrier to tumor infiltration can include tissues such as fascia, joint capsule, tendon, epineurium, and the vascular sheath. In general, the guidelines dictate that if a barrier to spread exists, the tumor should be removed outside of that barrier (ie, without violation). If there is no barrier to spread, the tumor is removed with a broad margin.

Based on these general guidelines, specific scenarios are described [28]. For superficial lesions, the tumor is removed with a wide margin where there is no barrier (ie, along the subcutaneous path) and at the barrier where a barrier is present (ie, fascia). For deep lesions, the tumor and pseudocapsule are removed with a wide margin along muscle. The resection of other structures and the desired margin for deep tumors depend on the presence or absence of a barrier instead of physical distance.

For most superficial sarcomas, a deep negative margin can be obtained by resecting the underlying fascia. Care should be taken to avoid violation of uninvolved compartments and inappropriate violation of fascia, because this may necessitate additional surgical resections, removal of a larger volume of tissue, and the addition of radiotherapy if not already required, all with the potential of associated negative functional consequences. Deep tumors by definition invade or are beneath the superficial fascia; therefore, they necessitate violation of the fascia investing the involved compartment. If a positive margin is obtained at the time of resection, a re-resection should be performed with the goal of obtaining a negative margin. Zagars and colleagues [9] from the M.D. Anderson Cancer Center reported on a series of 666 consecutive patients with localized extremity soft tissue sarcoma referred after macroscopic resection. All of the patients received adjuvant radiotherapy. Among the 295 patients who underwent re-resection, residual tumor was found in 46%; final negative margins were found in 87%. Local control was significantly improved at 15 years (82% versus 73%) in patients undergoing re-resection, as were metastasis-free and disease-free survival. These data highlight the importance of the final surgical margin for determining local control. If surgical resection with wide negative margins is not considered possible based on imaging, preoperative radiation therapy should be considered to improve the likelihood of achieving a margin-negative resection.

The intricacies of the general guidelines for surgical resection underscore the complexity of the surgical approach for soft tissue sarcomas, suggesting a need for these surgeries to be completed at centers with significant experience in the management of sarcoma. In a series of 4205 patients with operatively managed sarcoma, significantly lower rates of 30- and 90-day mortality, higher median survival, and lower amputation rates were found when surgery was performed at high-volume centers, even though significantly more high-grade tumors and tumors larger than 10 cm were managed at these centers [29]. An additional benefit present at most high-volume centers is the availability of a multidisciplinary sarcoma team. This team can help address and appropriately plan the therapy of patients with advanced or potentially technically challenging primary tumors.

Reconstruction

Determination of the appropriate surgical intervention is often dictated by the extent of local invasion on preoperative imaging. Instances in which amputation may be required or may be the preferred option include the involvement of major neurovascular structures by tumor, anticipated poor functional outcomes following adequate surgical resection and radiotherapy, and patient preference.

Although these general guidelines can assist in determining whether amputation is an appropriate option, they should not dictate therapy. In some instances, vascular reconstruction can be performed to effectively salvage a limb. Ghert and colleagues [30] reported on a series of 19 patients who underwent vascular resection and reconstruction as part of definitive surgery for soft tissue sarcoma of the extremities. Patients undergoing vascular reconstruction were more likely to experience wound complications (68% versus 32%), edema (87% versus 20%), and deep venous thrombosis (26% versus 0%) than matched controls. Amputation was also more common in the vascular reconstruction group (16% versus 3%); however, there was no significant difference in local or distant recurrence between the two groups, suggesting that vascular reconstruction can allow limb preservation in appropriately selected cases.

Significant defects of skin and soft tissue may result from the resection of large superficial extremity sarcomas. In this setting, the use of grafts and flaps may assist in wound closure. If a surgical defect is anticipated, the case should be discussed with a plastic surgeon before the definitive procedure to allow for determination of an appropriate closure technique and donor site. In addition, preoperative radiotherapy should be considered as an alternative to postoperative radiotherapy in this setting to minimize the potential for long-term complications of the combined therapy [31]. In general, patients with an anticipated need for extensive reconstruction should be referred to an institution with a multidisciplinary sarcoma team with experience and expertise in this area.

The role of radiotherapy for local control

Radiotherapy is frequently used as part of the multidisciplinary treatment of extremity sarcomas. Radiation can be used to improve the local control obtained with conservative surgery for soft tissue sarcomas, to improve the resectability of advanced tumors, and to treat unresectable disease. Radiation can be delivered with a variety of techniques, including external beam radiation and brachytherapy, and can be delivered preoperatively, intraoperatively, or postoperatively. The optimal timing (preoperative versus postoperative) and the type of radiotherapy (external beam versus brachytherapy) are controversial and may depend on the available technology, as well as patient and tumor characteristics.

The duration of therapy is different depending on the technique employed. External beam radiation is delivered Monday through Friday over the course of 6 to 7 weeks. Brachytherapy is usually employed postoperatively with treatment delivered over several hours or days. Brachytherapy for extremity sarcomas is technically challenging, and its use is often limited to referral centers with a multidisciplinary sarcoma team.

Radiation was first used in the definitive management of extremity sarcomas to provide an alternative to amputation when combined with conservative surgery [25,32]. In this setting, the wide excision of soft tissue sarcomas followed by adjuvant radiotherapy results in local control rates in excess of 80%. Since the initial trials demonstrating that wide excision and radiation were an acceptable treatment option for soft tissue sarcoma, the appropriate indications and timing for the delivery of radiotherapy have been clarified to some extent. In general, the use of radiotherapy is associated with an improvement in local control after surgical resection without any influence on overall survival or distant metastases.

External beam radiation can be delivered in the preoperative or postoperative setting. If radiation is to be delivered, there are several possible benefits of preoperative radiation versus postoperative radiation, even though local control appears to be similar with both approaches [33]. Preoperative radiotherapy may provide a higher likelihood of obtaining a margin-negative resection for large tumors or those in close proximity to vital structures. Radiation doses used preoperatively tend to be lower than those used postoperatively (typically, 50 Gy compared with 60 to 70 Gy). In addition, radiation fields tend to be smaller in the preoperative setting because postoperative treatment fields often include the entire tumor bed, surgical scars, and drain sites with additional margin. Taken together, these factors may explain the reduced long-term toxicity seen with the preoperative approach when compared with the postoperative approach [31]. In contrast, postoperative radiotherapy has less risk of surgical wound complications and allows selection of patients at the highest risk for recurrence based on surgical pathology. The decision of which sequencing to employ is best made after consideration of patient and tumor characteristics by a multidisciplinary sarcoma team.

In patients with large, marginally resectable lesions, a preoperative approach is typically preferred to improve the likelihood of a margin-negative resection and to allow a greater likelihood of function preservation. These important goals are generally an acceptable trade-off for an anticipated higher risk of wound complications. For patients in whom the risk of wound complications is prohibitively high, especially in smaller more readily respectable lesions, a postoperative approach may be preferred to decrease this risk while accepting an increased risk of late toxicity. For patients with small, superficial, or low-grade lesions or those with a questionable pathologic diagnosis, a postoperative approach may be preferred to allow a determination of the appropriateness of adjuvant radiotherapy.

An alternative method for delivering radiation at the time of surgery (intraoperatively) or shortly thereafter is brachytherapy, which involves placing catheters within the tumor bed at the time of surgery. Radioactive sources can then be placed in the catheters to deliver radiation to the tissues surrounding the resection cavity, typically after postoperative day 5 to minimize wound complications [34]. The radiation dose delivered with this technique can be supplemented with preoperative or postoperative external beam radiation if desired. This method has been found to be effective in providing excellent rates of local control for high-grade tumors; however, it does not appear to be effective in the management of low-grade tumors [34]. The major benefit of brachytherapy is that more normal surrounding tissue can be spared from radiation when compared with that exposed with external beam radiation. As described previously, brachytherapy is technically challenging and should only be used by practitioners familiar with its use in this setting.

Although radiation can enhance local control after surgical resection, several series support the argument that radiotherapy does not compensate for suboptimal resection. Local recurrence is significantly higher for patients who undergo a margin-positive resection even if they receive adjuvant radiotherapy [9,25]. Radiotherapy appears most beneficial for improving local control in the setting of a margin-negative resection; therefore, the use of adjuvant radiotherapy should not be seen as the alternative to a margin-negative resection, even if re-resection is required.

Although radiation is effective in improving local control after surgical resection, several series suggest that a subset of patients who have extremity sarcoma have adequate local control with surgical resection alone and do not benefit from radiotherapy [11,35–37]. The ability to accurately select patients at low risk of local recurrence after surgery would allow these patients to avoid the potential toxicity of radiotherapy. Pisters and colleagues [38] reported the results of a prospective trial of surgical therapy alone for T1 soft tissue sarcomas of the extremities or trunk that were resected with negative margins. In the 74 patients treated with surgery alone, 58% were high-grade lesions and 68% were superficial. The local recurrence rate at 10 years was 5.6%, and sarcoma-specific death occurred in 3.2%, suggesting that surgery alone is an appropriate option in selected patients. Pisters and colleagues suggested reserving radiotherapy for patients with final R1 resection and for patients with local recurrence. In contrast, a recent report from the Scandinavian Sarcoma Study Group in which records from 1093 patients with extremity and trunk wall sarcomas were reviewed failed to identify a subset of patients with extremity sarcoma that did not benefit from radiotherapy [39].

The exclusion of radiotherapy for patients with resected soft tissue sarcoma can be considered for patients with small low-grade lesions that are resected with widely negative margins (NCCN practice guidelines, www.NCCN.org). Patients with high-grade lesions, those with large lesions, and those with close or positive final margins should receive radiotherapy until more definitive data are available to make alternative recommendations. Within these guidelines, care should be taken to approach each individual patient with an understanding of the potential risks of radiation based on the location and size of the tumor, and one should weigh these risks with the expected gain in terms of local control.

Special considerations: distal extremities

Extremity sarcomas most often occur proximally at the hip and shoulder region. Distal extremity sarcomas present a unique challenge based on the anatomic and functional constraints. Because of the size and anatomy of the distal extremities, lesions involving the wrist, hand, ankle, or feet more frequently are in proximity to or involve vital neurovascular structures or muscles, joints, and tendons critical to function.

Similar to other extremity sarcomas, the evaluation of the extent of distal extremity lesions should be evaluated with MRI to assess the involvement of critical structures. MRI can be useful for biopsy planning and for evaluating the appropriateness of treatment options. Similar to other sites, biopsy should be carefully planned to avoid contamination of adjacent critical structures which would then need to be excised at the time of the definitive surgical procedure. Most often, an incisional biopsy is performed due to a perceived higher risk of contamination with core biopsies of lesions in these sites [40].

Because of the inability to achieve wide negative margins in many distal extremity sarcomas, most often, a combined modality approach is employed. Radiotherapy can be delivered pre- or postoperatively with the goal of enhancing local control from a definitive surgery. The preoperative radiotherapy approach allows the resection of less tissue adjacent to the tumor mass, potentially sparing critical structures, while also allowing a reduced dose of radiation to be delivered. This approach most likely provides the best functional outcome for patients when compared with definitive surgery followed by postoperative radiotherapy. Adjuvant radiotherapy is indicated in the setting of positive margins, close margins, or high-grade disease if not delivered preoperatively.

The use of surgery alone for patients with distal extremity lesions results in a higher rate of local recurrence if amputation is not employed. A series from Memorial Sloan-Kettering Cancer Center reviewed the outcomes of 50 patients managed with amputation or limited surgery for hand and foot sarcomas [41]. Local recurrences occurred in 32% of patients treated with limited surgery and in none of the patients undergoing amputation. Most of the local recurrences in this series occurred in patients with close or positive final resection margins.

Several small series have reported the ability to preserve function with limited surgery and radiotherapy while achieving acceptable recurrence rates for sarcomas of the hand and foot [42,43]. A recent series from the University of Florida reported on the outcomes of 23 patients with nonmetastatic sarcoma of the hand-wrist or foot-ankle complex treated with surgical resection and radiotherapy [44]. The patients in this series received preoperative (n = 7) or postoperative radiotherapy (n = 16) and were followed up for a median of 11 years. Seven of these patients had tumors greater than 5 cm, and 18 were high-grade lesions. Surgery was repeated until negative margins were obtained (n = 20) or until amputation (n = 3). The 10-year local regional control and ultimate limb salvage rates in these patients were both 91%. No patient required an amputation for toxicity. The risk of severe edema or fibrosis was 5%, with moderate limitation in the range of motion seen in 7%. These data support the use of limited surgery and radiotherapy for sarcomas of the hand-wrist and ankle-foot complex to obtain local control while maintaining a functional distal extremity.

Limited surgery alone should be avoided due to the higher risk of local recurrence unless the use of radiotherapy is expected to result in unacceptable toxicity. Amputation remains an acceptable treatment option for patients who decline conservative surgery and radiotherapy, in instances in which negative margins cannot be obtained, and when amputation is expected to have minimal functional consequences (ie, ray amputation). In some instances, limited surgery with reconstruction may lead to inferior functional outcomes when compared with amputation with prosthesis. In these instances, amputation may be preferred.

The definitive surgical procedure aims to excise the tumor, prior biopsy site, and an area of normal tissue with at least 2 cm of margin. Frequently, this goal is not achievable due to the proximity of critical structures. Reconstruction of resected tissues is critical to achieving a functional extremity, often requiring bone allografts or autografts, vascular reconstruction, tendon grafts, nerve grafts, and skin grafts [44]. In these instances, preoperative consultation with a multidisciplinary team including orthopedic oncology, plastic surgery, and radiation oncology facilitates operative planning.

Adjuvant chemotherapy

The high rates of eventual distant failure with high- and intermediate-grade sarcomas have led to an interest in delivering adjuvant chemotherapy to reduce the risk of distant failures. Several randomized trials and a meta-analysis have addressed the benefit of adjuvant chemotherapy in patients with sarcomas; however, its use remains controversial [45–49]. The Sarcoma

Meta-analysis Collaboration performed a meta-analysis of 14 randomized trials including 1568 patients with sarcoma to address the benefit of Adriamycin-based chemotherapy delivered in the adjuvant setting [45]. There was a significant improvement in distant relapse-free interval and in overall recurrence-free survival with the addition of Adriamycin-based adjuvant chemotherapy; however, there was no benefit in overall survival. The study has been criticized for the inclusion of multiple anatomic sites with differing prognoses and for the inclusion of patients at lower risk of distant failure.

An additional study published after the meta-analysis evaluated the role of chemotherapy (five cycles of epirubicin and ifosfamide) in 104 adult patients with grade 3 or 4 sarcomas measuring 5 cm or more involving the extremities or girdle [46]. Recurrent sarcomas were also included regardless of size. The disease-free survival was significantly improved with the addition of chemotherapy (48 versus 16 months), as was the median overall survival (75 versus 46 months). The absolute overall survival benefit of receiving chemotherapy at 4 years was 19%. The survival benefit has been questioned due to a similar metastatic rate in both arms.

Additional series evaluating the benefit of chemotherapy have tried to better define subsets of patients who might benefit from chemotherapy. A series of 101 patients with large, deep extremity synovial sarcomas from the Memorial Sloan-Kettering Cancer Center and UCLA found significantly improved disease-specific survival and distant recurrence-free survival with the addition of ifosfamide-based chemotherapy [47]. A similar series from the same institutions evaluated the effect of ifosfamide and Adriamycin-based chemotherapy in patients with resected high-grade, large, extremity liposarcomas. In that series, a benefit in disease-specific survival was found with the delivery of ifosfamide but not Adriamycin-based chemotherapy [48]. In contrast, a review of 674 patients with stage III soft tissue sarcoma of the extremities treated at Memorial Sloan-Kettering Cancer Center and M.D. Anderson Cancer Center suggested that the disease-specific survival benefits of chemotherapy do not persist beyond 1 year [49].

At this time, the role of chemotherapy for resected extremity soft tissue sarcomas is uncertain. Patients with a high risk of metastatic disease appear to benefit from chemotherapy. These patients include those with large, high-grade, and deep lesions. The recommendation to deliver chemotherapy must be individualized based on the risk of distant failure balanced with the risks of chemotherapy. In general, chemotherapy is often offered to young, healthy patients with high-risk tumors who are likely to tolerate the therapy well. Patients with medical comorbidities, specifically cardiac disease, may not be appropriate candidates for Adriamycin-based chemotherapy.

Neoadjuvant therapy

Chemotherapy has been evaluated as a mechanism to improve the resectability of locally advanced sarcomas when given alone or in combination with radiotherapy preoperatively. Rates of disease response obtained with the combination of radiation and chemotherapy delivered preoperatively are promising; however, the toxicity associated with this approach is currently limiting.

In an attempt to determine the role of neoadjuvant chemotherapy alone, the M.D. Anderson Cancer Center treated patients with locally advanced or high-grade extremity sarcoma (stage IIIB) with three cycles of preoperative doxorubicin, dacarbazine, cyclophosphamide, and ADIC. In a comparison with patient outcomes in historical randomized studies using postoperative chemotherapy, patients who received three cycles of preoperative doxorubicin, dacarbazine, cyclophosphamide, and ADIC had similar disease-free and overall survival [50]. Unfortunately, even when the patients considered as responders to the neoadjuvant regimen were analyzed, no significant benefit in local recurrence-free survival, distant metastasis-free survival, or overall survival could be demonstrated. The final results of a European Organization for Research and Treatment of Cancer trial randomizing patients to preoperative chemotherapy consisting of doxorubicin and ifosfamide versus local treatment alone are pending (www.clinicaltrials.gov).

One of the most successful regimens combining radiotherapy and chemotherapy in the neoadjuvant setting was first reported by DeLaney and colleagues [51]. In this single institution series, a preoperative chemotherapy regimen consisting of mesna, Adriamycin, ifosfamide, and dacarbazine (MAID) alternating with radiotherapy was delivered to patients with locally advanced high-grade extremity soft tissue sarcomas, followed by resection and additional adjuvant chemotherapy. With this intensive regimen, the 5-year local control, freedom from distant metastases, disease-free survival, and overall survival were improved (58% versus 87%) in a comparison with historical controls.

Based on the results obtained in this single institution series, a larger multi-institutional study was performed with the same regimen [52]. In that trial, 66 patients with large (>8 cm), high-grade extremity sarcomas received three cycles of neoadjuvant MAID chemotherapy alternating with radiotherapy and three cycles of adjuvant MAID chemotherapy. Although 3-year rates of disease-free, distant disease-free, and overall survival were encouraging (56.6%, 64.5%, and 75.1%, respectively), the toxicity was significant. Eighty-four percent of patients experienced a grade 4 toxicity (mainly hematologic), and two patients required an amputation for treatment-related toxicity.

A continuous infusion Adriamycin and concurrent radiotherapy regimen was tested at the M.D. Anderson Cancer Center as neoadjuvant therapy for patients with localized, potentially resectable intermediate- or high-grade soft tissue sarcoma [53]. In this series of 27 patients, dermatologic toxicity was dose limiting, occurring in 30% of patients at 17.5 $mg/m^2/wk$. Macroscopic complete resection was accomplished in all patients who underwent surgery (26 patients), and 50% of these patients had 90% or greater tumor necrosis on pathologic evaluation. These results are encouraging, especially the rates of pathologic response.

Currently, the neoadjuvant approach remains investigational based on the lack of randomized data supporting its use and the significant toxicity that results from this approach. It is possible that the combination of radiation and chemotherapy may allow limb preservation with superior long-term functional outcomes in the setting of locally advanced high- or intermediate-grade sarcomas that are large or that are located in proximity to or invading critical structures.

Recurrent disease

Patients with recurrent disease may present in a variety of ways ranging from an isolated local recurrence to an isolated metastasis to widely disseminated disease. Patients who present with a local recurrence should be evaluated and treated similarly as patients who present with a new primary [54]. Patients who present with an isolated metastasis can be considered for metastatectomy with or without pre- or postoperative chemotherapy or radiotherapy. In combination with evaluation and treatment for the primary site, if a local recurrence exists simultaneously, metastatectomy includes removal of limited disease to a single organ and regional nodal dissection if this site represents the single site of metastasis. Billingsley and colleagues [55] showed that if all lung metastases are removed, median survival is lengthened to 33 months as compared with a median survival of 11 months in patients with pulmonary metastases who do not undergo surgery. Patients who present with widely disseminated disease should be considered for a variety of palliative therapies, including surgery, chemotherapy, radiotherapy, embolization, and ablation procedures. Patients who present with widely disseminated disease who are symptomatic are most appropriate for the consideration of additional therapy. If asymptomatic, observation is also appropriate and may be the optimal approach in the correctly selected patient.

Follow-up evaluation

Limited evidence supports the efficacy of specific surveillance strategies, but experts agree that surveillance is prudent to identify recurrences that are still potentially curable and while the limb and function can still be salvaged [56–58]. NCCN guidelines attempt to establish a rational schedule while avoiding an overabundance of tests. These guidelines recommend that patients should be followed up with a history and physical examination every 3 to 6 months for 2 to 3 years, every 6 months for the next 2 years, and then annually (NCCN practice guidelines, www.NCCN.org). For stage I tumors, chest imaging (radiography or CT) should be performed every 6 to 12 months; for stage II and III tumors, chest imaging should be performed more frequently, every 3 to 6 months for 5 years and then annually. Periodic imaging with MRI or CT of the primary site should be considered if the combination of factors places the patient at increased risk for locoregional recurrence, especially if the location or depth of the lesion makes physical examination unreliable for this determination. Ultrasound, instead of MRI and CT, can also be considered as the mode of surveillance in these circumstances. After 10 years, the chance of local recurrence if the patient remains disease free becomes much smaller, and the requirement for surveillance imaging after this time point should be individualized.

Summary

For extremity sarcoma, limb salvage with the combination of function-preserving surgery and radiotherapy is the mainstay of treatment. The use of chemotherapy in the pre- or postoperative setting remains controversial and argues for an individualized approach to the patient and a multi-disciplinary approach by a dedicated team at a high-volume institution. The grade, depth, and histology of the sarcoma largely dictate the risk of the development of local recurrence and metastatic disease, but the loss of local control does not seem to determine the risk of metastatic disease. The addition of radiotherapy in the management of extremity sarcomas is a key development allowing function- and limb-preserving surgery with adequate rates of local control without an increase in the risk of systemic disease.

The anatomic site of the extremity sarcoma, proximal or distal, is associated with histologic subtypes that can be of vastly different biology and may determine a much different extent, sequence, and use of multimodality therapy for optimal outcomes. Given the complex factors associated with the determination of multimodality treatment coupled with the enormous heterogeneity and rarity of the disease, patients with extremity sarcomas should best be managed at high-volume specialized centers with multidisciplinary sarcoma teams.

References

[1] Jemal A, Siegel R, Ward E, et al. Cancer statistics, 2007. CA Cancer J Clin 2007;57:43–66.
[2] Mann GB, Lewis JJ, Brennan MF. Adult soft tissue sarcoma. Aust N Z J Surg 1999;69: 336–43.
[3] LeVay J, O'Sullivan B, Catton C, et al. Outcome and prognostic factors in soft tissue sarcoma in the adult. Int J Radiat Oncol Biol Phys 1993;27:1091–9.
[4] Vraa S, Keller J, Nielsen OS, et al. Prognostic factors in soft tissue sarcomas: the Aarhus experience. Eur J Cancer 1998;34:1876–82.
[5] Pisters PW, Leung DH, Woodruff J, et al. Analysis of prognostic factors in 1041 patients with localized soft tissue sarcomas of the extremities. J Clin Oncol 1996;14:1679–89.
[6] Coindre J, Terrier P, Bui N, et al. Prognostic factors in adult patients with locally controlled soft tissue sarcoma: a study of 546 patients from the French Federation of Cancer Centers Sarcoma Group. J Clin Oncol 1996;14:869–77.

[7] McKee MD, Liu DF, Brooks JJ, et al. The prognostic significance of margin width for extremity and trunk sarcoma. J Surg Oncol 2004;85:68–76.

[8] Gronchi A, Casali PG, Mariani L, et al. Status of surgical margins and prognosis in adult soft tissue sarcomas of the extremities: a series of patients treated at a single institution. J Clin Oncol 2005;23:96–104.

[9] Zagars GK, Ballo MT, Pisters PW, et al. Surgical margins and reresection in the management of patients with soft tissue sarcoma using conservative surgery and radiation therapy. Cancer 2003;97:2544–53.

[10] Gerrand CH, Wunder JS, Kandel RA, et al. The influence of anatomic location on functional outcome in lower-extremity soft-tissue sarcoma. Ann Surg Oncol 2004;11:476–82.

[11] Geer RJ, Woodruff J, Casper ES, et al. Management of small soft-tissue sarcoma of the extremity in adults. Arch Surg 1992;127:1285–9.

[12] Hunt K, Vorburger S, Cormier J. Surgical approaches to extremity sarcoma. In: Pollock R, editor. Soft tissue sarcomas. London: B.C. Decker; 2002. p. 89–109.

[13] Herr MJ, Harmsen WS, Amadio PC, et al. Epithelioid sarcoma of the hand. Clin Orthop Relat Res 2005;431:193–200.

[14] Zeytoonjian T, Mankin HJ, Gebhardt MC, et al. Distal lower extremity sarcomas: frequency of occurrence and patient survival rate. Foot Ankle Int 2004;25:325–30.

[15] Fong Y, Coit DG, Woodruff JM, et al. Lymph node metastasis from soft tissue sarcoma in adults: analysis of data from a prospective database of 1772 sarcoma patients. Ann Surg 1993;217:72–7.

[16] Rydholm A, Gustafson P, Rooser B, et al. Subcutaneous sarcoma: a population-based study of 129 patients. J Bone Joint Surg Br 1991;73:662–7.

[17] Vezeridis MP, Moore R, Karakousis CP. Metastatic patterns in soft-tissue sarcomas. Arch Surg 1983;118:915–8.

[18] Schwartz HS, Spengler DM. Needle tract recurrences after closed biopsy for sarcoma: three cases and review of the literature. Ann Surg Oncol 1997;4:228–36.

[19] Heslin MJ, Lewis JJ, Woodruff JM, et al. Core needle biopsy for diagnosis of extremity soft tissue sarcoma. Ann Surg Oncol 1997;4:425–31.

[20] Panicek DM, Gatsonis C, Rosenthal DI, et al. CT and MR imaging in the local staging of primary malignant musculoskeletal neoplasms: report of the Radiology Diagnostic Oncology Group. Radiology 1997;202:237–46.

[21] Schuetze SM. Utility of positron emission tomography in sarcomas. Curr Opin Oncol 2006; 18:369–73.

[22] Schuetze SM. Imaging and response in soft tissue sarcomas. Hematol Oncol Clin North Am 2005;19:471–87.

[23] McCarville MB, Christie R, Daw NC, et al. PET/CT in the evaluation of childhood sarcomas. AJR Am J Roentgenol 2005;184:1293–304.

[24] Hardin CA. Radical amputation for sarcoma of the extremities including postoperative resection of pulmonary metastasis. Ann Surg 1968;167:359–66.

[25] Rosenberg SA, Tepper J, Glatstein E, et al. The treatment of soft-tissue sarcomas of the extremities: prospective randomized evaluations of (1) limb-sparing surgery plus radiation therapy compared with amputation and (2) the role of adjuvant chemotherapy. Ann Surg 1982;196:305–15.

[26] Heslin MJ, Woodruff J, Brennan MF. Prognostic significance of a positive microscopic margin in high-risk extremity soft tissue sarcoma: implications for management. J Clin Oncol 1996;14:473–8.

[27] Stojadinovic A, Leung DH, Allen P, et al. Primary adult soft tissue sarcoma: time-dependent influence of prognostic variables. J Clin Oncol 2002;20:4344–52.

[28] Kawaguchi N, Ahmed AR, Matsumoto S, et al. The concept of curative margin in surgery for bone and soft tissue sarcoma. Clin Orthop Relat Res 2004;419:165–72.

[29] Gutierrez JC, Perez EA, Moffat FL, et al. Should soft tissue sarcomas be treated at high-volume centers? An analysis of 4205 patients. Ann Surg 2007;245:952–8.

[30] Ghert MA, Davis AM, Griffin AM, et al. The surgical and functional outcome of limb-salvage surgery with vascular reconstruction for soft tissue sarcoma of the extremity. Ann Surg Oncol 2005;12:1102–10.

[31] Davis AM, O'Sullivan B, Turcotte R, et al. Late radiation morbidity following randomization to preoperative versus postoperative radiotherapy in extremity soft tissue sarcoma. Radiother Oncol 2005;75:48–53.

[32] Yang JC, Chang AE, Baker AR, et al. Randomized prospective study of the benefit of adjuvant radiation therapy in the treatment of soft tissue sarcomas of the extremity. J Clin Oncol 1998;16:197–203.

[33] O'Sullivan B, Davis AM, Turcotte R, et al. Preoperative versus postoperative radiotherapy in soft-tissue sarcoma of the limbs: a randomised trial. Lancet 2002;359:2235–41.

[34] Pisters PW, Harrison LB, Leung DH, et al. Long-term results of a prospective randomized trial of adjuvant brachytherapy in soft tissue sarcoma. J Clin Oncol 1996;14:859–68.

[35] Karakousis CP, Emrich LJ, Rao U, et al. Limb salvage in soft tissue sarcomas with selective combination of modalities. Eur J Surg Oncol 1991;17:71–80.

[36] Khanfir K, Alzieu L, Terrier P, et al. Does adjuvant radiation therapy increase loco-regional control after optimal resection of soft-tissue sarcoma of the extremities? Eur J Cancer 2003; 39:1872–80.

[37] Baldini EH, Goldberg J, Jenner C, et al. Long-term outcomes after function-sparing surgery without radiotherapy for soft tissue sarcoma of the extremities and trunk. J Clin Oncol 1999; 17:3252–9.

[38] Pisters PW, Pollock RE, Lewis VO, et al. Long-term results of prospective trial of surgery alone with selective use of radiation for patients with T1 extremity and trunk soft tissue sarcomas. Ann Surg 2007;246:675–81 [discussion: 681–2].

[39] Jebsen NL, Trovik CS, Bauer HC, et al. Radiotherapy to improve local control regardless of surgical margin and malignancy grade in extremity and trunk wall soft tissue sarcoma: a Scandinavian Sarcoma Group Study. Int J Radiat Oncol Biol Phys 2008, in press.

[40] Ferguson PC. Surgical considerations for management of distal extremity soft tissue sarcomas. Curr Opin Oncol 2005;17:366–9.

[41] Owens JC, Shiu MH, Smith R, et al. Soft tissue sarcomas of the hand and foot. Cancer 1985; 55:2010–8.

[42] Johnstone PA, Wexler LH, Venzon DJ, et al. Sarcomas of the hand and foot: analysis of local control and functional result with combined modality therapy in extremity preservation. Int J Radiat Oncol Biol Phys 1994;29:735–45.

[43] Okunieff P, Suit HD, Proppe KH. Extremity preservation by combined modality treatment of sarcomas of the hand and wrist. Int J Radiat Oncol Biol Phys 1986;12:1923–9.

[44] Schoenfeld GS, Morris CG, Scarborough MT, et al. Adjuvant radiotherapy in the management of soft tissue sarcoma involving the distal extremities. Am J Clin Oncol 2006;29:62–5.

[45] Adjuvant chemotherapy for localised resectable soft-tissue sarcoma of adults: meta-analysis of individual data. Sarcoma Meta-analysis Collaboration. Lancet 1997;350:1647–54.

[46] Frustaci S, Gherlinzoni F, De Paoli A, et al. Adjuvant chemotherapy for adult soft tissue sarcomas of the extremities and girdles: results of the Italian randomized cooperative trial. J Clin Oncol 2001;19:1238–47.

[47] Eilber FC, Brennan MF, Eilber FR, et al. Chemotherapy is associated with improved survival in adult patients with primary extremity synovial sarcoma. Ann Surg 2007;246:105–13.

[48] Eilber FC, Eilber FR, Eckardt J, et al. The impact of chemotherapy on the survival of patients with high-grade primary extremity liposarcoma. Ann Surg 2004;240:686–95 [discussion: 695–7].

[49] Cormier JN, Huang X, Xing Y, et al. Cohort analysis of patients with localized, high-risk, extremity soft tissue sarcoma treated at two cancer centers: chemotherapy-associated outcomes. J Clin Oncol 2004;22:4567–74.

[50] Pisters PW, Patel SR, Varma DG, et al. Preoperative chemotherapy for stage IIIB extremity soft tissue sarcoma: long-term results from a single institution. J Clin Oncol 1997;15:3481–7.

[51] DeLaney TF, Spiro IJ, Suit HD, et al. Neoadjuvant chemotherapy and radiotherapy for large extremity soft-tissue sarcomas. Int J Radiat Oncol Biol Phys 2003;56:1117–27.

[52] Kraybill WG, Harris J, Spiro IJ, et al. Phase II study of neoadjuvant chemotherapy and radiation therapy in the management of high-risk, high-grade, soft tissue sarcomas of the extremities and body wall: Radiation Therapy Oncology Group Trial 9514. J Clin Oncol 2006; 24:619–25.

[53] Pisters PW, Patel SR, Prieto VG, et al. Phase I trial of preoperative doxorubicin-based concurrent chemoradiation and surgical resection for localized extremity and body wall soft tissue sarcomas. J Clin Oncol 2004;22:3375–80.

[54] Singer S, Antman K, Corson JM, et al. Long-term salvageability for patients with locally recurrent soft-tissue sarcomas. Arch Surg 1992;127:548–53 [discussion: 553–4].

[55] Billingsley KG, Burt ME, Jara E, et al. Pulmonary metastases from soft tissue sarcoma: analysis of patterns of diseases and postmetastasis survival. Ann Surg 1999;229(5):602–10 [discussion: 610–2].

[56] Whooley BP, Gibbs JF, Mooney MM, et al. Primary extremity sarcoma: what is the appropriate follow-up? Ann Surg Oncol 2000;7:9–14.

[57] Whooley BP, Mooney MM, Gibbs JF, et al. Effective follow-up strategies in soft tissue sarcoma. Semin Surg Oncol 1999;17:83–7.

[58] Kane JM III. Surveillance strategies for patients following surgical resection of soft tissue sarcomas. Curr Opin Oncol 2004;16:328–32.

ELSEVIER
SAUNDERS

SURGICAL
CLINICS OF
NORTH AMERICA

Surg Clin N Am 88 (2008) 559–570

Primary Breast Sarcoma

Ying Wei Lum, MD[a], Lisa Jacobs, MD[b],*

[a]*Department of Surgery, Johns Hopkins Hospital, 600 N Wolfe Street, Tower 110,*
Baltimore, MD 21287, USA
[b]*Department of Surgery & Oncology, Johns Hopkins Hospital, 600 N Wolfe Street,*
Osler 625, Baltimore, MD 21287, USA

Primary breast sarcomas are rare mesenchymal tumors accounting for 0.2% to 1% of all breast malignancies [1] and less than 5% of all soft tissue sarcomas [2]. The annual incidence has been estimated at approximately 44.8 new cases per 10 million women [3]. Since then, several reports have summarized single institution experience; however, due to the rarity of the disease, several important aspects of diagnosis and management are based on limited data. The pathologic classification of the disease remains controversial. Moreover, unlike epithelial breast cancers, there is still no consensus on the optimal treatment approach to these cases for primary and adjuvant therapy.

These tumors follow, and are similar to, other soft tissue sarcomas, and treatment approaches used for other sites should be applied to breast sarcomas as well. Although standard therapy used to consist of mastectomy with axillary dissection (similar to therapy for epithelial malignancies of the breast), there has been a shift in trend to perform wide local excision without axillary dissection similar to the treatment of soft tissue sarcomas in other locations. This change in philosophy has been primarily based on several retrospective studies over the last 2 decades. These studies have defined the natural history of the disease and provided useful information regarding local recurrence, distant recurrence, regional nodal involvement, and survival. Unfortunately, due to the limited sample size and variability in treatments used in most of these case series and reports, the role of adjuvant therapy remains undefined.

Etiology

The etiology of primary breast sarcomas is largely unknown. Silicone prostheses used in breast augmentation had previously been implicated as

---

* Corresponding author.
E-mail address: ljacob14@jhmi.edu (L. Jacobs).

0039-6109/08/$ - see front matter © 2008 Elsevier Inc. All rights reserved.
doi:10.1016/j.suc.2008.03.009   *surgical.theclinics.com*

a risk factor in the development of primary breast sarcomas; however, an analysis of SEER data from 1973 to 1990 looking at this relationship showed no such risk. There is evidence linking the development of breast sarcomas to patients who have been treated with external beam radiation for breast cancer or other malignancies in which the chest wall was included in the radiated field [4]. Angiosarcomas comprise a larger percentage of these cases linked to radiation exposure when compared with the other histopathologic subtypes [5,6]. The latency period between the development of breast sarcoma following radiotherapy is also shorter for angiosarcomas when compared with the other subtypes, that is, 8 years compared with 11 years [7,8].

Lymphedema, either of the breast or an extremity, resulting from axillary lymph node dissection or radiotherapy is another known risk factor, particularly for angiosarcomas. This correlation between chronic lymphedema and the development of angiosarcoma was described in 1948 by Stewart and Treves [9].

Clinical features

Primary breast sarcomas usually present in women with a peak incidence in the fourth to fifth decade (range, 16 to 81 years) [7,10–13]. The presenting feature is often a large, painless, and mobile mass [13–16]. They are equally distributed in both breasts but can rarely be bilateral [11,17]. These tumors are usually larger in size than epithelial breast cancers, with a median size of 5 to 6 cm (range, 2–40 cm) and should especially be suspected if associated with a rapid increase in size [7,11,13,18,19]. Other features, such as nipple discharge [18], nipple inversion [13], and skin changes [14], are rare but can occasionally occur. Angiosarcomas are an exception; they are often associated with skin discoloration, usually presenting with a bluish/purplish discoloration overlying the mass. There is evidence that patients with angiosarcoma tend to present at a younger age [10].

Pathology

Berg and colleagues [20] initially defined stromal sarcomas of the breast as a group of "mesenchymal malignant tumors with fibrous, myxoid and fatty components" and excluded malignant cystosarcoma phyllodes, lymphomas, and angiosarcomas; however, with a lack of consensus classification, other authorities have occasionally included various other histopathologic subtypes, including malignant or benign cystosarcoma phyllodes, angiosarcomas, and, occasionally, carcinosarcomas as well (Table 1). The most difficult distinction has been between cystosarcoma phyllodes compared with the other non-phyllodes sarcomas. Some investigators have reported a similar clinical course and survival for these two subtypes and,

Table 1
Major breast sarcoma studies

Study	Number of cases	Phyllodes tumors				Non-phyllodes tumors										Excluded	Included
		CS	CP	BCP	MCP	AS	FS	OS	LS	LMS	MFH	SC	SS	MTS	Others[a]		
Adem, et al [17]	25	–	–	–	–	+	+	+	–	+	–	–	–	–	+	CP,CS	–
Barrow, et al [25]	59	–	–	–	–	+	+	+	–	+	–	–	–	–	+	CP	–
Berg, et al [20]	25	–	–	–	–	–	+	+	+	–	–	–	–	–	–	MCP,AS,LP	–
Blanchard, et al [7]	55	–	–	–	–	+	+	+	+	+	+	–	+	–	+	–	DFP
Callery, et al [38]	32	–	–	–	–	–	+	–	–	+	+	–	–	–	–	AS	DFP
Christensen, et al [27]	68	–	–	±	+	+	–	+	+	+	+	–	+	–	–	–	–
Ciatto, et al [39]	70	–	–	–	+	+	–	–	+	+	+	–	+	+	–	–	–
Gutman, et al [11]	60	–	–	–	–	+	+	+	+	–	+	–	+	–	+	CP	–
McGowan, et al [22]	78	+	–	–	+	+	+	–	+	–	+	–	+	–	+	–	–
McGregor, et al [23]	58	+	+	–	–	+	+	–	+	+	+	–	+	–	+	–	DFP
North, et al [14]	25	–	–	–	–	+	+	–	+	–	+	+	+	–	+	–	–
Pandey, et al [15]	19	–	–	–	–	–	+	–	+	+	+	+	–	–	+	–	–
Pollard, et al [18]	25	–	–	–	–	+	+	–	+	–	+	–	–	–	+	–	–
Smola, et al [35]	8	–	–	–	–	–	–	–	–	–	–	+	–	–	+	CS,CP,DFP	–
Terrier, et al [12]	33	–	+	–	–	+	+	+	–	–	+	–	–	–	–	AS	–
Zelek et al [19]	83	–	–	–	–	+	–	+	–	–	+	+	–	–	+	–	–

Abbreviations: AS, angiosarcoma; BCP, borderline phyllodes tumors; CP, cystosarcoma phyllodes tumors; CP, cystosarcoma phyllodes; CS, carcinosarcoma; DFP, dermatofibrosarcoma protuberans; FS, fibrosarcoma; LMS, leiomyosarcoma; LP, lymphoma; LS, liposarcoma; MCP, malignant cystosarcoma phyllodes; MFH, malignant fibrous histiocytoma; MTS, mixed type sarcoma; OS, osteosarcoma; SC, spindle cell sarcoma; SS, stromal sarcoma.

[a] Other sarcomas include clear cell sarcoma, neurogenic sarcoma, alveolar soft part sarcoma, and rhabdomyosarcoma.

as such, deemed them similar [12,21–23]; however, given that cystosarcoma phyllodes tumors consist of mesenchymal cells with an epithelial component [24] (which is not present in other soft tissue sarcomas in other parts of the body) and also appear to arise from unique hormonally responsive stromal cells of the breast [16], they should be considered as a distinct clinicopathologic entity [17,18]. Although angiosarcomas were initially excluded from Berg's original description of true stromal sarcomas, it has been almost universally accepted that angiosarcomas are a histologic subtype of primary breast sarcomas [7,10,11,14,15,17,19,22,23,25]. In fact, angiosarcomas have in some series comprised the largest histologic subtype [7].

Primary breast sarcomas consist of a heterogeneous group as seen in soft tissue sarcomas in other parts of the body, including angiosarcoma, malignant fibrous histiocytoma, fibrosarcoma, stromal sarcoma, spindle cell sarcoma, liposarcoma, leiomyosarcoma, osteosarcoma, chondrosarcoma, and rhabdomyosarcoma. Of these, angiosarcomas [7,11,13–15,17], malignant fibrous histiocytoma [10,17–19,25], and stromal sarcoma [11] comprise the more common subtypes.

Prognostic factors

Angiosarcomas (occasionally referred as lymphangiosarcomas or hemangiosarcomas) have more commonly been shown to confer a more aggressive clinical course and are associated with a higher recurrence rate and lower overall survival [19,23,26,27]. Nevertheless, two studies from the M.D. Anderson Cancer Center [11,25] have shown a favorable prognosis for patients with angiosarcoma. The other histologic subtypes show minimal prognostic significance [12,19,23].

Other pathologic prognostic factors that have been studied include tumor grade, tumor size, cellular appearance, infiltrating borders, the number of mitoses, and stromal atypia [11,17]. Although not universally replicated, tumor grade [11,22] and size [11,17,18,25] have been more consistently shown to be predictive of outcome. Of the studies that have shown significance, evaluation of histologic grade showed that high-grade lesions were associated with a lower disease-free survival and overall survival [15,26,28–30]. Similarly, tumors less than 5 cm have been shown to be associated with better overall and disease-free survival [11,29]. These findings are similar to sarcomas found elsewhere in the body [31].

Diagnosis and work-up

The work-up is similar to that for other breast abnormalities. Imaging of all breast abnormalities should include diagnostic mammography, ultrasound, and, in some cases, breast MRI. Mammography of a primary breast sarcoma will usually demonstrate a soft tissue density that is nonspiculated [13,32]. Similarly, on ultrasound, the tumors appear as a solid mass with no shadowing. Although neither CT nor MRI has been studied specifically for primary breast sarcomas, their role in other extremity and retroperitoneal sarcomas has been established, and they could potentially be used in the evaluation of the patient with primary breast sarcoma. In fact, the National Comprehensive Cancer Center guidelines recommend baseline chest imaging because the lungs and chest wall can be common sites of recurrence. The role of positron emission tomography scanning is also unproven, but it may be useful in staging and possibly diagnosing breast sarcomas [33].

Because primary breast sarcomas are rare, the diagnosis is often missed on initial work-up and evaluation [11]. Biopsy of breast masses is best accomplished with core needle biopsy. The accuracy of fine-needle aspiration is often limited in establishing the histologic diagnosis of breast sarcomas. Core needle biopsy is preferred over excisional biopsy, but both methods are reliable and can provide sufficient tissue for histologic diagnosis and grading.

Staging

Size, histologic grade, and nodal or distant metastasis contribute to the staging of soft tissue sarcomas, including primary breast sarcomas (Box 1) [34]. Unlike epithelial breast cancers, nodal status is less informative, because metastases to regional lymph nodes are rare for sarcomas in general.

Management

Treatment for primary breast sarcoma should be accomplished through a multidisciplinary approach as is true for other soft tissue sarcomas. There are no consensus treatment guidelines or randomized controlled trials that have been specifically completed for breast sarcomas. Nevertheless, it is clear that surgery remains the mainstay of therapy. As with sarcomas in other locations, surgical management is becoming less aggressive with increased attempts at organ preservation.

Surgical management

Berg and colleagues initially published their series of breast sarcomas in which 9 of 13 patients who underwent wide local excision developed recurrence, whereas only 1 of 7 patients who had mastectomy had local failure [20]. Mastectomy was hence held as the gold standard. This opinion has been challenged over the last 2 decades, with the results from several retrospective series showing equivalent outcomes with wide local excision when negative margins can be achieved [7,11,19,22]. This finding is supported by the fact that, pathologically, sarcomas are rarely multicentric; however, in cases with large primary tumors, the overall cosmetic result is better

Box 1. Grade and tumor, node, metastasis (TNM) definitions

Tumor grade (G)
- GX: grade cannot be assessed
- G1: well differentiated
- G2: moderately differentiated
- G3: poorly differentiated
- G4: poorly differentiated or undifferentiated

Primary tumor (T)
- TX: primary tumor cannot be assessed
- T0: no evidence of primary tumor
- T1: tumor 5 cm or less in greatest dimension
- T1a: superficial tumor
- T1b: deep tumor
- T2: tumor 5 cm or larger in greatest dimension
- T2a: superficial tumor
- T2b: deep tumor

Regional lymph nodes (N)
- NX: regional lymph nodes cannot be assessed
- N0: no regional lymph node metastasis
- N1: regional lymph node metastasis (presence of positive nodes [N1] considered stage IV)

Distant metastasis (M)
- MX: distant metastasis cannot be assessed
- M0: no distant metastasis
- M1: distant metastasis

American Joint Committee on Cancer stage groupings

Stage I (tumor defined as low grade, superficial, and deep)
- G1, T1a, N0, M0
- G1, T1b, N0, M0
- G1, T2a, N0, M0
- G1, T2b, N0, M0
- G2, T1a, N0, M0
- G2, T1b, N0, M0
- G2, T2a, N0, M0
- G2, T2b, N0, M0

Stage II (tumor defined as high grade, superficial, and deep)
- G3, T1a, N0, M0
- G3, T1b, N0, M0
- G3, T2a, N0, M0

- G4, T1a, N0, M0
- G4, T1b, N0, M0
- G4, T2a, N0, M0

Stage III (tumor defined as high grade, large, and deep)
- G3, T2b, N0, M0
- G4, T2b, N0, M0

Stage IV (defined as any metastasis to lymph nodes or distant sites)
- Any G, any T, N1, M0
- Any G, any T, N0, M1

with mastectomy and reconstruction than with lumpectomy. Fig. 1 demonstrates a patient with a dermatofibrosarcoma protuberans resected with a lumpectomy. The excision resulted in a significant cosmetic defect with a marked discrepancy in breast size. Fig. 2 shows the same patient after mastectomy with deep inferior epigastric perforator flap reconstruction. A reduction and lift of the contralateral side will be completed at a later date for symmetry.

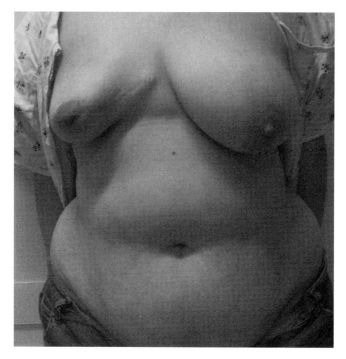

Fig. 1. Patient with dermatofibrosarcoma protuberans resected with lumpectomy.

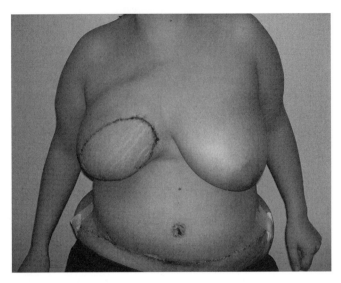

Fig. 2. Patient with dermatofibrosarcoma protuberans after mastectomy and deep inferior epigastric perforator flap reconstruction.

It is now widely accepted that axillary lymph node involvement in primary breast sarcoma is rare. When it does occur, the presence of axillary lymph node metastases reflects systemic dissemination of the disease rather than locoregional extension of the primary tumor. Furthermore, some of the reported axillary lymph node involvement in the literature is in series including carcinosarcomas (which, by definition, contain an epithelial component and should not be classified as primary breast sarcomas). Hence, axillary lymph node dissection is not routinely performed in the surgical management of primary breast sarcomas.

Controversy arises in the surgical management of tumors 5 cm or greater. A tumor size of 5 cm or greater has been demonstrated to be a reliable prognostic factor for recurrence [11]. Because local recurrence, in turn, is associated with a poor survival, there should be careful consideration of the choice of surgical management in patients with large primary tumors. There is little evidence to suggest that a larger operation (ie, mastectomy) for larger tumors confers any survival or disease-free advantage over a less extensive operation (eg, wide local excision) as long as negative margins are achieved [7,13,22,35]. In fact, margin status has been determined to be the single most important prognostic factor for treatment failure (both local and distant) [13,15]. Nevertheless, with the lack of definitive randomized results, some authorities remain hesitant to recommend less extensive surgery. The mentioned reasons favoring more extensive surgery include the presence of high-grade tumors; a large tumor to breast size ratio, which may compromise the feasibility of obtaining a wide circumferential margin; or the presence of deep seated tumors which are close to or involve the chest wall. Such cases would, in fact, require mastectomy including en bloc resection of chest wall [14–16].

Adjuvant therapy

The role of adjuvant therapy in the treatment of primary breast sarcomas remains undefined largely due to the limited sample size in prior retrospective series. Moreover, in many of these series, adjuvant therapy was provided to patients who presented with larger tumors, which probably inherently reflected more aggressive disease. There are several conflicting reports in the literature, with most showing no benefit or even a worse prognosis in patients treated with adjuvant therapy [7,14,18].

Nevertheless, a few reports show that adjuvant radiotherapy improves disease-free survival but not necessarily overall survival [36]. Furthermore, in two of the larger series in the literature, Barrow and colleagues from M.D. Anderson in the United States and Zelek and colleagues from the Institut Gustave-Roussy in France both drew extrapolations from the treatment principles of non-breast sarcomas and proposed that adjuvant radiotherapy be combined with wide local excision to improve local control. Currently, although there is no definitive evidence, adjuvant radiotherapy may be recommended to patients, especially if the primary tumor is larger than 5 cm, high grade, or resected with positive margins in a patient in whom repeat surgery is not possible [19,25].

The data on adjuvant chemotherapy are even less conclusive, with no studies completed to investigate drug regimens for breast sarcomas. Current regimens recommended include doxorubicin alone or in combination with ifosfamide based on data from other soft tissue sarcomas [37]. Similar to adjuvant radiotherapy, adjuvant chemotherapy has been recommended for patients with large (greater than 5 cm) or high-grade tumors [19].

Although neoadjuvant chemotherapy has been used with some success to downstage extremity sarcomas, there is some hesitation to recommend this for breast sarcomas, especially because the response rates are limited and not durable [19]. Furthermore, most breast sarcomas are usually amenable to surgical resection, albeit, with mastectomy if wide local excision is not feasible.

Prognosis

The 5-year overall survival rate for primary breast sarcomas is 50% to 66%, similar to that for other non-breast sarcomas [7,11,15,17,19,38]; however, the 5-year disease-free survival rate is lower and ranges between 33% and 52% [7,11,15,17,19], with most failures occurring within the first 15 months [11,17]. Local failure contributes to a high percentage of recurrent disease (up to one third of all patients in some series), further underscoring the importance of negative surgical margins. In cases of isolated local recurrence, salvage therapy can be performed with re-excision or completion mastectomy [15].

Primary breast sarcomas metastasize most commonly to the lung, bone, and liver. Other reported sites include the brain, skin, and subcutaneous tissue, and more rarely the spleen and adrenal glands [11,14,17]. In cases of metastatic disease, a multidisciplinary approach with all modalities including surgery for isolated disease, chemotherapy, and radiotherapy is required.

Summary

Primary breast sarcomas are rare malignancies of the breast for which treatment should be approached by a multidisciplinary team. Surgery remains the mainstay of therapy, with wide local excision conferring similar overall survival when compared with mastectomy, as long as negative margins of 2 to 3 cm can be obtained. Axillary dissection is not necessary with the low rate of nodal metastases. Adjuvant radiotherapy should be considered to assist in local control, especially in patients who have large or high-grade tumors. Adjuvant chemotherapy is limited to the high-risk group and consists of treatments most commonly used for soft tissue sarcomas in other locations. Adjuvant therapies used for epithelial malignancies of the breast such as anti-estrogens and chemotherapeutic agents are not useful in primary breast sarcomas.

References

[1] Geisler DP, Boyle MJ, Malnar KF, et al. Phyllodes tumors of the breast: a review of 32 cases. Am Surg 2000;66:360–6.
[2] Russell WO, Cohen J, Enzinger F, et al. A clinical and pathological staging system for soft tissue sarcomas. Cancer 1977;40:1562–70.
[3] May DS, Stroup NE. The incidence of sarcomas of the breast among women in the United States, 1973–1986. Plast Reconstr Surg 1991;87:193–4.
[4] Karlsson P, Holmberg E, Samuelsson A, et al. Soft tissue sarcoma after treatment for breast cancer–a Swedish population-based study. Eur J Cancer 1998;34:2068–75.
[5] Blanchard DK, Reynolds C, Grant CS, et al. Radiation-induced breast sarcoma. Am J Surg 2002;184:356–8.
[6] Huang J, Mackillop WJ. Increased risk of soft tissue sarcoma after radiotherapy in women with breast carcinoma. Cancer 2001;92:172–80.
[7] Blanchard DK, Reynolds CA, Grant CS, et al. Primary nonphylloides breast sarcomas. Am J Surg 2003;186:359–61.
[8] Brady MS, Garfein CF, Petrek JA, et al. Post-treatment sarcoma in breast cancer patients. Ann Surg Oncol 1994;1:66–72.
[9] Stewart FW, Treves N. Lymphangiosarcoma in postmastectomy lymphedema. Cancer 1948; 1:64–81.
[10] Ciatto S, Bonardi R, Cataliotti L, et al. Phyllodes tumor of the breast: a multicenter series of 59 cases. Coordinating Center and Writing Committee of FONCAM (National Task Force for Breast Cancer), Italy. Eur J Surg Oncol 1992;18:545–9.

[11] Gutman H, Pollock RE, Ross MI, et al. Sarcoma of the breast: implications for extent of therapy. The M.D. Anderson experience. Surgery 1994;116:505–9.

[12] Terrier P, Terrier-Lacombe MJ, Mouriesse H, et al. Primary breast sarcoma: a review of 33 cases with immunohistochemistry and prognostic factors. Breast Cancer Res Treat 1989;13:39–48.

[13] Shabahang M, Franceschi D, Sundaram M, et al. Surgical management of primary breast sarcoma. Am Surg 2002;68:673–7 [discussion: 677].

[14] North JH Jr, McPhee M, Arredondo M, et al. Sarcoma of the breast: implications of the extent of local therapy. Am Surg 1998;64:1059–61.

[15] Pandey M, Mathew A, Abraham EK, et al. Primary sarcoma of the breast. J Surg Oncol 2004;87:121–5.

[16] Moore MP, Kinne DW. Breast sarcoma. Surg Clin North Am 1996;76:383–92.

[17] Adem C, Reynolds C, Ingle JN, et al. Primary breast sarcoma: clinicopathologic series from the Mayo Clinic and review of the literature. Br J Cancer 2004;91:237–41.

[18] Pollard SG, Marks PV, Temple LN, et al. Breast sarcoma: a clinicopathologic review of 25 cases. Cancer 1990;66:941–4.

[19] Zelek L, Llombart-Cussac A, Terrier P, et al. Prognostic factors in primary breast sarcomas: a series of patients with long-term follow-up. J Clin Oncol 2003;21:2583–8.

[20] Berg JW, Decrosse JJ, Fracchia AA, et al. Stromal sarcomas of the breast: a unified approach to connective tissue sarcomas other than cystosarcoma phyllodes. Cancer 1962; 15:418–24.

[21] Lattes R. Sarcomas of the breast. Int J Radiat Oncol Biol Phys 1978;4:705–8.

[22] McGowan TS, Cummings BJ, O'Sullivan B, et al. An analysis of 78 breast sarcoma patients without distant metastases at presentation. Int J Radiat Oncol Biol Phys 2000;46:383–90.

[23] McGregor GI, Knowling MA, Este FA. Sarcoma and cystosarcoma phyllodes tumors of the breast–a retrospective review of 58 cases. Am J Surg 1994;167:477–80.

[24] Ward RM, Evans HL. Cystosarcoma phyllodes: a clinicopathologic study of 26 cases. Cancer 1986;58:2282–9.

[25] Barrow BJ, Janjan NA, Gutman H, et al. Role of radiotherapy in sarcoma of the breast–a retrospective review of the M.D. Anderson experience. Radiother Oncol 1999;52:173–8.

[26] Merino MJ, Carter D, Berman M. Angiosarcoma of the breast. Am J Surg Pathol 1983;7: 53–60.

[27] Christensen L, Schiodt T, Blichert-Toft M, et al. Sarcomas of the breast: a clinico-pathological study of 67 patients with long term follow-up. Eur J Surg Oncol 1988;14: 241–7.

[28] Rosen PP, Kimmel M, Ernsberger D. Mammary angiosarcoma: the prognostic significance of tumor differentiation. Cancer 1988;62:2145–51.

[29] Jones MW, Norris HJ, Wargotz ES, et al. Fibrosarcoma-malignant fibrous histiocytoma of the breast: a clinicopathological study of 32 cases. Am J Surg Pathol 1992;16:667–74.

[30] Donnell RM, Rosen PP, Lieberman PH, et al. Angiosarcoma and other vascular tumors of the breast. Am J Surg Pathol 1981;5:629–42.

[31] Grobmyer SR, Brennan MF. Predictive variables detailing the recurrence rate of soft tissue sarcomas. Curr Opin Oncol 2003;15:319–26.

[32] Elson BC, Ikeda DM, Andersson I, et al. Fibrosarcoma of the breast: mammographic findings in five cases. AJR Am J Roentgenol 1992;158:993–5.

[33] Bakheet SM, Powe J, Ezzat A, et al. F-18 FDG whole-body positron emission tomography scan in primary breast sarcoma. Clin Nucl Med 1998;23:604–8.

[34] Greene FL, Fritz AG, Balch CM, et al. Soft tissue sarcoma. In: American Joint Committee on Cancer, editor. AJCC Cancer Staging Manual. 6th edition. New York: Springer; 2002. p. 193–7.

[35] Smola MG, Ratschek M, Amann W, et al. The impact of resection margins in the treatment of primary sarcomas of the breast: a clinicopathological study of 8 cases with review of literature. Eur J Surg Oncol 1993;19:61–9.

[36] Johnstone PA, Pierce LJ, Merino MJ, et al. Primary soft tissue sarcomas of the breast: local-regional control with postoperative radiotherapy. Int J Radiat Oncol Biol Phys 1993;27: 671–5.

[37] Sarcoma Meta-analysis Collaboration. Adjuvant chemotherapy for localised resectable soft-tissue sarcoma of adults: meta-analysis of individual data. Sarcoma meta-analysis collaboration. Lancet 1997;350:1647–54.

[38] Callery CD, Rosen PP, Kinne DW. Sarcoma of the breast: a study of 32 patients with reappraisal of classification and therapy. Ann Surg 1985;201:527–32.

[39] Ciatto S, Bonardi R, Cataliotti L, et al. Sarcomas of the breast: a multicenter series of 70 cases. Neoplasma 1992;39:375–9.

ELSEVIER
SAUNDERS

SURGICAL
CLINICS OF
NORTH AMERICA

Surg Clin N Am 88 (2008) 571–582

Truncal Sarcomas and Abdominal Desmoids

Jacqueline M. Garonzik Wang, MD[a],
Steven D. Leach, MD[b],*

[a]Department of Surgery, Johns Hopkins University School of Medicine,
600 N. Wolfe St./Osler 603, Baltimore, MD 21287, USA
[b]Oncology and Cell Biology, Johns Hopkins Medical Institution, Broadway Research Bldg,
Room 471, Baltimore, MD 21287, USA

This article gives a brief overview of the common histologies observed in truncal sarcomas and reviews the fundamental principles of diagnosis and treatment. Although the behavior of most cancers varies, depending on their site of origin, sarcomas generally behave similarly regardless of derivation. Therefore, many of the principles outlined in the previous articles are applicable to the epidemiology, diagnosis, and treatment of truncal sarcomas. Because of the rarity of sarcomas, the available information regarding them has been extrapolated from data that include extremity sarcomas and sarcomas of other anatomic locations. Furthermore, because only 17.9% of sarcomas originate in the trunk [1], definitive epidemiologic, diagnostic, and therapeutic information often is lacking.

Diagnosis is based on tissue biopsy with pathologic determination. Imaging, such as plain film radiographs, CT, and MRI, is most useful when planning operative treatment. Surgical resection with wide margins is the initial standard of treatment; however a multimodal approach including radiotherapy and chemotherapy often is favored. Consequently, it is often recommended that patients who have truncal or other soft tissue sarcomas be treated in a tertiary care center where a multidisciplinary approach can be facilitated [2].

This article also provides a general review of abdominal desmoids. Abdominal desmoids are unique entities similar to truncal sarcomas but with a unique set of management principles. These lesions are benign, slow-growing tumors of myofibroblast origin that can be locally aggressive. Despite

---

* Corresponding author.
E-mail address: stleach@jhmi.edu (S.D. Leach).

doi:10.1016/j.suc.2008.04.001
surgical.theclinics.com

the lack of metastatic potential, these lesions have a very high local recurrence rate, making definitive treatment a challenge. Desmoids also have been seen in association with familial adenomatous polyposis (FAP) syndrome, suggesting a genetic link to the adenomatous polyposis coli (*APC*) mutation. Other risk factors include trauma and estrogen exposure. Although surgery remains the primary treatment, operative planning often is complicated by the involvement of visceral vasculature. Furthermore, intra-abdominal trauma, such as surgery, is a risk factor for disease progression in patients who have FAP [3]. Therefore other treatment modalities and regimens are currently under active investigation.

Truncal sarcomas

History and clinical findings

Like sarcoma in other anatomic locations, truncal sarcoma often presents as a slow-growing, painless mass. Patients' symptoms often are secondary to the compressive nature of the tumor. Lesions often are quite large on presentation. Lawrence and colleagues [1] surveyed 5800 patients who had sarcomas and found that almost half waited at least 4 months after symptomatic presentation before undergoing an adequate initial work-up. Twenty percent waited at least 6 months after their first evaluation before appropriate diagnoses were made. Truncal sarcomas, like all other sarcomas, are associated with a variety of carcinogenic agents and hereditary syndromes. Chlorophenols, Thorotrast, arsenic, and radiation are just a few of the many agents that have been linked to subsequent sarcoma formation. Likewise, genetic syndromes such as Li-Fraumeni syndrome, retinoblastoma, von Reckinghausen's disease, and Gardner's syndrome are associated with the development of soft tissue sarcomas.

Diagnosis

Biopsy often is the first diagnostic modality used. The performing physician should include sarcoma as part of the differential diagnosis to ensure proper sampling techniques that do not hamper future diagnostic or treatment options. Although fine-needle biopsy often is the modality of choice for sampling other masses, its use is limited with soft tissue sarcomas. Often this technique does not provide an adequate sample for accurate diagnosis, especially in centers with little experience in the evaluation of sarcoma cytology. Core-needle biopsy is the preferred initial sampling method. If a core biopsy is insufficient or impossible, the next diagnostic step is incisional biopsy. Whenever possible, incisional biopsies should be performed by the surgeon performing the definitive resection and in a manner that allows the resulting scar to be excised at the time of the definitive surgery. To avoid tumor dissemination at the time of biopsy, no flaps should be raised, nor should any tissue planes disrupted. Also, it is imperative to avoid hematoma formation, because this also carries a risk of expanding the field containing tumor cells.

Pathology

Histologic tumor types are similar to those seen in sarcomas arising in other anatomic locations (Box 1), with desmoids being a unique and very common subtype often found in this location. Although histologic class is an important prognosticator in extremity and head and neck sarcomas, its role is less relevant in truncal sarcomas, because wide local resection with negative margins is achieved more easily, given the greater tissue surface area and lack of major vital structures [4]. Furthermore, tumor behavior varies not only among tumor types but also within individual types. Because grade often plays a more important role, it has been including in the staging of soft tissue sarcomas [5].

Imaging

Radiographic evaluation is useful in determining the extent of disease and following disease progression, both before and after definitive treatment. As mentioned in other articles, CT scan and MRI are the most useful imaging modalities for evaluating soft tissue sarcomas [6] (see the article by Fadul and Fayad, elsewhere in this issue). A CT scan also can help determine if the patient has evidence of metastatic disease. MRI gives the clinician detailed information regarding the anatomic extent of the tumor and about nerve, and bony involvement and allows detailed operative planning [5]. Angiography rarely is needed, but it may be helpful if there is concern about vascular invasion.

Box 1. Types of truncal sarcomas

Angiosarcoma
Leiomyosarcoma
Malignant fibrous histiocytoma
Neurofibrosarcoma
Rhabdomyosarcoma
Desmoid[a]
Fibrosarcoma
Liposarcoma
Mesenchymoma
Osteosarcoma
Synovial sarcoma

---

[a] Benign lesion, but locally infiltrative and frequently recurs.

Staging

Soft tissue sarcomas are staged using a modified TNM system, which includes grade (GTNM), Current staging, however, does not distinguish between well-differentiated and moderately differentiated tumors. The absence of this distinction may represent an inadequacy of the staging system, because some data suggest that moderately differentiated tumors have a worse prognosis than well-differentiated lesions [7]. In 1998 the T staging was subdivided further to consider the location of the lesion in relationship to the superficial fascia. The location of the lesion is designated as "a" if it is entirely above and "b" if below the fascia of the abdominal wall. This differentiation provides additional prognostic information to the staging system. An "a" lesion has a better prognosis than a "b" lesion of similar size and grade.

Treatment

En bloc resection with wide margins is the treatment of choice for all sarcomas, including truncal sarcomas [1,4,5]. If adequate margins are not achieved, local recurrence is common. Lymphadenectomy is reserved for situations in which clinical or radiographic evidence of nodal involvement exists, because nodal metastasis is rare [4]. Several histologic subtypes are associated with an increased risk of nodal spread, however, and evaluation of possible nodal disease should be emphasized when dealing with epithelioid sarcoma, rhabdomyosarcoma, clear cell sarcoma, and angiosarcoma. Radiotherapy sometimes is recommended if residual disease, positive or narrow margins, or high-grade tumor is present [4]. Neoadjuvant chemotherapy and/or radiotherapy have been recommended if preoperative imaging suggests that negative surgical margins may be difficult to obtain. Overall, a paucity of literature exists defining the role of radiation and chemotherapy, and this lack is exacerbated further by the rarity of soft tissue sarcomas. Two randomized, controlled trials demonstrated an increased local control rate with adjuvant radiation therapy, however [8,9]. This benefit is most apparent in high-grade lesions [8]. Further, radiation therapy has been shown to improve local control and limb sparing in extremity sarcoma, and these data often have been extrapolated to truncal sarcomas [8]. In a randomized, controlled trial performed at Memorial-Sloan Kettering Cancer Center, adjuvant brachytherapy did improve local control after resection of soft tissue sarcomas, but this benefit was limited to patients who had high-grade lesions [9]. In a recently published Scandinavian prospective trial, adjuvant radiotherapy prevented local recurrence irrespective of grade, location, or margin status, with benefit most pronounced in high-grade lesions [10]. Surgery is still the modality of choice, however, because vital intra-abdominal and spinal structures often represent dose-limiting factors for radiotherapy. Further, no studies have shown a definitive benefit from chemotherapy alone, and its use therefore should be limited to metastatic and unresectable disease or clinical trials. Hence, local control is accomplished best with surgical resection and wide margins, with the possible addition of radiation for large or highly invasive tumors.

Because these tumors are rare, patients may receive better and more appropriate treatment at high-volume centers. Gutierrez and colleagues [2] reviewed cases registered in Florida between 1981 and 2001 and showed that patients treated at a high-volume center (defined as one with an operative volume above the sixty-seventh percentile) had lower short-term and long-term mortality, with 30-day mortality rates of 0.7% versus 1.5% ($P = .028$) and 90-day mortality rates of 1.6% versus 3.6% ($P = .001$). This benefit was observed even though tumors treated at the high-volume centers were larger and of higher grade.

There are more options for reconstruction following the resection of truncal sarcomas than for sarcomas arising in other anatomic sites, because of the lack of adjacent vital structures, the increased surface area, and the ability to use prosthetic material and/or pedicled or free flaps. If the anticipated defect is large, involvement of a plastic surgery team during both the resection and reconstruction planning is imperative to provide the patient with an optimal cancer operation and optimal functional and cosmetic outcomes.

Prognosis

Multiple studies suggest that tumor grade, margin status, and tumor size are important independent variables in patient prognosis [11,12]. Overall survival for truncal sarcomas seems to fall between that observed for extremity and retroperitoneal sarcomas. Singer and colleagues found that the overall 15-year survival rate for extremity soft tissue sarcomas was 68.4%, compared with 59.5% for truncal and 50% for retroperitoneal sarcomas [11]. In this study tumor grade was extremely important in predicting survival: the 12-year survival rate was 92% for low-grade sarcomas, 75% for intermediate grade sarcomas, and 43% for high-grade sarcomas [11]. Also, prognosis was influenced by tumor size, with tumors smaller than 5 cm having a 70% 12-year survival rate and tumors greater than 5 cm having a 49.5% 12-year survival rate. Singer and colleagues [11] also examined how surgical outcome affected survival. Overall survival was 67% with negative microscopic margins, compared with 49% for positive margins.

Patterns of recurrence

One of the unfortunate characteristics of sarcomas in general is their propensity for recurrence. Although there are exceptions, recurrence occurs in a predictable manner. In most cases recurrence occurs locally, most often in the resection bed itself. Local recurrence rates have been reported to be as high as 40% to 50% and to be linked to inadequate margins and aggressive histopathology [12,13]. A review performed at Brigham and Women's hospital showed that 67% of patients who had locally recurrent soft tissue sarcoma were able to undergo re-resection with reasonable survival rates [14]. Radiotherapy is an option for patients not receiving adjuvant therapy as initial treatment. If the patient did receive prior external beam radiation, brachytherapy may still represent a suitable treatment option.

As in other sarcomas, metastatic disease most commonly occurs in the lung. Pulmonary metastases are seen in as many as 20% of trunk and extremity soft tissue sarcomas [15]. For isolated pulmonary metastases, surgical resection is a feasible option if the patient is a good surgical candidate. Survival rates after pulmonary metastectomy for isolated pulmonary metastases range from 23% to 50% [15–17]. For multifocal metastatic disease or metastases to unresectable sites, chemotherapy often is the only treatment option. Doxorubicin is the most commonly used chemotherapeutic agent. Although other combination therapies have been tested, doxorubicin thus far is the safest and most effective [18,19] (see the article by Thornton, elsewhere in this issue).

Follow-up

Because local recurrence is common with truncal sarcomas, close follow-up is recommended. Patients should return at least every 3 months for the first 2 years and then be seen bi-annually for another 5 years. Physical examination, laboratory studies, and imaging are warranted to rule out recurrence. Chest radiographs combined with CT scanning are performed routinely bi-annually for 2 to 3 years to rule out disease recurrence and to evaluate for possible pulmonary metastasis [3].

Desmoid tumors

Abdominal desmoids, also known as "aggressive fibromatosis," are soft tissue lesions that behave similarly to other truncal soft tissue sarcomas but have unique characteristics. These tumors, like other soft tissue sarcomas, present as slow-growing, indolent masses. Unlike typical sarcomas however, these tumors rarely metastasize. They also frequently recur locally [20]. Diagnosis and radiographic evaluation are essentially identical to that of other truncal soft tissue sarcomas.

Most desmoid tumors arise sporadically, but a small percentage (~5%) occurs in association with FAP syndrome [21]. There is some association between abdominal desmoids and pregnancy. A small percentage of desmoids arise from cesarean section scars after pregnancy. These findings have linked desmoid proliferation to hormonal stimulation, specifically estrogen.

Desmoids are classified as either abdominal or extra-abdominal. Because this article focuses solely on truncal lesions, it chiefly reviews abdominal desmoids. Furthermore, abdominal desmoids are far more common than extra-abdominal desmoids. Abdominal desmoids are categorized further as superficial or intra-abdominal tumors [22]. Most of the intra-abdominal lesions are seen in association with FAP. These lesions are associated with mutations in the *APC* gene that are found in patients who have FAP. Multiple *APC* germline mutations have been described and potentially linked to desmoid proliferation in this patient population. These tumors usually are found in the mesentery, and their growth and compression of neighboring structures can lead to significant morbidity and sometimes even death in these patients [23].

Myofibroblasts have been targeted as the cells responsible for desmoid development, but why the myofibroblasts proliferate and develop into a desmoid is unclear. Some data link desmoid proliferation to estrogen, which may explain the higher incidence in women of reproductive age [24]. Tissue injury, such as trauma and/or surgery, also has been implicated in tumor development [21,25].

The natural history of desmoid lesions is unpredictable. Although most are indolent and slow growing, some lesions are aggressive [21]. There are some reports of spontaneous regression, but such occurrences are mainly in women and are associated with chemical or surgical menopause [26]. Most lesions are indolent and have benign-appearing histology, but local growth and compression have caused significant morbidity. Involvement of abdominal vessels and organs often complicates management. Furthermore, the lesions often recur despite surgical intervention [21].

The diagnostic work-up is similar to that of other soft tissue sarcomas, but a thorough familial history should be elicited to identify high-risk individuals. Physical examination may yield an incidental slow-growing mass or an expanding and symptomatic lesion. Mass lesions arising in old abdominal and caesarean scars should raise the suspicion for a desmoid tumor [23]. Because they grow in an indolent manner, these lesions can be very large at presentation. Occasionally the patient presents with paresthesias or pain secondary to adjacent nerve compression [26]. Intra-abdominal desmoids also can present with abdominal pain and obstructive symptoms secondary to adjacent visceral compression. If an abdominal desmoid is suspected, CT and MRI can delineate the extent of the lesion and aid in surgical planning [22]. Table 1 outlines a staging system described by Church and colleagues [22] in 2005 that helps predict tumor behavior in a manner that guides therapeutic intervention.

Although surgical resection with wide local margins has been the reference standard for definitive treatment of abdominal desmoids, few randomized, clinical trials have compared different treatment strategies. This comparison is complicated by the varying clinical courses of these tumors. It is not clear if the treatment algorithm should be identical for both stable lesions and locally compressive lesions. Nonetheless, all patients who have intra-abdominal desmoids should have a complete work-up for FAP because of the association between these entities [22]. In 2006, Latchford

Table 1
Staging of intra/transabdominal desmoid tumors

Stage	Description	Treatment
I	Asymptomatic, not growing	Simple observation or nontoxic ("prophylactic") therapy (ie, NSAIDs). Resection if found incidentally during surgery
II	Symptomatic, <10 cm in maximum diameter, not growing	Resection (method of choice). If unresectable, use combination therapy (ie, tamoxifen or raloxifene + NSAIDs).
III	Symptomatic, 10–20 cm in maximum diameter, or asymptomatic and slowly growing	Active treatment. Therapy includes NSAIDs, tamoxifen, relaxifene and vinblastine/methotrexate. Anti-sarcoma therapy (adriamycin/dacarbazine) when less toxic therapy is effective.
IV	Symptomatic, >20 cm, or rapid growth, or complicated	Urgent therapy, which includes surgery (often major exenterative surgery), anti-sarcoma chemotherapy, and radiation

Abbreviations: NSAIDS, nonsteroidal anti-inflammatory drugs.
Data from Church J, Berk T, Boman BM, et al. Staging intra-abdominal desmoid tumors in familial adenomatous polyposis: a search for a uniform approach to a troubling disease. Dis Colon Rectum 2005;48:1528–34; with permission.

and colleagues proposed a treatment algorithm and guidelines for abdominal desmoids (Fig. 1) [20]. Observation is an acceptable option for small, asymptomatic, stable lesions that are not near vital structures. These lesions should be followed with serial imaging to ensure that they do not grow. This method is supported by evidence that a small percentage of lesions regress. Others, however, argue that regression is rare and that these lesions should be resected prophylactically despite their stability and small size.

Multiple pharmacologic therapies have been suggested for abdominal desmoids, but their use is limited by the infrequency of this disease and the lack of good clinical trials. Therefore surgery remains the standard approach. In one series, medical therapy was used as the initial treatment for intra-abdominal disease or multicentric disease [21,24]. Nonsteroidal anti-inflammatory drugs, such as sulindac and indomethacin, and anti-estrogens, such as tamoxifen, have been suggested as options for pharmacologic treatment [21,27]. Despite the lack of randomized, controlled trials, observational studies show that about 50% of patients who have desmoid tumors have some response to these pharmacologic agents. Without randomization, however, it is difficult to assess whether this response is truly secondary to medical therapy. In some studies, up to 50% of patients who had desmoids had stable disease without surgical or pharmacologic intervention [28]. Despite the lack of data, nontoxic pharmacologic therapy is encouraged both pre- and postoperatively in patients who are at risk for recurrence or who have advanced disease [21].

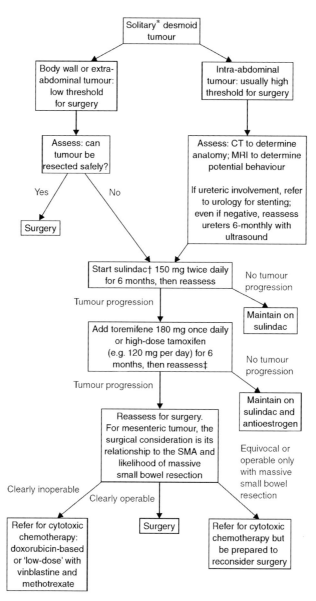

Fig. 1. Proposed algorithm for the treatment of complicated lesions. (*From* Latchford AR, Strut NJH, Neale K, et al. A 10-year review of surgery for desmoid disease associated with familial adenomatous polyposis. Br J of Surg 2006;93:1262; with permission.)

More recently, cytotoxic pharmacologic agents have been considered in the treatment of desmoids. Indications for cytotoxic therapy often include failure of noncytotoxic regimens and unresectable, inoperable, or persistent disease [21,23,24]. Cytotoxic drugs can be used in a neoadjuvant setting to aid in future resectability. Multiple chemotherapeutic regimens have been suggested, but clinical trials have yet to determine a definitive regimen. Combinations of methotrexate, doxorubicin, vinblastine, dacarbazine, and/or cyclophosphamide have been recommended [22,24]. The response to doxorubicin-based chemotherapy has been as high as 50%, but excessive toxicity often limits its use clinically [24].

Surgical intervention remains a mainstay of therapy. Abdominal wall lesions that are accessible (< 10 cm in diameter) should be resected early to achieve negative margins more readily and to limit the potential soft tissue defect requiring reconstruction [21,24]. Surgical intervention for intra-abdominal lesions often is complicated by tumoral involvement of neighboring visceral, mesenteric, or vascular structures, however, and it has been suggested that resection itself can be associated with more aggressive recurrence [3]. For this reason, debulking surgery is not recommended [29]. Consequently, surgical resection of intra-abdominal lesions is indicated only in selected clinical circumstances, that is, in lesions that are causing potentially correctable complications such as small bowel obstruction, in lesions that do not involve vital structures, in rapidly growing lesion that threatens nearby structures, or when pharmacologic management has failed [23,24].

Another therapeutic option is radiation therapy used alone or in combination with other therapeutic interventions. Radiotherapy also can be used in the adjuvant or neoadjuvant setting. Inoperable lesions have been rendered resectable following radiation therapy in combination with chemotherapy [28]. Definitive data are lacking, however, and radiation enteritis has limited its use in truncal and intra-abdominal lesions [21,22]. Newer treatment modalities such as radiofrequency ablation, imaging-guided chemical ablation, and gene transfer therapy also have been reported. Evidence in support of these treatment methods is very limited, and they are not recommended as first-line therapies [22].

Despite these treatment options, desmoids are locally infiltrative lesions that recur frequently. Surgery with wide negative margins still is the best treatment to prevent recurrence. Positive margins nearly double the recurrence rate [29]. Even with negative margins, recurrence rates as low as 10% and as high as 75% are reported [12,20,22,24]. Surgery itself may lead to recurrence in some instances, because tissue trauma has been linked to tumor growth [3]. Although randomized, controlled trials regarding the treatment of recurrence are lacking, re-operation is still a mainstay of treatment, and adjuvant and alternative methods of therapy may be helpful in limiting further tumor progression.

Summary

Truncal sarcomas and abdominal desmoids are lesions that often are slow growing and indolent in nature with locally infiltrative features. Local compression of visceral structures can cause significant morbidity and mortality. Surgical resection with negative margins is the treatment of choice. Because vital visceral organs and local infiltration often make achieving negative margins difficult, other therapeutic modalities have been suggested. Randomized, controlled trials demonstrating that these therapies provide significant survival benefit have not yet been performed. Further research is needed to determine the optimal treatment plan for individual scenarios. It is clear that surgical resection is the treatment of choice for appropriate lesions not involving visceral structures or their associated blood supply. Treatment for more complicated lesions is not straightforward. For these lesions the algorithm proposed by Latchford and colleagues [20] is useful in initial treatment planning (see Fig. 1). Because the recurrence rate remains high regardless of therapy, close follow-up is imperative.

Acknowledgments

The authors thank Dr. Frank Giardello for helpful suggestions in the preparation of this article.

References

[1] Lawrence W Jr, Donegan WL, Natarajan A, et al. Adult soft tissue sarcomas: a pattern of care survey of the American College of Surgeons. Ann Surg 1987;205:349–59.

[2] Gutierrez JC, Perez EA, Moffat FL, et al. Should soft tissue sarcomas be treated at high-volume centers? An analysis of 4205 patients. Ann Surg 2007;245:952–8.

[3] Lynch HT, Fitzgibbons R Jr. Surgery, desmoid tumors, and familial adenomatous polyposis: a case report and literature review. Am J Gastroenterol 1996;91:2598–601.

[4] Malawer MM, Sugarbaker P. Musculoskeletal cancer surgery: treatment of sarcomas and allied diseases. 1st edition. New York: Springer; 2002, Chapter 8, Management of truncal sarcoma. p. 165–78.

[5] Cameron JL. Current surgical therapy. 8th edition. Philadelphia: Elsevier Mosby; 2004.

[6] Arca MJ, Sondak VK, Chang AE, et al. Diagnostic procedures and pre-treatment evaluation of soft tissue sarcomas. Semin Surg Oncol 1994;10:323–31.

[7] Myhre-Jensen O, Kaae S, Madsen EH, et al. Histopathological grading in soft-tissue tumours. Relation to survival in 261 surgically treated patients. Acta Pathol Microbiol Immunol Scand 1983;91(2):145–50.

[8] Yang JC, Chang AE, Baker AR, et al. Randomized prospective study of the benefit of adjuvant radiation therapy in the treatment of soft tissue sarcomas of the extremity. J Clin Oncol 1998;16:197–203.

[9] Pisters PW, Harrison LB, Leung DH, et al. Long-term results of a prospective randomized trial of adjuvant brachytherapy in soft tissue sarcoma. J Clin Oncol 1996;14:859–68.

[10] Jebsen NL, Trovik CS, Bauer HCF, et al. Radiotherapy to improve local control regardless of surgical margin and malignancy grade in extremity and trunk wall soft tissue sarcoma: a Scandinavian Sarcoma Group study. Int J Radiat Oncol Biol Phys 2008, in press.

[11] Singer S, Corson JM, Demetri GD, et al. Prognostic factors predictive of survival for truncal and retroperitoneal soft-tissue sarcoma. Ann Surg 1995;221:185–95.

[12] Hayry P, Scheinin TM. The desmoid (Reitamo) syndrome: etiology, manifestations, pathogenesis, and treatment. Curr Probl Surg 1988;25:225–320.

[13] Stojadinovic A, Hoos A, Karpoff HM, et al. Soft tissue tumors of the abdominal wall: analysis of disease pattern and treatment. Arch Surg 2001;136:70–9.

[14] Singer S, Antman K, Corson JM, et al. Long-term salvageability for patients with locally recurrent soft-tissue sarcomas. Arch Surg 1992;127:548–53.

[15] Brennan MF. The surgeon as a leader in cancer care: lessons learned from the study of soft tissue sarcoma. J Am Coll Surg 1996;182:520–9.

[16] McCormack P. Surgical resection of pulmonary metastases. Semin Surg Oncol 1990;6: 297–302.

[17] Choong PF, Pritchard DJ, Rock MG, et al. Survival after pulmonary metastasectomy in soft tissue sarcoma: prognostic factors in 214 patients. Acta Orthop Scand 1995;66:561–8.

[18] Borden EC, Amato DA, Rosenbaum C, et al. Randomized comparison of three Adriamycin regimens for metastatic soft tissue sarcomas. J Clin Oncol 1987;5:840–950.

[19] Edmonson JH, Ryan LM, Blum RH, et al. Randomized comparison of doxorubicin alone versus ifosfamide plus doxorubicin or mitomycin, doxorubicin, and cisplatin against advanced soft tissue sarcomas. J Clin Oncol 1993;11:1269–75.

[20] Latchford AR, Strut NJH, Neale K, et al. A 10-year review of surgery for desmoid disease associated with familial adenomatous polyposis. Br J Surg 2006;93:1258–64.

[21] Sakorafas GH, Nissotakis C, Peros G. Abdominal desmoid tumors. Surg Oncol 2007;16: 131–42.

[22] Church J, Berk T, Boman BM, et al. Staging intra-abdominal desmoid tumors in familial adenomatous polyposis: a search for a uniform approach to a troubling disease. Dis Colon Rectum 2005;48:1528–34.

[23] Sturt JNH, Clark SK. Current ideas in desmoid tumors. Fam Cancer 2006;5:275–85.

[24] Lopez R, Kemalyan N, Mosely HS, et al. Problems in diagnosis and management of desmoid tumors. Am J Surg 1990;159:450–3.

[25] Reitamo JJ, Scheinin TM, Hayry P. The desmoid syndrome: new aspects in the cause, pathogenesis and treatment of the desmoid tumour. Am J Surg 1986;151:230–7.

[26] Hansmann A, Adolph C, Vogel T, et al. High-dose tamoxifen and sulindac as first line treatment for desmoid tumors. Cancer 2004;100:612–20.

[27] Church JM. Desmoid tumors in patients with familial adenomatous polyposis. Seminars in Colon and Rectal Surgical Oncology 2003;1:11–5.

[28] Moslein G, Dozois RR. Desmoid tumors associated with familial adenomatous polyposis. Perspective in Colon and Rectal Surgery 1998;10:109–26.

[29] Ballo MT, Zagars GK, Pollack A. Desmoid tumor: prognostic factors and outcome after surgery, radiation therapy, or combined surgery and radiation therapy. J Clin Oncol 1999; 17:158–67.

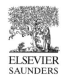

SURGICAL
CLINICS OF
NORTH AMERICA

Surg Clin N Am 88 (2008) 583–597

Management of Retroperitoneal Sarcomas

Matthew T. Hueman, MD[a],
Joseph M. Herman, MD, MSc[b],
Nita Ahuja, MD[c],*

[a]The Johns Hopkins University School of Medicine, 600 North Wolfe Street, Blalock 665,
Baltimore, MD 21287, USA
[b]The Johns Hopkins University School of Medicine, 401 North Broadway,
Weinberg 1440–Oncology, Baltimore, MD 21231, USA
[c]The Johns Hopkins University School of Medicine, 1650 Orleans Street, CRB1-342,
Baltimore, MD 21231, USA

Retroperitoneal sarcomas are relatively rare tumors that are expected to compose approximately 15% of the 9220 cases of soft tissue sarcoma anticipated in the United States in 2007 [1]. Retroperitoneal sarcomas present specific therapeutic challenges because of their location and frequent intimate association with several structures in the retroperitoneum. This proximity to major vessels, visceral organs, axial skeleton, and neural structures may significantly impair the ability to perform a margin-negative resection, which is the single potentially curative treatment approach in patients who have localized disease [2,3]. Even in the setting of a complete resection, local recurrence is common. For this reason, several adjuvant therapies have been evaluated. In this article, the authors describe the presentation, evaluation, and management of patients who have retroperitoneal sarcomas.

Natural history

Most patients who have a retroperitoneal sarcoma present with an abdominal mass [2], although neurologic symptoms, pain, early satiety, and obstructive gastrointestinal symptoms are also seen as presenting symptoms in some patients [4]. Because of the typically silent nature of these tumors until they are large enough to present as an abdominal mass, most retroperitoneal sarcomas are large when diagnosed. In a single institution series of more than

* Corresponding author.
E-mail address: nahuja@jhmi.edu (N. Ahuja).

0039-6109/08/$ - see front matter © 2008 Elsevier Inc. All rights reserved.
doi:10.1016/j.suc.2008.03.002 *surgical.theclinics.com*

500 patients who had primary and recurrent retroperitoneal sarcomas, 71% of primary retroperitoneal sarcomas were greater than 10 cm in size at diagnosis, with an additional 23% measuring between 5 and 10 cm in size [2].

Approximately 11% of patients who have a primary retroperitoneal sarcoma also present with metastatic disease, with the lung and liver representing the most common site of metastasis [2]. Retroperitoneal sarcomas can occur over a broad age range, but typically present in the sixth decade [5] with a slight male predominance [2]. Approximately two thirds of cases are of high-grade histology, with liposarcomas and leiomyosarcomas representing the most common histologic findings [2]. Dedifferentiation to leiomyosarcoma or rhabdomyosarcoma or a less-differentiated liposarcoma may also be seen with retroperitoneal liposarcomas and may be associated with worse outcomes, including increased rates of recurrence, increased rates of metastases, and worse survival compared with well-differentiated tumors [6,7]. Recurrent liposarcomas may also commonly present with dedifferentiation after initial presentation as a well-differentiated liposarcoma and are associated with worse outcomes compared with their differentiated counterparts [7].

Although histologic subclassification may provide prognostic information, patients who have tumors of similar histologic appearance can have quite different clinical courses. The use of microarray technology to evaluate gene expression profiles in biopsy or surgical specimens may provide insight into the pathogenesis of these tumors, allow further subclassification or prognostication, or assist in the identification of therapeutic targets. A recent series evaluating microarray in 49 lipomatous samples generated a 142-gene predictor of tissue class that was able to predict histology based on expression profiles with 86% accuracy [8]. This technology may someday be used in a method analogous to that used currently in the management of patients who have breast cancer to prognosticate and to determine the appropriateness of adjuvant therapies.

In general, outcomes after therapy for retroperitoneal sarcoma are inferior to those obtained with extremity soft tissue sarcomas, likely because of several factors, including the location of the tumors, inability to obtain negative margins, the size and extent at diagnosis, and the inability to provide adequate adjuvant therapy because of the proximity to sensitive structures. Local recurrence-free survival rates of 59% at 5 years have been reported at high-volume centers [2]. Tumor characteristics that predict a higher risk for local recurrence include higher histologic grade and liposarcoma histology [2,3].

In patients presenting with localized primary disease, distant metastases are more likely to occur in patients who have high-grade tumors or a positive resection margin [2]. Histologic grade clearly affects the likelihood of survival in patients who have retroperitoneal sarcoma, with patients with high-grade histologic findings having a median survival of 33 months compared with 149 months for low-grade histologic findings [2].

A recent review of the Surveillance, Epidemiology, and End Results (SEER) database was performed over a 29-year period from 1973 to 2001 and evaluated the incidence of, the use of radiotherapy in, and the relation of demographic factors to retroperitoneal sarcoma during this period [9]. In reviewing the SEER database, Porter and colleagues [9] were able to show that over this 29-year period, the incidence of retroperitoneal sarcomas has remained the same, at approximately 2.7 cases per 10 cases [6]; the percentage of patients receiving radiotherapy is relatively low at approximately 25.9%, most radiotherapy is delivered adjuvantly (85.5%) and only a small amount is delivered before surgery (4.7%) and during surgery (5.1%); and that patients who underwent radiotherapy were, on average, 5 years younger than those who underwent surgery alone. Interestingly, geographic location was a statistically significant factor governing the use of adjuvant radiotherapy, presumably reflecting individual and institutional practice patterns in the absence of definitive randomized data supporting a conclusive benefit. Finally, they estimated that the overall resection rate was approximately 70% and increased from 54.8% during 1973 to 1978 to 78.5% during 1996 to 2001. A limitation to this paper utilizing SEER dataset is that it does not include the percentage of patients with an initial presentation of metastatic disease, the margin status of those resected (R0 or R1) and whether that influenced referral for radiotherapy, and the disease-free and overall survival rates of these patients. Overall, the conclusion of this review of the SEER database is that prospective trials evaluating the use and timing of radiotherapy in this uncommon disease might require a significant change in current practice patterns should level 1 evidence support the benefit of radiotherapy.

Diagnosis and evaluation

Retroperitoneal sarcomas account for approximately one third of all retroperitoneal masses [10]. Although most extravisceral large masses in the retroperitoneum represent a retroperitoneal sarcoma, a differential diagnosis, including lymphoma, testicular neoplasm, germ cell tumor, desmoids, functioning and nonfunctioning adrenal masses, renal tumor, pancreatic tumor, and gastrointestinal stromal tumor, should be considered [4,11,12]. If visceral invasion is present, the differential should include tumors of these organs and site-directed endoscopy with or without biopsy, if feasible, to evaluate for intraluminal evidence of involvement (eg, stomach, duodenum, pancreas, colon), should be performed.

History and physical examination should be focused to narrow the differential diagnosis and in an attempt to determine the extent of disease; with appropriate attention to this component of the evaluation, many of the previously mentioned differential diagnoses can be eliminated and direct further studies. Symptoms suggestive of lymphoma include the classic B symptoms of unexplained fever, drenching night sweats, and weight loss in addition to the symptoms of unexplained pruritus and alcohol-induced pain at the sites of disease. For patients who have testicular neoplasm included in the differential diagnosis, the physical examination should include testicular examination for masses and consideration for testicular ultrasound. In addition, if a testicular neoplasm or germ cell tumor is included in the differential diagnosis, initial laboratory studies should include serum tumor markers, such as alpha fetoprotein (AFP), β-human chorionic growth hormone (β-HCG), and lactate dehydrogenase (LDH). LDH may also be elevated in patients who have lymphomas and should not be considered diagnostic of a testicular or germ cell tumor in this setting.

The initial diagnostic evaluation of patients who are suspected of having retroperitoneal sarcoma should include a contrast enhanced CT of the abdomen and pelvis to evaluate the size and extent of the lesion. The use of oral and intravenous contrast is necessary to allow adequate visualization of the surrounding vascular structures, visceral organs, and skeletal structures for the assessment of resectability [5,13]. The CT appearance of liposarcomas typically includes fat density components, but other retroperitoneal sarcoma histologic findings can be difficult to distinguish from other retroperitoneal tumors [14]. MRI of the abdomen has been evaluated as a method of staging; however, MRI often does not add additional information to that obtained with contrast-enhanced CT of the abdomen. In the situation of inability to deliver CT contrast, MRI may provide an alternative modality to assess local disease extent [13].

The performance of biopsy for these lesions in the preoperative setting is controversial if there is a low index of suspicion for other tumors based on the initial evaluation; however, if neoadjuvant therapy is used, histologic verification is usually necessary. In this event, a CT-guided core biopsy is the preferred diagnostic approach [11]. As pointed out in a review by Windham and Pisters [12], surgical exploration rather than biopsy is recommended by some as the most appropriate next step for a retroperitoneal mass suspected of being a sarcoma. The authors believe that a reasonable approach, as proposed by Windham and Pisters [12], is to perform a percutaneous biopsy only when the diagnosis may change the preoperative therapy, such as using neoadjuvant imatinib mesylate for gastrointestinal stromal tumors (see the article by Hueman and Schulick, Management of Gastrointestinal Stromal Tumors, elsewhere in this issue) or primary chemotherapy for lymphoma, and otherwise proceed to the operating room as the next appropriate step [12]. The authors certainly stress that a negative biopsy does not argue for a period of observation and should not delay operative intervention. Additionally, if distant metastases are present and surgical therapy is not being considered for primary management, a biopsy of the primary tumor or a metastatic site may be required for alternative therapy to be administered. In the situation of an incidental note of a suspected retroperitoneal sarcoma at the time of abdominal surgery, a biopsy should be performed before resection to avoid the potentially morbid and unnecessary resection of a chemotherapy-sensitive tumor, such as a germ cell tumor or lymphoma [11].

Chest imaging is typically performed to evaluate for the presence of lung metastases. This can include a plain radiograph or CT of the chest. Because of the increased likelihood of distant metastases in patients who have high-grade tumors, some advocate a plain chest radiograph in patients who have low-grade tumors and a low risk for lung metastases and chest CT in patients who have high-grade tumors and a higher likelihood of lung metastases [5]. Retroperitoneal sarcomas are staged according to the American Joint Committee on Cancer (AJCC) sarcoma staging system. If present in a retroperitoneal location, sarcomas are considered deep for the purposes of staging (Table 1).

Table 1
American joint committee on cancer staging for soft tissue sarcomas

Grade				
GX	Grade cannot be assessed			
G1	Well differentiated			
G2	Moderately differentiated			
G3	Poorly differentiated			
G4	Undifferentiated			
Primary tumor				
TX	Primary tumor cannot be assessed			
T0	No evidence of primary tumor			
T1	Tumor ≤ 5 cm in greatest dimension			
T1a	Superficial tumor			
T1b	Deep tumor			
T2	Tumor >5 cm in greatest dimension			
T2a	Superficial tumor			
T2b	Deep tumor			
Regional lymph nodes				
NX	Regional lymph nodes cannot be assessed			
N0	No regional lymph node metastases			
N1	Regional lymph node metastases			
Distant metastases				
MX	Distant metastases cannot be assessed			
M0	No distant metastases			
M1	Distant metastases			
Stage grouping				
Stage I	G1-2	T1a, 1b, 2a, 2b	N0	M0
Stage II	G3-4	T1a, T1b, T2a	N0	M0
Stage III	G3-4	T2b	N0	M0
Stage IV	Any G	Any T	N1	M0
	Any G	Any T	Any N	M1

Deep indicates invading fascia (retroperitoneal and visceral lesions and most head and neck lesions are considered deep). Superficial indicates above and not invading the superficial fascia.
    Abbreviation: G, grade.
    Data from Greene F, Page D, Norrow M. AJCC cancer staging manual. 6th edition. New York: Springer; 2002.

Management

As described previously, disease control outcomes for retroperitoneal sarcoma are inferior to those obtained for sarcomas at other locations for a variety of reasons, including the difficulty to obtain wide negative surgical margins, higher rates of unresectability, higher rates of margin-positive resection, and difficulty in delivering adjuvant therapies (eg, radiotherapy). Patients who present with a retroperitoneal sarcoma should ideally be evaluated by members of a multidisciplinary sarcoma team experienced in the management of these tumors, especially if a multimodality approach is considered. Recent evidence from a series of more than 4000 patients who had sarcomas, including retroperitoneal sarcomas, supports improved outcomes when patients are managed at high-volume centers [15].

Surgical management

Surgical resection is considered the only potentially curative treatment modality, and complete surgical resection with negative margins remains the goal of therapy for most patients (Fig. 1). The likelihood of a margin-negative surgical resection depends on several factors, including invasion of adjacent visceral organs, vascular structures, and skeletal structures.

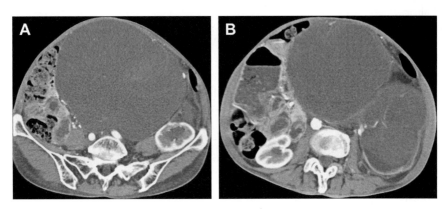

Fig. 1. Figs. 1 through 5 are of the same patient who had the primary tumor seen here in this figure of a CT image in December 2005. (*A*) Retroperitoneal sarcoma pictured on this CT image involves the left kidney. Final pathologic examination revealed this mass to be a dedifferentiated liposarcoma requiring left nephrectomy and adrenalectomy, distal pancreatectomy and splenectomy, and transverse colectomy for microscopic- and gross margin–negative resection. The patient opted for no adjuvant therapy after her primary resection. She had a recurrence by June 2007 and declined operative therapy until she developed a high-grade small bowel obstruction in February 2008. She underwent R1 resection of her recurrent liposarcoma (now well differentiated) and underwent intraoperative radiotherapy with a plan for adjuvant postoperative radiotherapy. (*B*) CT image is of the same patient in December 2005 before resection. Retroperitoneal sarcomas can be challenging because they often involve major midline structures. In this image, the retroperitoneal mass is pushing the aorta to the left of the midline. Ultimately, the mass was able to be resected without a vascular resection.

Other operative findings that may alter the intended surgical approach include the presence of peritoneal metastases or the presence of distant metastatic disease [5].

Complete resection rates vary by series but typically range from 54% to 88% [2,16–19]. Disease control outcomes are clearly linked to the completeness of resection in surgical series, with inferior outcomes noted after incomplete resection or margin-positive resection. In general, macroscopically incomplete resection is not thought to extend overall survival compared with no resection [2,5].

The surgical approach is important to increase the likelihood of a margin-negative resection which offers the best chance of local control. Although the approach may differ depending on the location and extent of the tumor, in general, a midline incision followed by medial visceral rotation is performed to provide adequate exposure of the tumor bed and surrounding anatomy [5]. Ideally, dissection then proceeds outside the limits of the pseudocapsule in an effort to increase the likelihood of obtaining a margin-negative resection, although this may frequently require resection of surrounding vasculature or visceral organs [5].

Resection of surrounding visceral organs is frequently required to obtain sufficient margin on the tumor (see Fig. 1). Rates of resection of visceral organs at the time of resection of retroperitoneal sarcomas vary significantly by series from approximately 34% to 75% [2,16,17,19]. Because disease control outcomes depend significantly on the adequacy of resection, this approach has also been extended to the setting of vascular involvement.

Favorable local control rates with acceptable morbidity have been reported in a series evaluating arterial and venous resection in this setting, highlighting the importance of an aggressive surgical approach [20]. In this series of 141 patients who had retroperitoneal sarcomas, 17.7% underwent surgery for tumors with vascular involvement. The vessels involved included the aorta, inferior vena cava, superior mesenteric vein, and iliac vessels (see Fig. 1B). Resection of the tumor and vasculature included ligation, vessel repair, reimplantation, or bypass grafting in these patients. Morbidity in this series was 36%; however, operative mortality was 4%, which compares favorably with other surgical series. A complete resection was performed in 60% of patients, with margin-negative resection accomplished in 40% of patients. Local control rates with this approach were 82.4% with 5-year survival rates of 66.7% in patients in whom a margin-negative resection was obtained. These results highlight the importance of an aggressive surgical approach in patients who have retroperitoneal sarcomas.

Multimodality therapy

Because of the high rates of local recurrence after surgical resection of retroperitoneal sarcomas, especially with high-grade tumors or with margin-positive resection, the addition of radiotherapy has been evaluated as a mechanism to improve local control. Unlike extremity sarcomas, radiotherapy dose is often limited by the anatomic constraints of the abdominal compartment, primarily because of the proximity of several radiosensitive structures to the tumor bed, such as bowel, kidney, and neural structures (see the article by Kaushal and Citrin, The Role of Radiation Therapy in the Management of Sarcomas, elsewhere in this issue for even further details).

In general, radiotherapy may be delivered before surgery, during surgery, or after surgery with a variety of techniques. These techniques include standard external beam radiation delivered before or after surgery, which typically targets the tumor or tumor bed with additional margin for suspected microscopic disease. In addition, such techniques as brachytherapy and intraoperative radiotherapy can be performed in conjunction with surgical resection and may be delivered in combination with external beam radiotherapy as a method to escalate radiation dose locally (Fig. 2).

In most centers, radiotherapy is often reserved for patients who have high-grade lesions or in patients in whom a margin-positive resection is anticipated. The goal of therapy is to allow a margin-negative resection, which would result in better local control and improved survival. Typically, if

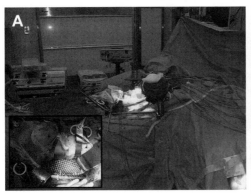
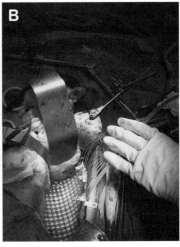

Fig. 2. (*A*) Intraoperative photograph of the patient seen in Fig. 1 is at the time of her recurrence and resection in March 2008, right after the successful gross margin–negative resection during the intraoperative radiotherapy portion of the case (see Figs. 3–5). The catheters emanating from the iridium source can be seen entering the patient's abdomen and, in the picture inset, into the tumor bed. (*B*) Close-up photograph of the tumor bed in the retroperitoneum, after resection of her recurrence. The retractors are holding lead shields to help protect intra-abdominal structures during the delivery of intraoperative radiation (15 Gy was delivered during surgery with a plan for adjuvant radiotherapy after successful postoperative recovery). At the left side of the photograph, the most medial retractor is holding the duodenal stump at the fourth portion. The tumor involved the distal duodenum and proximal jejunum right at the ligament of Treitz and caused a proximal high-grade small bowel obstruction.

external radiotherapy is planned, a preoperative approach is preferred to decrease the risk for toxicity, to minimize the additional normal tissue that must be irradiated, and to improve the likelihood of a margin-negative resection. Unfortunately, because of the relative rarity of these tumors, most series reported regarding the benefit and toxicity of radiotherapy are small prospective series or retrospective. Without the benefit of completed randomized trials, treatment recommendations are currently based primarily on the few prospective trials, several retrospective series, and consensus guidelines. The American College of Surgeons Oncology Group (ACOSOG) initiated a phase III randomized trial (Z9031) to address the role of preoperative radiotherapy in patients who have primary retroperitoneal sarcoma, which, despite a "call to arms" eloquently articulated in a recent editorial [21], closed prematurely because of lack of accrual. The early closure of this trial because of low accrual is emblematic of the difficulty of studying retroperitoneal sarcomas; some have suggested that not only the low incidence of this disease but preconceived opinions of the best therapy limit our ability to randomize patients to receiving adjuvant therapy or not [21].

Perhaps the best evidence supporting efficacy of preoperative radiotherapy is a recent report of long-term data from 72 patients who had intermediate- or high-grade retroperitoneal sarcoma treated with preoperative radiotherapy in two prospective series [22]. Most patients (89%) completed preoperative radiotherapy, and almost 90% of patients who completed preoperative radiotherapy underwent laparotomy with curative intent; of those patients who underwent laparotomy, 95% had a macroscopically complete (R0 or R1) resection [16]. Patients who received preoperative radiotherapy had a 5-year disease free survival rate of 46% and a 5-year survival rate of 50%, and those who completed preoperative radiotherapy and underwent a macroscopically complete resection had a 5-year local recurrence-free survival rate of 60%. These results compare favorably with historical data.

In regard to chemotherapy, there is similar uncertainty regarding the benefit of chemotherapy delivered in the neoadjuvant setting with the intent of improving resectability (see the article by Thornton, Chemotherapeutic Management of Soft Tissue Sarcoma, elsewhere in this issue for further detail on the use of chemotherapy in the treatment of retroperitoneal sarcoma). Few series evaluating neoadjuvant chemotherapy have included patients who have retroperitoneal sarcomas. Meric and colleagues [23] reported a series of retrospectively identified patients treated with neoadjuvant adriamycin- or ifosfamide-based chemotherapy with the intent of evaluating radiographic response and impact on surgical management. In this series, 23 of the 65 included patients had potentially resectable retroperitoneal sarcomas. At the time of surgery, 17% of the patients who had retroperitoneal sarcoma were deemed to have unresectable disease, and none of the patients who experienced tumor regression experienced a response significant enough to result in organ salvage. Based on these results, the use of neoadjuvant chemotherapy should be advocated only in the setting of a clinical trial.

The use of adjuvant chemotherapy in the management of sarcomas at any site to reduce the risk for distant disease failure is also controversial. Several prospective trials evaluating adjuvant chemotherapy in patients who have sarcomas have been completed but have not shown consistent evidence of disease-free survival or overall survival benefit.

To attempt to answer the question of the potential benefit of adjuvant chemotherapy in patients who have localized soft tissue sarcoma, the Sarcoma Meta-analysis Collaboration conducted a meta-analysis of 14 randomized trials of doxorubicin-based adjuvant chemotherapy in adult patients [24]. Patients with a variety of primary sites were included in this analysis. An absolute survival benefit of 4% at 10 years was appreciated in the chemotherapy group; however, this benefit seemed to be attributable to a benefit in patients who had extremity sarcomas.

The rarity of retroperitoneal sarcomas has further complicated efforts to determine the appropriateness of chemotherapy. It is unlikely that a large randomized trial addressing this question is going to be completed in the near future. The use of adjuvant chemotherapy in this setting would be an extrapolation from the controversial data supporting the use of adjuvant chemotherapy in extremity sarcomas.

A final option for multimodality treatment of retroperitoneal sarcomas is the combination of radiation and chemotherapy. This approach was recently reported in a phase I trial in which 35 patients who had resectable intermediate- or high-grade retroperitoneal sarcoma underwent neoadjuvant therapy with weekly doxorubicin and escalating doses of external radiotherapy to a maximum dose of 50.4 Gy in addition to a 15-Gy intraoperative radiotherapy boost [25]. Progression prevented surgical resection in 6 of the patients, but a gross total resection was performed in 26 of the 29 patients who underwent surgery. Toxicity with this approach was primarily observed in the highest radiation dose group, with 18% of patients developing grade 3 or 4 nausea. One patient died of multisystem organ failure in the postinduction period. One patient who had a pelvic tumor developed ureteral strictures. Overall, it was deemed that this approach was tolerable. The efficacy of this approach has not been reported.

Unresectable disease

The management of unresectable sarcoma should be tailored to the individual patient depending on the patient's overall functional status, extent of disease, and symptoms. Options, such as neoadjuvant therapy with the attempt to render disease resectable, are possible. Alternative options include a palliative approach. Palliative options can include supportive care, surgical therapy, radiotherapy, and chemotherapy.

The role of surgery for palliating intra-abdominal sarcomas has been evaluated in a series from Memorial Sloan Kettering Cancer Center (MSKCC) [26]. These investigators report on 112 patients who underwent

156 palliative procedures for intra-abdominal sarcomas. Most frequently, these procedures were performed to palliate gastrointestinal obstruction or pain. Complications occurred in 29% of cases, with a periprocedural mortality rate of 9%. Complications were more common in patients presenting with gastrointestinal obstruction. The median duration of symptom relief in this series was 150 days, with hepatobiliary symptoms, pain, and bleeding most effectively palliated. Although it is clear from these data that palliation can be achieved with surgical intervention in a subset of patients who have intra-abdominal sarcomas, there is a significant possibility of morbidity and mortality, which should be considered. It is clear from these data that patient selection for surgical palliation is critical in providing acceptable outcomes.

Some evidence exists that incomplete resection might provide a survival benefit for patients who have retroperitoneal sarcomas, specifically in patients who have liposarcomas, the most common histologic subtype (comprising 40% of all retroperitoneal sarcomas, in most series). In fact, it has been suggested that retroperitoneal liposarcomas might represent a histologic subtype for which a more aggressive surgical approach, including multiple resections for recurrent disease and incomplete resections, might be justified [12]. It is possible that the benefit obtained with aggressive local therapy in this histologic subtype may be attributable in large part to the lower rate of distant metastasis in patients who have liposarcomas (7%) compared with the rate of metastasis in patients who have other subtypes (15%–34%), coupled with the fact that these patients often die of local failure [27–29]. Shibata and colleagues [29] reported a retrospective series from the MSKCC in 2001 of 55 patients who had retroperitoneal liposarcomas: 43 cases were incompletely resected and 12 cases were unresected. In these patients, incomplete resection was an independent factor for increased survival compared with patients who had unresected tumors (median survival: 26 months versus 4 months; $P < .0001$); this benefit was more pronounced in patients who had primary versus recurrent tumors. As previously noted, however, macroscopically incomplete resection in retroperitoneal sarcomas is not thought to extend overall survival compared with no resection [2,5]. In a retrospective earlier review in 1998 of prospectively gathered data at the same institution (MSKCC), Lewis and colleagues [2] showed that patients who had any histologic subtype of retroperitoneal sarcoma and underwent incomplete resection fared just as poorly as those patients who presented with initially unresectable disease and did much worse than those patients who underwent complete resection. Although incomplete resection may or may not provide a survival benefit, Shibata and colleagues [29] did show that palliation of symptoms was achieved in most (75%) patients who had the specific histologic subtype of retroperitoneal liposarcoma undergoing incomplete resection.

Given that most patients who have retroperitoneal liposarcomas succumb from complications of local recurrence, it is tempting to entertain that even incomplete resection may provide some survival benefit. This

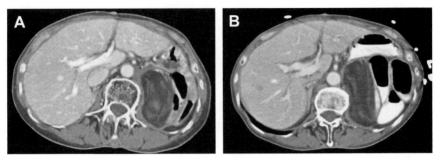

Fig. 3. (*A*) CT image is of the same patient after resection, shown here with the recurrence seen in June 2007. The patient has had a recurrence in less than 2 years but continues to be without evidence of metastatic disease, which is characteristic of liposarcomas. (*B*) Patient was reluctant to undergo additional operative or adjuvant therapy. This CT image is of the same patient seen in a July 2007 image. The mass is slightly bigger and starting to push midline structures again.

enthusiasm for even incomplete resection of liposarcoma providing pallia-tive and possible survival benefits should be tempered by the fact that these benefits may not be seen in all grades of liposarcoma. Dedifferentiated liposarcomas not only have a higher local recurrence rate (80%) than well-differentiated liposarcomas in the setting of microscopic and gross mar-gin-negative resections but exhibit a higher rate of distant metastasis (up to 30%) [30]. In consideration of all these points, the authors believe that in the appropriately selected symptomatic patients (particularly in a patient pre-senting with primary and not recurrent disease), surgeons at high-volume centers should consider operative intervention even if a liposarcoma is con-sidered incompletely resectable.

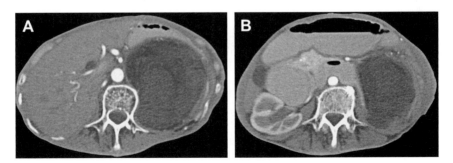

Fig. 4. (*A*) Patient decided to not undergo additional therapy and remained relatively asymp-tomatic until this CT image seen in February 2008, when she presented with a high-grade partial small bowel obstruction at the ligament of Treitz. This CT image shows dramatic enlargement of the retroperitoneal liposarcoma recurrence when compared with Fig. 2. (*B*) This CT image in February 2008 shows the high-grade small bowel obstruction associated with the enlarging re-current left upper quadrant retroperitoneal sarcoma. After much discussion and failed attempt at nonoperative management of her small bowel obstruction, the patient elected to undergo an attempt at resection of the liposarcoma recurrence.

Recurrent disease

Local recurrence is common for retroperitoneal sarcomas, a situation that presents therapeutic challenges (Fig. 3). For lesions that are deemed resectable, this remains the preferred treatment modality at the time of local recurrence (Fig. 4). The likelihood of obtaining a margin-negative resection is significantly lower at the time of local recurrence and at subsequent recurrences [2]. In general, primary resections result in complete resections in as many as 80% of patients, whereas complete resection of recurrent disease occurs in 57% of patients, with lower rates at subsequent recurrences [2]. As in the primary disease setting, complete resection of recurrent disease is associated with improved survival [2], and this should be the intended goal if surgical therapy is chosen (Fig. 5).

If adjuvant therapy was not delivered at the time of the initial resection, this remains an option in the recurrent disease setting (see Fig. 2). Similar to the primary disease setting, options for additional therapy include neoadjuvant or adjuvant radiotherapy and chemotherapy. In the setting of unresectable local recurrence, palliative radiotherapy or chemotherapy may also be considered to relieve local symptoms.

Follow-up evaluation

In general, patients who have high-grade tumors should undergo frequent clinical and imaging surveillance to evaluate for recurrent disease. Surveillance imaging should include CT of the chest, abdomen, and pelvis

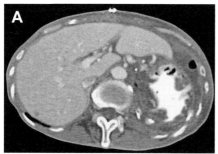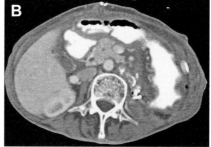

Fig. 5. (*A*) CT image in March 2008 is of the same patient after resection of the recurrent liposarcoma. The stomach has moved into the space previously occupied by the recurrent mass. The patient underwent intraoperative radiation brachytherapy to the tumor bed with a plan for postoperative adjuvant radiotherapy. (*B*) CT image in March 2008 shows resolution of the small bowel obstruction caused by the recurrent mass. The final pathologic examination revealed a well-differentiated recurrent liposarcoma with grossly negative but microscopically positive margins. The patient required an en bloc resection of a portion of the distal duodenum and proximal jejunum along with the recurrent liposarcoma, with a duodenal fourth portion stump and duodenojejunostomy at the second portion of the duodenum.

at intervals of every 3 to 6 months for the first 2 years for low- and high-grade lesions, followed by biannual evaluations in patients who have high-grade tumors and annual evaluations in patients who have low-grade tumors [11].

Summary

Retroperitoneal sarcomas present a therapeutic challenge based on their location, extent of invasion at diagnosis, and propensity for local recurrence. Surgical therapy remains the only potentially curative treatment option; however, even with aggressive surgical approaches, local recurrence remains a common type of failure. For patients who have high-grade lesions, distant metastatic disease may also limit survival. Optimizing disease control while minimizing the morbidity of therapy remains the primary goal of management. Inclusion of patients in randomized trials addressing the use of adjuvant therapies may provide better evidence of the most appropriate management for these patients.

References

[1] Jemal A, Siegel R, Ward E, et al. Cancer statistics, 2007. CA Cancer J Clin 2007;57(1):43–66.

[2] Lewis JJ, Leung D, Woodruff JM, et al. Retroperitoneal soft-tissue sarcoma: analysis of 500 patients treated and followed at a single institution. Ann Surg 1998;228(3):355–65.

[3] Heslin MJ, Lewis JJ, Nadler E, et al. Prognostic factors associated with long-term survival for retroperitoneal sarcoma: implications for management. J Clin Oncol 1997;15(8):2832–9.

[4] Raut CP, Pisters PW. Retroperitoneal sarcomas: combined-modality treatment approaches. J Surg Oncol 2006;94(1):81–7.

[5] Katz MH, Choi EA, Pollock RE. Current concepts in multimodality therapy for retroperitoneal sarcoma. Expert Rev Anticancer Ther 2007;7(2):159–68.

[6] Binh MB, Guillou L, Hostein I, et al. Dedifferentiated liposarcomas with divergent myosarcomatous differentiation developed in the internal trunk: a study of 27 cases and comparison to conventional dedifferentiated liposarcomas and leiomyosarcomas. Am J Surg Pathol 2007;31(10):1557–66.

[7] Fabre-Guillevin E, Coindre JM, Somerhausen Nde S, et al. Retroperitoneal liposarcomas: follow-up analysis of dedifferentiation after clinicopathologic reexamination of 86 liposarcomas and malignant fibrous histiocytomas. Cancer 2006;106(12):2725–33.

[8] Singer S, Socci ND, Ambrosini G, et al. Gene expression profiling of liposarcoma identifies distinct biological types/subtypes and potential therapeutic targets in well-differentiated and dedifferentiated liposarcoma. Cancer Res 2007;67(14):6626–36.

[9] Porter GA, Baxter NN, Pisters PW. Retroperitoneal sarcoma: a population-based analysis of epidemiology, surgery, and radiotherapy. Cancer 2006;106(7):1610–6.

[10] Thomas JM. Retroperitoneal sarcoma. Br J Surg 2007;94(9):1057–8.

[11] Demetri GD, Benjamin RS, Blanke CD, et al. NCCN Task Force report: management of patients with gastrointestinal stromal tumor (GIST)—update of the NCCN clinical practice guidelines. J Natl Compr Canc Netw 2007;5(Suppl 2):S1–29 [quiz: S30].

[12] Windham TC, Pisters PW. Retroperitoneal sarcomas. Cancer Control 2005;12(1):36–43.

[13] Tzeng CW, Smith JK, Heslin MJ. Soft tissue sarcoma: preoperative and postoperative imaging for staging. Surg Oncol Clin N Am 2007;16(2):389–402.

[14] Cohan RH, Baker ME, Cooper C, et al. Computed tomography of primary retroperitoneal malignancies. J Comput Assist Tomogr 1988;12(5):804–10.

[15] Gutierrez JC, Perez EA, Moffat FL, et al. Should soft tissue sarcomas be treated at high-volume centers? An analysis of 4205 patients. Ann Surg 2007;245(6):952–8.

[16] Dalton RR, Donohue JH, Mucha P Jr, et al. Management of retroperitoneal sarcomas. Surgery 1989;106(4):725–32 [discussion: 732–3].

[17] Kilkenny JW 3rd, Bland KI, Copeland EM 3rd. Retroperitoneal sarcoma: the University of Florida experience. J Am Coll Surg 1996;182(4):329–39.

[18] van Dalen T, Hoekstra HJ, van Geel AN, et al. Locoregional recurrence of retroperitoneal soft tissue sarcoma: second chance of cure for selected patients. Eur J Surg Oncol 2001;27(6):564–8.

[19] Gronchi A, Casali PG, Fiore M, et al. Retroperitoneal soft tissue sarcomas: patterns of recurrence in 167 patients treated at a single institution. Cancer 2004;100(11):2448–55.

[20] Schwarzbach MH, Hormann Y, Hinz U, et al. Clinical results of surgery for retroperitoneal sarcoma with major blood vessel involvement. J Vasc Surg 2006;44(1):46–55.

[21] Kane JM 3rd. At the crossroads for retroperitoneal sarcomas: the future of clinical trials for this "orphan disease." Ann Surg Oncol 2006;13(4):442–3.

[22] Pawlik TM, Pisters PW, Mikula L, et al. Long-term results of two prospective trials of preoperative external beam radiotherapy for localized intermediate- or high-grade retroperitoneal soft tissue sarcoma. Ann Surg Oncol 2006;13(4):508–17.

[23] Meric F, Hess KR, Varma DG, et al. Radiographic response to neoadjuvant chemotherapy is a predictor of local control and survival in soft tissue sarcomas. Cancer 2002;95(5):1120–6.

[24] Adjuvant chemotherapy for localised resectable soft-tissue sarcoma of adults: meta-analysis of individual data. Sarcoma Meta-analysis Collaboration. Lancet 1997;350(9092):1647–54.

[25] Pisters PW, Ballo MT, Fenstermacher MJ, et al. Phase I trial of preoperative concurrent doxorubicin and radiation therapy, surgical resection, and intraoperative electron-beam radiation therapy for patients with localized retroperitoneal sarcoma. J Clin Oncol 2003;21(16):3092–7.

[26] Yeh JJ, Singer S, Brennan MF, et al. Effectiveness of palliative procedures for intra-abdominal sarcomas. Ann Surg Oncol 2005;12(12):1084–9.

[27] Jaques DP, Coit DG, Hajdu SI, et al. Management of primary and recurrent soft-tissue sarcoma of the retroperitoneum. Ann Surg 1990;212(1):51–9.

[28] McGrath PC, Neifeld JP, Lawrence W Jr, et al. Improved survival following complete excision of retroperitoneal sarcomas. Ann Surg 1984;200(2):200–4.

[29] Shibata D, Lewis JJ, Leung DH, et al. Is there a role for incomplete resection in the management of retroperitoneal liposarcomas? J Am Coll Surg 2001;193(4):373–9.

[30] Singer S, Antonescu CR, Riedel E, et al. Histologic subtype and margin of resection predict pattern of recurrence and survival for retroperitoneal liposarcoma. Ann Surg 2003;238(3):358–70 [discussion: 370–1].

[31] Greene F, Page D, Norrow M. AJCC cancer staging manual. 6th edition. New York: Springer; 2002.

ELSEVIER
SAUNDERS

SURGICAL
CLINICS OF
NORTH AMERICA

Surg Clin N Am 88 (2008) 599–614

Management of Gastrointestinal Stromal Tumors

Matthew T. Hueman, MD[a], Richard D. Schulick, MD[b],*

[a]*The Johns Hopkins University School of Medicine, 600 North Wolfe Street, Blalock 665, Baltimore, MD 21287, USA*
[b]*The Johns Hopkins University School of Medicine, 1650 Orleans Street, Cancer Research Building I, Room 442, Baltimore, MD 21231–1000, USA*

A gastrointestinal stromal tumor (GIST) is a rare mesenchymal malignancy of the gastrointestinal (GI) tract. Malignant GISTs were first defined as a separate entity from a collection of nonepithelial malignancies of the GI tract in the 1980s and 1990s based on pathologic and clinical behavior. The discovery of activating KIT mutations as a near-uniform occurrence in these tumors greatly influenced the classification [1] and therapeutic management of these tumors. In this article, the authors describe the management of GISTs, concentrating on surgical management and targeted therapies.

Pathologic findings

A GIST is a mesenchymal tumor of the GI tract and is thought to derive from the interstitial cells of Cajal [2], innervated cells associated with Aurbach's plexus. In general, GISTs can be subtyped into spindle-cell (70% of cases), epithelioid (20% of cases), or mixed morphology based on their microscopic appearance [1], although the prognostic relevance of this classification is unclear. Immunohistochemical staining for several markers, including KIT, CD34, ACAT2, S100, DES, and keratin, can be helpful in establishing a diagnosis, although KIT positivity is the classic finding for GISTs and is in present in 95% of cases [1,3]. The differential diagnosis for submucosal lesions of the GI tract is large and includes such pathologic findings as intraabdominal fibromatosis, leiomyoma, schwannoma, inflammatory fibroid polyp, and leiomyosarcoma [4]. The use of immunohistochemical stains, as

---

* Corresponding author.
E-mail address: rschulick@jhmi.edu (R.D. Schulick).

doi:10.1016/j.suc.2008.03.001

described previously, can assist in differentiating GISTs from the potential alternative diagnoses.

Perhaps the most important pathologic factor for GISTs relating to therapeutic management is the presence of well-described mutations in the KIT or platelet-derived growth factor receptor (PDGFR) α-tyrosine kinase receptors. The KIT receptor is a transmembrane tyrosine kinase receptor and is closely related to the PDGFR [5]. Activation of KIT by its ligand stem-cell factor results in activation of downstream signaling pathways [6]. Several mutations in various portions of the KIT receptor have been described in GISTs that result in constitutive activation of the receptor and activation of downstream signaling [7].

PDGFR α-mutations have also been found in GISTs that do not contain KIT mutations and may provide an alternative pathway for activation [8]. These mutations also seem to render the PDGFR α-receptor constitutively active. Mutations in PDGFR-α seem to be significantly less frequent than activating KIT mutations; however, the presence of these mutations also has significant therapeutic implications.

Presentation and natural history

Approximately 5000 new GIST cases are expected in the United States annually [1]. The mean age at diagnosis for patients who have GISTs is 63 years, with a slightly higher risk in men, especially African-American men [9]. A separate familial syndrome that includes GISTs, hyperpigmentation, and dysphagia has been described; however, the phenotypic and molecular characteristics of these tumors seem otherwise similar to sporadic GISTs [10,11].

GISTs can occur in any tubular organ of the GI tract and, less frequently, in nontubular portions of the GI tract, such as the mesentery or omentum [12]. Most commonly, GISTs occur in the stomach (50%) (Figs. 1 and 2), small bowel (25%) (Fig. 3), and colorectum (10%) [9,13,14]. Patients who have GISTs typically present with symptoms relating to an enlarging abdominal mass (see Fig. 1), bleeding (see Fig. 3), or obstruction, although incidental note of a GIST at the time of endoscopy or surgery for another cause is not uncommon. GISTs tend to originate in the wall of the primary site and may grow to protrude into the lumen (see Fig. 3C) or toward the serosa (see Fig. 2A, B). Luminal extension may be associated with ulceration and hemorrhage (see Fig. 3C).

At the time of presentation, as many as half of patients who have a GIST have distant metastases [14]. Of patients who have metastatic disease, nearly two thirds have hepatic involvement. Isolated hepatic metastatic disease is common in patients with hepatic involvement. Extra-abdominal metastases and lymph node metastases at presentation are rare [14].

The most favorable subset for disease outcomes seems to be patients who have completely resected localized disease. Even in the setting of complete resection, however, recurrence is relatively common. In completely resected patients in whom no targeted adjuvant therapy is delivered, approximately 40% experience a recurrence [14]. Isolated local recurrences account for one third of these recurrences, and distant metastases alone account for nearly half of these recurrences. Positive resection margins are associated with a higher risk for local recurrence.

A more malignant phenotype of GIST has been described to occur in approximately 30% of cases [15], characterized by a high risk for local recurrence, peritoneal spread, and development of hepatic metastasis [7]. Because of this clinical heterogeneity, attempts have been made to define risk categories to predict which patients are likely to exhibit a more malignant course.

Risk stratification

GISTs include a wide range of tumors with variable prognosis. Several pathologic factors have been noted to be prognostic of significance, including mitotic index, size, and primary location. The National Institutes of Health (NIH) consensus workshop for GISTs first reported a risk stratification schema based on size and mitotic count in the hope of better defining groups of patients expected to exhibit an aggressive clinical course [1]. The risk stratification divided tumors into very low-, low-, intermediate-, and high-risk categories based on size (<2 cm, 2–5 cm, 5–10 cm, and >10 cm) and on the number of mitoses per 50 high-power fields (HPFs), typically reported as less than 5, 5 to 10, or greater than 10.

Since the NIH consensus risk stratification was published, several other negative prognostic factors have been described, including male gender, incomplete resection, nongastric tumor location, high tumor cellularity, and high Ki-67 count [16,17]. In addition, several molecular characteristics, such as immunophenotype, have been described, which also can assist in determining prognosis, including specific deletions in the KIT gene [18,19]. Importantly, these observations that molecular phenotype provides prognostic information have been extended to series of patients receiving adjuvant targeted therapy [20,21].

Evaluation

If possible, patients who have a GIST should be evaluated in a multidisciplinary clinic with expertise in sarcomas. The initial evaluation of patients who have a GIST should include a history and physical examination aimed at determining any symptoms or signs of local or metastatic disease. Imaging evaluation should include CT of the chest and abdomen. If not already completed, endoscopy with or without endoscopic ultrasound sometimes is of benefit [22]. The use of CT is important not only for evaluation of the size and location of the mass but to plan the operative approach. Endoscopic evaluation allows a confirmation of the appearance of the mass and biopsy if indicated.

The classic CT appearance of a GIST is a well-defined tumor with a heterogeneous rim of soft tissue [23]. Central fluid attenuation is not uncommon. If metastatic disease is obvious on CT imaging, it is often seen in the liver or peritoneum, with ascites being a rare manifestation. Small GIST tumors (<5 cm) often have a sharper tumor margin and homogeneous tumor density (see Fig. 2), whereas larger lesions (>10 cm) are more likely to have a more irregular border and inhomogeneous density (see Fig. 1) [24].

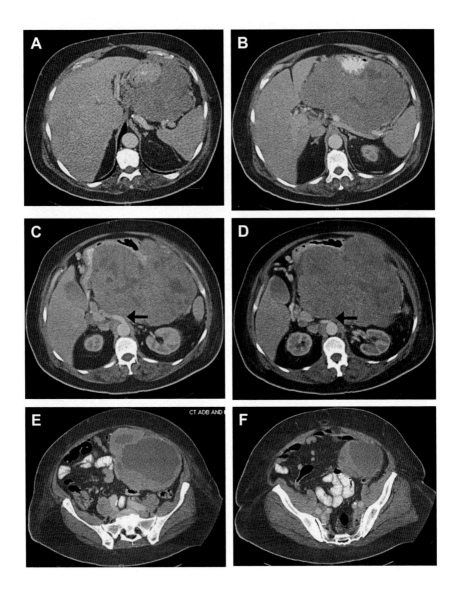

Several series have evaluated whether the radiographic or endoscopic appearance of presumed GISTs can predict final histology (GIST versus other histologies) and factors associated with recurrence and disease progression. By correlating imaging and endoscopic appearance with final pathologic findings, characteristics have been defined that may allow for a more accurate determination of histology and better preoperative stratification into risk groups. Although features like invasion into surrounding structures and evidence of dissemination are known to be correlated with malignant behavior, these series have identified additional characteristics, such as size larger than 5 cm, lobulated border, heterogeneous enhancement, mesenteric fat infiltration, ulceration, presence of regional adenopathy, exophytic growth pattern, hemorrhage, necrosis, and cyst formation [25–27].

Positron emission tomography (PET) scanning has also been used to evaluate the extent of disease in patients who have a GIST; however, to date, it has played more of a role in the assessment of response to therapy. Fluorodeoxyglucose (FDG) uptake in GIST tumors may rapidly decrease after initiation of targeted therapy, with complete metabolic responses reported within 1 week of initiation of therapy [28]. The patients experiencing the rapid metabolic response often proceed to a significant anatomic response to therapy. Although PET seems to be useful in assessment of response to therapy, it is currently not accepted as standard of care in the staging of patients who have a GIST.

Fig. 1. These CT images are of a 70-year-old white man who presented with early satiety and abdominal pain and show an extremely large isolated 25-cm (anteroposterior) × 20-cm (cephalocaudad) left upper quadrant mass, a presumptive GIST. The patient underwent partial gastrectomy with radical tumor excision and Billroth I reconstruction. Final pathologic examination revealed a margin-negative strongly c-KIT– and CD34-expressing GIST with a generally low mitotic rate but with evidence of necrosis and small sections with a mitotic rate between 5 and 10 mitoses per 50 HPFs. In combination with its size, evidence of necrosis, and intermediate mitotic rate, the patient was believed to be at high risk for recurrence and, after a prolonged postoperative course complicated by a pulmonary embolism, is undergoing adjuvant imatinib therapy. (A) CT image shows the cephalad extent of the extremely large GIST tumor, which, during surgery, was determined to be an exophytic posterior gastric GIST. The GIST had numerous 1-cm large veins throughout its superficial surface, making resection with minimal blood loss challenging. (B) CT image shows the heterogeneous nature of the mass and its mass-producing effect, as it is pushing the stomach anteriorly, pancreas (and splenic vein) posteriorly, and left lateral segment of the liver laterally. (C) CT image shows this heterogeneous mass pushing the stomach anteriorly and the duodenum laterally. The black arrow points to the close relation of the mass to the celiac axis but highlights that these tumors do not generally invade but rather push other structures. (D) CT image is similar to CT image in C and reveals a heterogeneous lobulated mass. The black arrow in this image points to the close relation of the mass to the superior mesenteric artery and highlights the technical difficulty these masses can cause when they distort critical anatomy. (E) CT image shows central attenuation consistent with central necrosis and reveals that this large left upper quadrant gastric GIST extended into the pelvis and displaced intestines. (F) CT image shows the extent of this left upper quadrant mass as it continues into the pelvis.

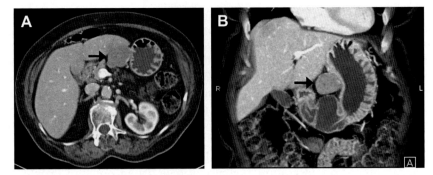

Fig. 2. These CT images are of a 63-year-old African-American woman who presented with nonspecific abdominal pain. After a thorough workup, the patient was found to have a presumptive 4.4-cm gastric GIST, as seen on these images. She was referred to our institution because of concern that the exophytic gastric mass involved the gastroesophageal junction. She underwent exploratory laparotomy and local gastrectomy and made a routine and complete recovery; during surgery, the GIST, as is characteristic, was seen to be located on a narrow stalk (well away from the gastroesophageal junction on the lesser curve), and a partial gastrectomy without tumor spillage was easily performed. The final pathologic examination revealed a strongly and diffusely c-KIT– and CD34-expressing GIST that was 5.5 cm in largest diameter and had six mitoses per 50 HPFs. It was recommended that she undergo adjuvant imatinib therapy. (*A*) Black arrow points to the gastric GIST, which is anterior and on the lesser curve. The mass extended more cephalad and could be easily confused as involving the gastroesophageal junction on axial CT. (*B*) Black arrow points to the gastric GIST, which on this coronal view on three-dimensional CT, clearly reveals the exophytic mass to be on the lesser curve, well away from the gastroesophageal junction.

The use of biopsy for a suspected GIST is controversial, and should be considered based on the concern for alternative diagnoses. If the lesion is accessible through an endoscopic approach, this is the preferred modality for biopsy [22]. Alternatively, if the lesion is small and surgical removal is expected to result in minimal morbidity, surgical removal may be an appropriate alternative. If neoadjuvant therapy is considered, pathologic diagnosis is usually required before initiation of therapy.

Management

Surgical resection is the preferred treatment for GISTs, and as with sarcomas in general, is thought to be the only potentially curative treatment approach. Once the diagnosis or presumed diagnosis of GIST is made and pretreatment evaluation is completed, an assessment of operability should be made. For patients who have localized, technically resectable disease, surgical therapy is the appropriate initial therapy. For patients who have locally advanced disease that is deemed unresectable or marginally resectable, targeted therapy, as discussed later in this section, should be considered in an attempt to render the tumor resectable [22]. In general, radiation and cytotoxic chemotherapy are ineffective in GISTs and are only used in refractory disease for palliative purposes.

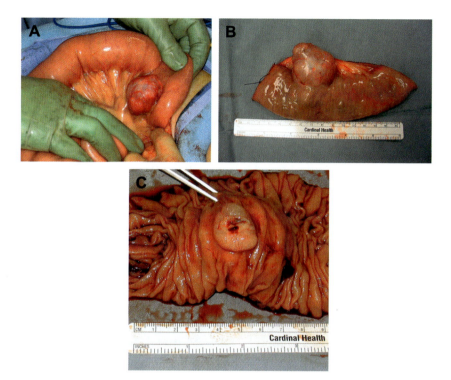

Fig. 3. These intraoperative photographs are of a 50-year-old white woman who twice presented with hemodynamically significant hemorrhage requiring transfusion. On her initial presentation, despite upper and lower endoscopy in addition to wireless capsule endoscopy, a source could not be found. She presented again with GI bleeding before her workup for an occult source was completed and was found to have an isolated proximal jejunal mass on CT scan of her abdomen. The photographs show a proximal jejunum GIST, which measured approximately 4.4 cm, is exophytic, and has an intraluminal component. The patient underwent an upper midline exploratory laparotomy with segmental small bowel resection and reanastomosis and did not have another bleeding episode, recovering without difficulty. The final pathologic examination revealed a 4.5-cm c-KIT– and CD34-expressing GIST with less than five mitoses per 50 HPFs. Given that it was a less than 5-cm GIST with a low mitotic rate, it was not recommended that the patient undergo adjuvant imatinib therapy. Follow-up CT scans as long as 1 year out do not reveal a recurrence. (*A*) Intraoperative photograph reveals the in vivo exophytic jejunal GIST on the mesenteric border. The GIST was only approximately 10 cm from the ligament of Treitz. (*B*) Ex vivo intraoperative photograph of the segmental small bowel resection reveals grossly negative margins. (*C*) Ex vivo intraoperative photograph of the intraluminal component of the small intestinal GIST; this was the source of this patient's two hemodynamically significant GI bleeds that both required transfusion.

Surgical management

At the time of surgery, the abdomen should be explored to evaluate for any evidence of peritoneal dissemination or liver involvement, because these are the predominant sites of metastases and eventual recurrence. The tumor should be carefully dissected to avoid tumor rupture because of a risk for dissemination. Typically, avoidance of tumor rupture and resection with a negative margin are most easily performed if the tumor and pseudocapsule are resected with a margin.

Options for resection approach depend on the location of the primary tumor and the pattern of growth, but peritumoral resections—as opposed to segmental resections—should be avoided because of a higher risk for recurrence [29]. Because of the low risk for lymph node involvement, a routine lymphadenectomy in patients who have clinically localized disease is not advocated. The final goal of surgery is complete tumor resection with a negative margin and an intact pseudocapsule. In the event of a margin-positive resection, additional surgery should be considered and weighed against the potential morbidity of the procedure.

For GIST of the esophagus, esophagectomy with complete resection of involved surrounding tissue is one approach [30]. Some have advocated enucleation or "esophageal-sparing wide local excision" to minimize morbidity while providing adequate local control, especially for smaller lesions less than 2 cm. This disease site remains controversial, because esophageal GISTs are limited to enucleation or esophagectomy; segmental resections, such as in small intestine and gastric GISTs, are not technically feasible in the esophagus. No definitive recommendations can be made because the literature supporting each approach is derived from small case series. GISTs of the duodenum are typically located in the second and third portions of the duodenum and may require partial duodenal resection or, more commonly, pancreaticoduodenectomy [31]. Most gastric tumors can be resected with local resection, with major gastrectomy reserved for lesions involving the pylorus or gastroesophageal junction [32].

Laparoscopic approaches have more recently been investigated in the management of GISTs, and several small series have reported outcomes with this approach. Novitsky and colleagues [33] recently reported outcomes from a prospective database of 50 patients treated with laparoscopic resection for GISTs with 36 months of follow-up. In this series, the surgical pproach varied significantly depending on the location of the tumor, but in all cases, abdominal exploration was performed before resection to rule out hepatic or peritoneal metastases with the use of intraoperative ultrasound to evaluate suspicious hepatic lesions. Intraoperative flexible endoscopy was used to assist in accurately locating the tumor and planning the most appropriate technique for resection. Three patients underwent a segmental resection, and 47 patients underwent a local resection. GISTs were never directly manipulated with laparoscopic instruments to minimize the risk for rupture. Seventy-eight percent of tumors in this series were located in the proximal stomach. Mean estimated blood loss in this series was 85 mL, with a mean operative time of 135 minutes. There was no conversion to open procedures, tumor rupture, or postoperative mortality. At 36 months after follow-up, 96% of patients were alive and disease-free. Four of the 50 patients experienced disease recurrence, in every case, involving the liver.

Pathologic evaluation revealed a mean of 5 mitotic figures per 50 HPFs with 18% of specimens having 10 or more mitotic figures per 50 HPFs. Although the use of adjuvant imatinib is not clearly described in this series, the results are certainly promising.

Additional series have reported outcomes with a laparoscopic approach, each with acceptable morbidity and disease control rates [34–37]. Although the technique seems to be safe and effective with GISTs, there are concerns regarding increased risk for tumor rupture or spillage. In addition, to reduce the potential for rupture or morbidity with this approach, many advocate limiting the use of laparoscopic resection to small GISTs, such as those measuring less than 2 cm in size [22].

Targeted therapy in advanced disease

Before the introduction of targeted therapy, there were few effective therapeutic options for patients who have GISTs. The introduction of imatinib mesylate, however, a small-molecule inhibitor of KIT and PDGFR-α, has provided an effective therapeutic option for many patients in whom no such option previously existed. Several studies have now been completed in patients who have advanced GISTs, evaluating the benefit of imatinib mesylate. The results of several trials that have evaluated the benefit of imatinib, and the most appropriate dose are summarized here.

Dose of imatinib mesylate

A multicenter randomized trial of imatinib at a dose of 400 or 600 mg/d in patients who had advanced GISTs was reported in 2002 [38]. In this trial, 147 patients were randomized to one of the two doses of imatinib with crossover possible to 600 mg/d for patients in the 400-mg/d dose arm. At a follow-up of 9 months, no patient developed a complete response, 53.7% of patients developed a partial response, and 27.9% of patients had stable disease. There was no difference in the rate or duration of response between the two arms of the study.

The Sarcoma Intergroup trial evaluated the benefit of higher dose imatinib [39]. This trial randomized 716 patients who had GISTs with documented expression of KIT to imatinib at 400 or 800 mg/d. At a median follow-up of 14 months, there was no difference in response rates or survival between the arms of this study.

The European Organization for Research and Treatment of Cancer (EORTC), Italian Sarcoma Group, and Australasian Gastrointestinal Trials Group also evaluated low- or high-dose imatinib in patients who had metastatic GISTs [40]. In this trial, 946 patients were randomized to imatinib at a dose of 400 mg delivered once or twice daily. More dose reduction and treatment interruptions were required in the twice-daily arm, with no significant difference in response rates. Overall, 5% of patients developed a complete response, 47% developed a partial response, and 32% had stable disease. Overall survival in the study was 85% to 86% at 1 year and 69% to 74% at 2 years. Despite the similarities in these measures, progression-free survival was significantly longer in the higher dose arm. Patients who progressed on 400 mg/d were allowed to cross over to the 800-mg/d dose arm. After crossover, 18% of patients were alive and progression-free at 1 year [41]. The benefit in progression-free survival with high-dose imatinib seen in this study was later found to correlate with the presence of activating mutations in exon 9 of KIT [42].

Duration of targeted therapy and predictors of response

The optimal duration and scheduling of imatinib in patients who have advanced GISTs is unknown. This question was addressed in a study of the French Sarcoma Group, which randomized patients who had stable disease, a partial response, or a complete response after 1 year of imatinib at a dose of 400 mg/d to interruption of therapy until progression or continuation until intolerance [43]. Patients who progressed after interruption were restarted on therapy with imatinib. In this series 8 of the 26 patients in the continuous imatinib arm compared with 26 of 32 patients in the interrupted imatinib arm experienced disease progression. Twenty-four of the 26 patients in the interrupted imatinib arm responded to the reintroduction of imatinib. These results suggest that in patients who have advanced disease and experience an ongoing response to therapy, imatinib should be continued indefinitely.

Several series have attempted to define prognostic factors to help identify patients who are likely to respond to targeted therapies. A review of 934 patients who had advanced GISTs treated in a randomized trial with imatinib mesylate determined that patients who developed resistance within 3 months of initiating therapy were more likely to have lung metastases without liver metastases, low hemoglobin, and a high granulocyte count [44]. Early resistance occurred in only 12% of patients included in this trial. Late resistance to imatinib, defined as resistance after 3 months of therapy, occurred more frequently and was associated with a high baseline granulocyte count and primary site location. Patients with resistance that developed after 3 months of therapy were more likely to have a high baseline granulocyte count, large tumor, and nongastric primary and to have been initiated on a lower dose of imatinib (400 mg/d compared with 400 mg twice daily). These results provide some insight into factors predictive for resistance to imatinib; however, perhaps more exciting are series evaluating molecular predictors of response.

An evaluation of tumors from patients who had GISTs treated with imatinib in a phase II clinical trial found correlations with the type of mutation and response to therapy [21]. Patients who had a GIST with exon 11 mutations in KIT had an 83.5% response rate to imatinib compared with a 47.8% response rate for patients who had a GIST with exon 9 mutations. Patients who had a GIST with no KIT mutation had a 0% response rate to imatinib. In addition to better response rates, patients who had GIST tumors with exon 11 mutations also had improved overall survival compared with patients who had exon 9 mutations or no activating mutations. These findings were later confirmed in an additional series of patients who had GISTs included in EORTC trials [42].

Sunitinib as an alternative to imatinib

Because progression eventually occurs in a significant number of patients who have GISTs treated with imatinib, additional targeted inhibitors have been evaluated as therapy after imatinib resistance. A randomized placebo-controlled trial of sunitinib, a multitarget tyrosine kinase inhibitor, was performed in 312 patients who had imatinib-resistant GISTs [45]. Patients enrolled in this trial received sunitinib at a dose of 50 mg/d for 4 weeks, followed by 2 weeks of rest for each 6-week cycle. Randomization was unblinded early because of a significant benefit in the sunitinib arm of the trial. The median time to tumor progression was 27.3 weeks in the sunitinib arm compared with 6.4 weeks with placebo. Overall survival was also improved in the sunitinib arm, but median survival had not been reached at the time of the report. Only 13 patients in the series were intolerant to sunitinib, and adverse events were reported to be mild or moderate in most cases. These data provide evidence that additional targeted therapy may be of significant benefit for patients who have advanced GISTs after development of imatinib resistance. Sunitinib is now approved by the US Food and Drug Administration (FDA) for patients who have an imatinib-resistant GIST or intolerance to imatinib.

Targeted therapy as adjuvant therapy

Targeted therapy has also been evaluated in the context of adjuvant therapy. Nilsson and colleagues [46] recently reported on a series of 23 patients who had high-risk GISTs. In this series, all patients underwent a complete resection, followed by the delivery of imatinib at a dose of 400 mg/d for 1 year. The mean follow-up for these patients was 40 months. A historical group matched for risk category, tumor size, and proliferative index was selected for comparison. Only 1 patient in the imatinib treatment group developed recurrent disease compared with 67% of patients in the control group. Although this series is small, it is important evidence that imatinib may play a role in the adjuvant therapy of GIST.

Preliminary findings of an American College of Surgeons Oncology Group (ACOSOG) placebo-controlled randomized trial evaluating the efficacy of imatinib in the adjuvant setting for completely resected GISTs have been reported, with promising results [47]. At the time of the report of these data, 708 patients who had a completely resected KIT-expressing GIST measuring more than 3 cm had been randomized to placebo versus imatinib at a dose of 400 mg/d for 1 year. Crossover was allowed for patients in the placebo arm at the time of progression. Accrual in this study was halted at interim analysis based on the preliminary results. At a median follow-up of 1.2 years in recurrence-free patients, the 1-year relapse-free survival rate was 97% in the imatinib arm and 83% in the placebo arm. Although survival data were immature in this presentation of the data, patients are to be followed for up to 10 years on this protocol.

Several additional trials are completed or ongoing that should provide evidence for the role of imatinib as adjuvant therapy [48]. ACOSOG Z9000 is a single-arm trial evaluating the role of adjuvant imatinib mesylate at a dose of 400 mg/d administered orally in patients who have high-risk disease. Safety data from this study have been reported in abstract form; however, efficacy data have yet to be reported [49]. The EORTC is randomizing patients who have intermediate- or high-risk GISTs to 2 years of imatinib versus placebo. A trial performed by the Scandinavian Sarcoma Group is evaluating 12 versus 36 months of imatinib as adjuvant therapy in patients who have high-risk disease.

Targeted therapy as neoadjuvant therapy

In some instances, surgical resection at the time of initial diagnosis may be deemed inappropriate because of metastatic disease or the extent of local invasion and the expected morbidity of the required surgical approach. In those instances, neoadjuvant therapy with imatinib may be considered with periodic reassessment to determine operability [22]. Several small series and case reports have presented the results of this approach, which seems to be promising [50–52]. Response rates as high as 76% have been documented with neoadjuvant imatinib [51], with approximately one quarter of primary and recurrent lesions converting to resectable lesions [52]. Long-term disease control has been documented in patients undergoing complete resection after response to neoadjuvant therapy for locally advanced disease [52,53].

Current recommendations for targeted therapy (National Comprehensive Cancer Network guidelines)

Based on the data summarized previously, current recommendations for imatinib therapy in patients who have metastatic GISTs include continuous delivery at a stable dose until progression or intolerance occurs. A higher daily dose of imatinib may be more appropriate in the subset of patients with activating KIT mutations in exon 9. At the time of disease progression, options include increasing the dose of imatinib or moving to alternative therapies, such as sunitinib. For unresectable GISTs, neoadjuvant imatinib may be delivered with periodic evaluations for determination of resectability and the appropriateness of intervention.

For patients who have completely resected GISTs, adjuvant imatinib may be considered after a complete resection, although the optimal duration of therapy is unknown and the most appropriate patient subset for which adjuvant therapy is beneficial is unknown. For incomplete resections in which additional surgical therapy is not considered an option, adjuvant imatinib may also be delivered. Patients who have recurrent disease should also be considered for imatinib therapy. Common toxicities associated with chronic administration of imatinib include mild to moderate nausea, edema, and rash [43].

Summary

A GIST is a rare tumor with a complex natural history. Surgical management is the mainstay of therapy, with margin-negative resection being the optimal surgical outcome. Targeted therapy with tyrosine kinase inhibitors has revolutionized the care of these patients, providing improved outcomes for patients who have completely resected tumors and resulting in prolonged responses in patients who have advanced disease. With ongoing advancements in the field, it is possible that targeted therapy may be selected in the future based on the specific mutation exhibited in each GIST and the resulting expected response rates. Newer tyrosine kinase inhibitors and targeted agents are being developed with the hope of providing improved response rates or alternative therapies for patients progressing on established agents.

References

[1] Fletcher CDM, Berman JJ, Corless C, et al. Diagnosis of gastrointestinal stromal tumors: a consensus approach. Hum Pathol 2002;33(5):459–65.

[2] Kindblom LG, Remotti HE, Aldenborg F, et al. Gastrointestinal pacemaker cell tumor (GIPACT): gastrointestinal stromal tumors show phenotypic characteristics of the interstitial cells of Cajal. Am J Pathol 1998;152(5):1259–69.

[3] Sarlomo-Rikala M, Kovatich AJ, Barusevicius A, et al. CD117: a sensitive marker for gastrointestinal stromal tumors that is more specific than CD34. Mod Pathol 1998;11(8): 728–34.

[4] Kirsch R, Gao ZH, Riddell R. Gastrointestinal stromal tumors: diagnostic challenges and practical approach to differential diagnosis. Adv Anat Pathol 2007;14(4):261–85.

[5] Qiu FH, Ray P, Brown K, et al. Primary structure of c-kit: relationship with the CSF-1/ PDGF receptor kinase family—oncogenic activation of v-kit involves deletion of extracellular domain and C terminus. EMBO J 1988;7(4):1003–11.

[6] Blume-Jensen P, Claesson-Welsh L, Siegbahn A, et al. Activation of the human c-kit product by ligand-induced dimerization mediates circular actin reorganization and chemotaxis. EMBO J 1991;10(13):4121–8.

[7] Corless CL, Fletcher JA, Heinrich MC. Biology of gastrointestinal stromal tumors. J Clin Oncol 2004;22(18):3813–25.

[8] Heinrich MC, Corless CL, Duensing A, et al. PDGFRA activating mutations in gastrointestinal stromal tumors. Science 2003;299(5607):708–10.

[9] Tran T, Davila JA, El-Serag HB. The epidemiology of malignant gastrointestinal stromal tumors: an analysis of 1,458 cases from 1992 to 2000. Am J Gastroenterol 2005;100(1): 162–8.

[10] Robson ME, Glogowski E, Sommer G, et al. Pleomorphic characteristics of a germ-line KIT mutation in a large kindred with gastrointestinal stromal tumors, hyperpigmentation, and dysphagia. Clin Cancer Res 2004;10(4):1250–4.

[11] Li FP, Fletcher JA, Heinrich MC, et al. Familial gastrointestinal stromal tumor syndrome: phenotypic and molecular features in a kindred. J Clin Oncol 2005;23(12):2735–43.

[12] Miettinen M, Sobin LH, Sarlomo-Rikala M. Immunohistochemical spectrum of GISTs at different sites and their differential diagnosis with a reference to CD117 (KIT). Mod Pathol 2000;13(10):1134–42.

[13] Rubin BP, Heinrich MC, Corless CL. Gastrointestinal stromal tumour. Lancet 2007; 369(9574):1731–41.

[14] DeMatteo RP, Lewis JJ, Leung D, et al. Two hundred gastrointestinal stromal tumors: recurrence patterns and prognostic factors for survival. Ann Surg 2000;231(1):51–8.

[15] Miettinen M, El-Rifai W, HL Sobin L, et al. Evaluation of malignancy and prognosis of gastrointestinal stromal tumors: a review. Hum Pathol 2002;33(5):478–83.

[16] Rutkowski P, Nowecki ZI, Michej W, et al. Risk criteria and prognostic factors for predicting recurrences after resection of primary gastrointestinal stromal tumor. Ann Surg Oncol 2007;14(7):2018–27.

[17] Wu TJ, Lee LY, Yeh CN, et al. Surgical treatment and prognostic analysis for gastrointestinal stromal tumors (GISTs) of the small intestine: before the era of imatinib mesylate. BMC Gastroenterol 2006;6:29.

[18] Martin J, Poveda A, Llombart-Bosch A, et al. Deletions affecting codons 557-558 of the c-KIT gene indicate a poor prognosis in patients with completely resected gastrointestinal stromal tumors: a study by the Spanish Group for Sarcoma Research (GEIS). J Clin Oncol 2005;23(25):6190–8.

[19] Andersson J, Bumming P, Meis-Kindblom JM, et al. Gastrointestinal stromal tumors with KIT exon 11 deletions are associated with poor prognosis. Gastroenterology 2006;130(6): 1573–81.

[20] Chirieac LR, Trent JC, Steinert DM, et al. Correlation of immunophenotype with progression-free survival in patients with gastrointestinal stromal tumors treated with imatinib mesylate. Cancer 2006;107(9):2237–44.

[21] Heinrich MC, Corless CL, Demetri GD, et al. Kinase mutations and imatinib response in patients with metastatic gastrointestinal stromal tumor. J Clin Oncol 2003;21(23):4342–9, 10.1200/JCO.2003.04.190.

[22] Demetri GD, Benjamin RS, Blanke CD, et al. NCCN Task Force report: management of patients with gastrointestinal stromal tumor (GIST)—update of the NCCN clinical practice guidelines. J Natl Compr Canc Netw 2007;5(Suppl 2):S1–29 [quiz: S30].

[23] Burkill GJ, Badran M, Al-Muderis O, et al. Malignant gastrointestinal stromal tumor: distribution, imaging features, and pattern of metastatic spread. Radiology 2003;226(2): 527–32.

[24] Ghanem N, Altehoefer C, Furtwangler A, et al. Computed tomography in gastrointestinal stromal tumors. Eur Radiol 2003;13(7):1669–78.

[25] Chun HJ, Byun JY, Chun KA, et al. Gastrointestinal leiomyoma and leiomyosarcoma: CT differentiation. J Comput Assist Tomogr 1998;22(1):69–74.

[26] Horton KM, Juluru K, Montogomery E, et al. Computed tomography imaging of gastrointestinal stromal tumors with pathology correlation. J Comput Assist Tomogr 2004;28(6): 811–7.

[27] Levy AD, Remotti HE, Thompson WM, et al. Gastrointestinal stromal tumors: radiologic features with pathologic correlation. Radiographics 2003;23(2):283–304, 456 [quiz: 532].

[28] Heinicke T, Wardelmann E, Sauerbruch T, et al. Very early detection of response to imatinib mesylate therapy of gastrointestinal stromal tumours using 18fluoro-deoxyglucose-positron emission tomography. Anticancer Res 2005;25(6C):4591–4.

[29] Aparicio T, Boige V, Sabourin JC, et al. Prognostic factors after surgery of primary resectable gastrointestinal stromal tumours. Eur J Surg Oncol 2004;30(10):1098–103.

[30] Blum MG, Bilimoria KY, Wayne JD, et al. Surgical considerations for the management and resection of esophageal gastrointestinal stromal tumors. Ann Thorac Surg 2007;84(5): 1717–23.

[31] Winfield RD, Hochwald SN, Vogel SB, et al. Presentation and management of gastrointestinal stromal tumors of the duodenum. Am Surg 2006;72(8):719–22 [discussion: 722–3].

[32] Wayne JD, Bell RH Jr. Limited gastric resection. Surg Clin North Am 2005;85(5):1009–20, vii.

[33] Novitsky YW, Kercher KW, Sing RF, et al. Long-term outcomes of laparoscopic resection of gastric gastrointestinal stromal tumors. Ann Surg 2006;243(6):738–45 [discussion: 745–7].

[34] Choi SM, Kim MC, Jung GJ, et al. Laparoscopic wedge resection for gastric GIST: long-term follow-up results. Eur J Surg Oncol 2007;33(4):444–7.

[35] Lai IR, Lee WJ, Yu SC. Minimally invasive surgery for gastric stromal cell tumors: intermediate follow-up results. J Gastrointest Surg 2006;10(4):563–6.

[36] Hindmarsh A, Koo B, Lewis MP, et al. Laparoscopic resection of gastric gastrointestinal stromal tumors. Surg Endosc 2005;19(8):1109–12.

[37] Nishimura J, Nakajima K, Omori T, et al. Surgical strategy for gastric gastrointestinal stromal tumors: laparoscopic vs. open resection. Surg Endosc 2007;21(6):875–8.

[38] Demetri GD, von Mehren M, Blanke CD, et al. Efficacy and safety of imatinib mesylate in advanced gastrointestinal stromal tumors. N Engl J Med 2002;347(7): 472–80, 10.1056/NEJMoa020461.

[39] Benjamin RS, Rankin C, Fletcher C, et al. Phase III dose-randomized study of imatinib mesylate (STI571) for GIST: Intergroup S0033 early results. Proceedings of the American Society for Clinical Oncology 2003;22 [abstract 3271].

[40] Verweij J, Casali PG, Zalcberg J, et al. Progression-free survival in gastrointestinal stromal tumours with high-dose imatinib: randomised trial. Lancet 2004;364(9440):1127–34.

[41] Zalcberg JR, Verweij J, Casali PG, et al. Outcome of patients with advanced gastro-intestinal stromal tumours crossing over to a daily imatinib dose of 800 mg after progression on 400 mg. Eur J Cancer 2005;41(12):1751–7.

[42] Debiec-Rychter M, Dumez H, Judson I, et al. Use of c-KIT/PDGFRA mutational analysis to predict the clinical response to imatinib in patients with advanced gastrointestinal stromal tumours entered on phase I and II studies of the EORTC Soft Tissue and Bone Sarcoma Group. Eur J Cancer 2004;40(5):689–95.

[43] Blay JY, Le Cesne A, Ray-Coquard I, et al. Prospective multicentric randomized phase III study of imatinib in patients with advanced gastrointestinal stromal tumors comparing interruption versus continuation of treatment beyond 1 year: the French Sarcoma Group. J Clin Oncol 2007;25(9):1107–13.

[44] Van Glabbeke M, Verweij J, Casali PG, et al. Initial and late resistance to imatinib in advanced gastrointestinal stromal tumors are predicted by different prognostic factors: a European Organisation for Research and Treatment of Cancer-Italian Sarcoma Group-Australasian Gastrointestinal Trials Group study. J Clin Oncol 2005;23(24): 5795–804, 10.1200/JCO.2005.11.601.

[45] Demetri GD, van Oosterom AT, Garrett CR, et al. Efficacy and safety of sunitinib in patients with advanced gastrointestinal stromal tumour after failure of imatinib: a randomised controlled trial. Lancet 2006;368(9544):1329–38.

[46] Nilsson B, Sjolund K, Kindblom LG, et al. Adjuvant imatinib treatment improves recurrence-free survival in patients with high-risk gastrointestinal stromal tumours (GIST). Br J Cancer 2007;96(11):1656–8.

[47] DeMatteo RP, Owzar K, Maki RG, et al. Adjuvant imatinib mesylate increases recurrence free survival (RFS) in patients with completely resected localized primary gastrointestinal stromal tumor (GIST): North American Intergroup Phase III trial ACOSOG Z9001. Proceedings of the American Society for Clinical Oncology 2007 [abstract 10079].

[48] Available at: http://www.clinicaltrials.gov. Accessed November 1, 2007.

[49] DeMatteo RP, Antonescu CR, Chadaram V, et al. Adjuvant imatinib mesylate in patients with primary high risk gastrointestinal stromal tumor (GIST) following complete resection: safety results from the U.S. Intergroup Phase II trial ACOSOG Z9000. Proceedings of the American Society for Clinical Oncology 2005;23(16S).

[50] Bumming P, Andersson J, Meis-Kindblom JM, et al. Neoadjuvant, adjuvant and palliative treatment of gastrointestinal stromal tumours (GIST) with imatinib: a centre-based study of 17 patients. Br J Cancer 2003;89(3):460–4.

[51] Scaife CL, Hunt KK, Patel SR, et al. Is there a role for surgery in patients with "unresectable" cKIT+ gastrointestinal stromal tumors treated with imatinib mesylate? The American Journal of Surgery. Papers from the Southwestern Surgical Congress, presented at the 55th annual meeting in Tucson, Arizona, April 27–30, 2003. 2003/12 2003;186(6):665–9.

[52] Andtbacka RH, Ng CS, Scaife CL, et al. Surgical resection of gastrointestinal stromal tumors after treatment with imatinib. Ann Surg Oncol 2007;14(1):14–24.

[53] Gutierrez JC, Perez EA, Moffat FL, et al. Should soft tissue sarcomas be treated at high-volume centers? An analysis of 4205 patients. Ann Surg 2007;245(6):952–8.

ELSEVIER
SAUNDERS

SURGICAL
CLINICS OF
NORTH AMERICA

Surg Clin N Am 88 (2008) 615–627

Pediatric Soft Tissue Sarcomas

David M. Loeb, MD, PhD[a,b,*],
Katherine Thornton, MD[b,c], Ori Shokek, MD[b,d]

[a]*Oncology and Pediatrics, Sidney Kimmel Comprehensive Cancer Center,
Johns Hopkins University, Bunting-Blaustein Cancer Research Building, Room 2M51,
1650 Orleans Street, Baltimore, MD 21231, USA*
[b]*Musculoskeletal Tumor Program, Sidney Kimmel Comprehensive Cancer Center,
Johns Hopkins University, Bunting-Blaustein Cancer Research Building, Room 2M51,
1650 Orleans Street, Baltimore, MD 21231, USA*
[c]*Oncology, Sidney Kimmel Comprehensive Cancer Center, Johns Hopkins University,
Bunting-Blaustein Cancer Research Building, Room 1M88,
1650 Orleans Street, Baltimore, MD 21231, USA*
[d]*Radiation Oncology and Molecular Radiation Sciences, Sidney Kimmel Comprehensive
Cancer Center, Johns Hopkins University, Weinberg 1440,
401 North Broadway, Baltimore, MD 21231, USA*

Soft tissue sarcomas in children are relatively rare. Approximately 850 to 900 children and adolescents are diagnosed each year with rhabdomyosarcoma (RMS) or one of the non-RMS soft tissue sarcomas (NRSTS). Of these, 350 are cases of RMS. RMS is the most common soft tissue sarcoma in children 14 years old and younger, and NRSTS is more common in adolescents and young adults. Infants also get NRSTS, but their tumors constitute a distinctive set of histologies, including infantile fibrosarcoma and malignant hemangiopericytoma, not seen in adolescents. Surgery is a major therapeutic modality for all pediatric soft tissue sarcomas, and radiation can play a role in the local therapy for these tumors. RMS is always treated with adjuvant chemotherapy, whereas chemotherapy is reserved for the subset of NRSTS that are high grade or unresectable. This review discusses the etiology, biology, and treatment of pediatric soft tissue sarcomas, including new approaches to therapy aimed at improving the dismal prognosis of patients who have recurrent and metastatic disease.

* Corresponding author. Sidney Kimmel Comprehensive Cancer Center, Johns Hopkins University, Bunting-Blaustein Cancer Research Building, Room 2M51, 1650 Orleans Street, Baltimore, MD 21231.
E-mail address: loebda@jhmi.edu (D.M. Loeb).

0039-6109/08/$ - see front matter © 2008 Elsevier Inc. All rights reserved.
doi:10.1016/j.suc.2008.03.008 *surgical.theclinics.com*

Rhabdomyosarcoma

Epidemiology

RMS is the most common soft tissue sarcoma among children less than 15 years old, with an incidence of 4.6 per million per year [1]. This represents 50% of all soft tissue sarcomas in this age range. It is slightly more common in boys than in girls, with a ratio of 1.1:1. RMS is slightly more common in white children than in black children less than 5 years old (1.1:1) but is more common in black children than in white children 5 years of age or older (1.2:1). Over the past 30 years, the incidence of RMS in the pediatric age group has been constant [1].

Etiology

Little is known about the etiology of RMS. A few cases are associated with Li-Fraumeni syndrome (caused by germline mutations in p53) [2] or with neurofibromatosis (caused by mutations in NF1) [3]. There also is a weak association with congenital anomalies, especially in boys [4]. These tumors sometimes are seen as second malignant neoplasms after radiation therapy.

Molecular and cellular biology

There are two major histologic variants of RMS—embryonal and alveolar. Other, minor, histologic types include spindle cell, botryoid, and pleomorphic. Embryonal RMS is named for its resemblance to immature skeletal muscle, accounts for 60% of RMS cases in patients less than 20 years of age, and tends to arise in the head and neck region, orbits, and genitourinary region (including bladder and prostate). Alveolar RMS, named for its resemblance to normal lung parenchyma, arises predominantly in the head and neck region and the extremities [3]. Histologically, RMS is a small round blue cell tumor, characterized by expression of muscle-specific antigens, such as desmin and MyoD, and by the presence of eosinophilic rhabdomyoblasts on standard pathologic staining.

Alveolar RMS is characterized by the presence of one of two recurrent chromosomal translocations: t(2;13)(q35;q14), seen in 55% of cases, or t(1;13)(p36;q14), seen in 22% of cases [5]. These fuse the FKHR gene on chromosome 13 with PAX 3 (chromosome 2) or PAX 7 (chromosome 1). In each case, the DNA-binding domain of the PAX gene is fused to the transactivation domain of the FKHR gene. Disruption of PAX genes leads to abnormal muscle development [6], suggesting a causal relationship between the translocation and the development of malignancy. The PAX3-FKHR translocation seems to carry a poorer prognosis than PAX7-FKHR [7].

Recurrent translocations have not been identified in cases of embryonal RMS. As the age of molecular medicine is begun, there is a movement toward redefining the subtypes of RMS as "translocation associated" and "non–translocation associated," allowing a disease classification based on objective molecular data rather than on subjective histologic appearance.

Clinical description

Signs and symptoms at the time of diagnosis depend on the location of the primary tumor. In general, patients present with a painless mass, although involvement of cortical bone causes pain, orbital tumors may present with proptosis, and genitourinary tumors often present with hematuria. Head and neck primaries account for 29% of cases of embryonal RMS and for 22% of alveolar RMS. Extremity primaries account for 39% of cases of alveolar RMS but only 6% of embryonal cases. In contrast, 28% of cases of embryonal RMS arise in the genitals, bladder, and prostate whereas only 3% of alveolar cases arise in these areas [5].

Evaluation and management

The initial evaluation of patients who have RMS involves determining a patient's stage and clinical group. A biopsy is required for diagnosis, and because clinical grouping of RMS is based in part on the extent of surgery, an excisional biopsy is preferred. When complete excision of the tumor is not feasible, an incisional biopsy is still necessary to confirm the diagnosis. Staging usually consists of a CT scan of the chest, abdomen, and pelvis; a bone scan; and bone marrow aspirates and biopsies (Fig. 1). The role of positron emission tomographic (PET) scanning in the evaluation of RMS patients remains controversial. A retrospective study of the usefulness of PET scans in the staging of patients who had RMS from Memorial Sloan-Kettering Cancer Center showed that a negative PET excluded

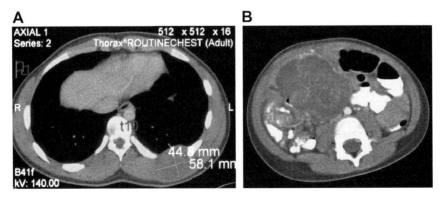

Fig. 1. CT appearance of RMS. (*A*) Chest CT from a 16-year-old-boy who presented with a "lump on the back." (*B*) Abdominal CT with intravenous and oral contrast from a 5-year-old girl who presented with abdominal pain and constipation.

disease in 21 of 23 cases where a CT or MRI was equivocal, but PET failed to show disease in 10 other sites where it was clearly visualized by CT, MRI, or bone scan (and confirmed clinically) [8]. Thus, a prospective study is necessary to definitively determine the value of PET in the evaluation of patients who have RMS.

RMS is staged using a disease-specific TNM staging system (Table 1). Unique to this system is the recognition that some sites of disease (orbit, head and neck, and biliary tract, for example) carry an inherent more favorable prognosis [9]. In addition to staging, a clinical group is assigned to each patient (Table 2), based on the extent of initial resection, margin status, lymph node involvement, and distant spread. Intergroup Rhabdomyosarcoma Study Group (IRSG) studies have demonstrated that clinical group is one of the most important predictors of treatment failure [10], further emphasizing the important role the initial surgery plays in overall patient outcome. After assignment of a stage and clinical group, this information is combined to categorize patients as low, intermediate, or high risk (Table 3), which determines the specific treatment course.

Because of the importance of clinical group in determining treatment and prognosis, and because of the dependence of clinical grouping on the initial surgery, adherence to appropriate surgical principles is critical. The basic principle of wide and complete resection with a surrounding envelope of normal tissue should be followed whenever and wherever possible, as long as sacrifice of surrounding normal tissue does not result in unacceptable loss of function or is not feasible.

Table 1
TNM staging of rhabdomyosarcoma

Stage	Sites	T	Size	N	M
1	Orbit Head and neck Genitourinary/not bladder or prostate Biliary tract	T_1 or T_2	a or b	N_0 or N_1 or N_x	M_0
2	Bladder or prostate Extremity Cranial parameningeal Other	T_1 or T_2	a	N_0 or N_x	M_0
3	Bladder or prostate Extremity Cranial parameningeal Other	T_1 or T_2	a b	N_1 N_0 or N_1 or N_x	M_0 M_0
4	All	T_1 or T_2	a or b	N_0 or N_1	M_1

Abbreviations: a, ≤ 5 cm in diameter; b, >5 cm in diameter, N_0, regional lymph nodes not involved; N_1, regional nodes clinically involved with neoplasm; N_x, clinical status of regional nodes unknown; M_0, no distant metastasis; T1, confined to anatomic site of origin; T2, extension or fixation to surrounding tissue.

Table 2
Rhabdomyosarcoma clinical group definitions

Group	Definition
Group I	Localized disease completely resected
Group IIa	Gross total resection with microscopic residual disease
Group IIb	Regionally involved lymph nodes, completely resected with the primary
Group IIc	Regional disease with involved nodes, totally resected with microscopic residual disease or histologic evidence of involvement of the most distant lymph node in the dissection
Group III	Incomplete resection
Group IV	Distant metastases

Pathologic confirmation of clinically positive lymph nodes is essential, because this has a direct impact on the extent of radiotherapy. There is little literature available on the role of sentinel lymph node identification and biopsy in patients who have RMS, but this approach may be helpful in RMS of the extremities [11], where the current Children's Oncology Group (COG) recommendation is for aggressive regional lymph node sampling. Prophylactic regional node dissection is not recommended, but staging ipsilateral retroperitoneal lymph node dissection is required for all boys 10 years of age or older who have paratesticular RMS or patients less than 10 years old who have radiographically positive nodes.

If the initial surgical procedure is a biopsy or an excision designed for a benign tumor, the question of pretreatment re-excision often arises. Wide re-excision is the current recommendation in such cases, unless this results in unacceptable loss of function or an unacceptable cosmetic result. If this re-excision is performed before administration of chemotherapy, it results in a lower clinical group and a more favorable prognosis. In patients for whom local radiotherapy is the primary local treatment modality, a residual persistent mass is common and is not associated with patient outcome [12]. For that reason, second-look surgeries are not routinely recommended.

The treatment of RMS has evolved over time, driven primarily by national cooperative group studies under the auspices of the IRSG. The success of this approach is evident from comparing survival of patients who

Table 3
Risk stratification in rhabdomyosarcoma

Histology	Clinical group	Stage	Risk group
Embryonal	I, II, III	1	Low
Embryonal	I, II	2, 3	Low
Embryonal	III	2, 3	Intermediate
Embryonal	IV	4	High
Alveolar	I, II, III	1, 2, 3	Intermediate
Alveolar	IV	4	High

have had RMS treated in successive IRSG studies. From IRS-I through IRS-IV there has been steady improvement in patient outcomes (Fig. 2).

Guidelines for the use of local radiotherapy depend on clinical group. Analysis of clinical group I patients treated in the first four IRSG studies showed a significant benefit to the use of radiotherapy for patients who had alveolar histology in local control and overall survival [13]. Radiotherapy for clinical group II patients has been used routinely in the IRS studies with local and regional failure rates of 8% and 4% at 5 years [14]. Good local control has been reported historically with radiotherapy for clinical group III patients also, with a local failure rate of only 13% at 5 years on IRS-IV [15]. Some cooperative groups have attempted to minimize the impact of local therapy by withholding radiotherapy in clinical group III patients who had favorable response to chemotherapy or patients whose disease is resected after induction chemotherapy, but this approach is associated with unfavorable local control and decreased survival [16,17].

As with other high-grade solid tumors, successful treatment of RMS requires systemic chemotherapy, which is used to treat distant metastases or prevent the progression of micrometastases to overt disease. The specifics of systemic chemotherapy vary depending on risk stratification. For low-risk patients, current standard therapy consists of four cycles of vincristine, actinomycin, and cyclophosphamide (VAC) followed by four cycles of vincristine and actinomycin for the lowest-risk patients and 12 cycles of vincristine and actinomycin for the patients who have slightly higher-risk tumors. For intermediate-risk patients, standard treatment consists of 14 cycles of VAC. Currently, the COG is conducting a clinical trial comparing this with 14 cycles of alternating VAC and vincristine and irinotecan. For high-risk patients, the current COG protocol treats patients with an admixture of chemotherapy cycles including vincristine and irinotecan; vincristine, doxorubicin, and cyclophosphamide; and ifosfamide and etoposide, with

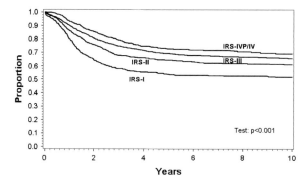

Fig. 2. Survival IRS-I through IRS-IV. Improvement in survival with successive clinical trials. The overall survival curves for each IRS study are shown. (*Courtesy of* W. Meyer, University of Oklahoma, Oklahoma City, OK; with permission.)

a total of 20 cycles of therapy. Because of the dismal prognosis for patients presenting with metastatic RMS, autologous peripheral blood stem cell transplant has been used; however, its role is not established and its use should be reserved for clinical trials.

Nonrhabdomyosarcoma soft tissue sarcomas

Epidemiology

The incidence of soft tissue sarcomas in children younger than 20 years of age is 11.0 per million, representing 7.4% of cancer cases in this age group [1]. Approximately 60% of these are NRSTS. These tumors are rare in younger children and become more common with increasing patient age, and in older adolescents these tumors are more common than RMS, although no single histology accounts for more than 15% of all cases [1].

Etiology

There are no known causes, or even risk factors, for the development of NRSTS in children or adolescents.

Molecular and cellular biology

There is a wide variety of histologic tumor types grouped under the umbrella term, NRSTS. These correspond to the various normal cell types that develop from mesenchymal cells (Table 4). The International Classification

Table 4
Histologic subtypes of nonrhabdomyosarcoma soft tissue sarcomas in pediatric patients

Histology	Normal counterpart	Incidence
Fibrosarcoma	Fibroblast	0.6
Infantile fibrosarcoma	Fibroblast	0.2
Malignant fibrous histiocytoma	Fibroblast	0.8
Dermatofibrosarcoma protuberans	Fibroblast	1.0
Malignant peripheral nerve sheath tumor	Schwann cell	0.6
Kaposi's sarcoma	Blood vessels	0.1
Liposarcoma	Adipocyte	0.1
Leimyosarcoma	Smooth muscle	0.3
Synovial sarcoma	Synovial cells	0.7
Hemangiosarcoma	Blood vessels	0.2
Malignant hemangiopericytoma	Vessel pericytes	0.1
Alveolar soft part sarcoma		0.1
Chondrosarcoma	Chondrocytes	0.1

Incidence is age-adjusted rate per million for patients less than 20 years old.
From Gurney J, Young JL Jr, Roffers SD, et al. Cancer incidence and survival among children and adolescents: United States SEER Program 1975–1995. Vol NIH Pub. 99-4649. Bethesda (MD): National Cancer Institute, SEER Program; 1999.

of Childhood Cancer subdivides pediatric NRSTS into four categories: (1) the fibrosarcoma category, (2) Kaposi's sarcoma, (3) the "other specified" soft tissue sarcomas (including synovial sarcoma, angiosarcoma, and hemangiopericytoma; leiomyosarcoma; liposarcoma; and extraosseous Ewing's sarcoma), and (4) "unspecified" soft tissue sarcomas [1]. These categories are useful for epidemiology but ultimately have no bearing on treatment or prognosis.

Many of the NRSTS tumors have a characteristic chromosomal alteration that, along with distinctive histology, allows for definitive diagnosis (Table 5). In at least one such case, the t(17;22) found in dermatofibrosarcoma protuberans, the characteristic translocation provides a target for tumor-directed treatment. This translocation puts the platelet-derived growth factor (PDGF) β-chain under the control of the constitutively active collagen type Ia promoter, resulting in autocrine stimulation of the PDGF receptor. Inhibition of this receptor with imatinib mesylate resulted in an objective response in nine of nine patients in a recently published study from Australia [18]. It is hoped that future research will allow the development of additional therapies targeted at the molecular abnormalities that cause these cancers.

Clinical description

Typically, NRSTS presents with a painless mass that is found by a patient or a patient's parents. Usually, these masses are slow growing, and

Table 5
Cytogenetic abnormalities in soft tissue sarcomas

Diagnosis	Cytogenetic abnormality	Genes involved
Alveolar RMS	t(2;13) or t(1;13)	FKHR on chromosome 13 and PAX3 (chromosome 2) or PAX7 (chromosome 1)
Infantile fibrosarcoma	t(12;15)	TEL (ETV6) on chromosome 12 and NTRK3 (TRKC) on chromosome 15
Dermatofibrosarcoma Protuberans	t(17;22)	PDGF β-chain on chromosome 17 and collagen type Ia on chromosome 22
Synovial sarcoma	t(X;18)	SYT on chromosome 18 and SSX-1 or SSX-2 on the X chromosome
Liposarcoma	t(12;16)	FUS gene on chromosome 16 and CHOP gene on chromosome 12
Myxoid chondrosarcoma	t(9;22)	EWS on chromosome 22 and TEC gene on chromosome 9
Alveolar soft part sarcoma	t(X;17)	Unidentified genes, esp. at chromosome band 17q25

symptoms, if any, are the result of compression or invasion of normal structures and, therefore, vary by tumor location. Orbital tumors, for example, may cause proptosis, whereas intra-abdominal tumors may cause abdominal fullness, constipation, back pain, or early satiety.

Evaluation and management

The evaluation of a soft tissue mass in a child begins with careful imaging of the primary tumor, usually with an MRI. This provides superior anatomic definition, may be helpful in distinguishing benign from malignant tumors, and provides the necessary information regarding proximity to surrounding neurovascular structures that allow appropriate surgical planning by an orthopedic or surgical oncologist. A CT scan of the chest, abdomen, and pelvis is an important part of the evaluation for metastatic disease. [18]Fluorodeoxyglucose-PET scan is gaining in importance for diagnostic purposes and for evaluating response to therapy [19,20].

A biopsy is necessary to establish the diagnosis. In most cases, a core needle biopsy is adequate to obtain diagnostic tissue, and the accuracy of core needle biopsies is excellent, with a high sensitivity and specificity [21–23]. Combined with low morbidity, this is the diagnostic procedure of choice. It is recommended that biopsies be obtained by a trained orthopedic surgical oncologist or radiologist and preferably at a multidisciplinary sarcoma treatment center. The biopsy site should be chosen so that the track lies in the field of future en bloc resection [24]. If a core needle biopsy does not provide a diagnosis, a surgical biopsy becomes necessary.

Surgery remains the mainstay of treatment for NRSTS. The goal of surgical excision is complete removal of the mass with a margin of surrounding normal tissue. In general, a 1-cm margin is considered acceptable, and closer margins should prompt consideration of re-excision. When tumors abut critical neurovascular structures, complete resection risks compromising the integrity of distal structures. Under these conditions, adequate resection may not be possible, and such patients require adjuvant chemotherapy or radiation therapy. Local control rates with limb-sparing surgery for extremity sarcomas, with judicious use of adjuvant radiation therapy, approach 95%, equivalent to what was once obtained with amputation [25,26]. Accordingly, amputation should be reserved for cases of major artery or nerve involvement, sufficiently extensive bone involvement such that removal of the entire bone is required, or recurrence after previous resection with adjuvant radiation therapy.

The role of adjuvant (or neoadjuvant) therapy in the management of NRSTS is still a matter of investigation. It generally is believed that the usefulness of chemotherapy and radiation therapy depends on a patient's risk for relapse and sarcoma-specific death. A nomogram for predicting 12-year sarcoma-specific death rates has been devised based on prospectively collected data from 2136 consecutive adult patients who had soft tissue sarcoma treated at Memorial Sloan-Kettering Cancer Center (Fig. 3) [27]. Prognostic variables, including patient age, tumor size, histologic grade, histologic subtype, and tumor location, were incorporated into the nomogram. The nomogram has been validated using an independent group of patients treated at University of California, Los Angeles and found to provide accurate prognostic information [28]. A study attempting to validate the nomogram for use in a pediatric population found that death rate was underestimated and that the majority of this effect was the result of an increased prognostic importance of tumor size in the pediatric population [29].

Retrospective studies of pediatric NRSTS have identified a similar group of important prognostic factors, including localized versus metastatic disease, extent of tumor resection, maximal tumor diameter, and tumor grade. A retrospective analysis of NRSTS patients treated at St. Jude Children's Research Hospital suggested three risk subgroups: (1) patients who had grossly resected localized tumors, with a predicted 5-year survival of 89%; (2) patients who had initially unresected localized tumors, with a predicted 5-year survival of 56%; and (3) patients who had metastatic tumors, with a predicted 5-year survival of 15% [30]. This study, however, did not incorporate tumor grade or tumor size in its prognostic subgroups. The current COG NRSTS protocol is designed in part to test a similar risk stratification

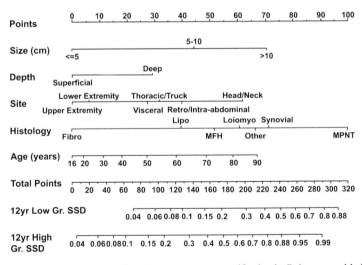

Fig. 3. Postoperative nomogram for 12-year sarcoma-specific death. Points are added up for size (second line), depth (third line), site (fourth line), histology (fifth line), and patient age (sixth line). A line drawn down from the point total to the low-grade or high-grade line reveals the likelihood of sarcoma-specific death in 12 years. Fibro, fibrosarcoma; GR, grade; Lipo, liposarcoma; leiomyo, leiomyosarcoma; MFH, malignant fibrous histiocytoma; MPNT, malignant peripheral-nerve tumor; SSD, sarcoma-specific death. (*From* Kattan MW, Leung DH, Brennan MF. Postoperative nomogram for 12-year sarcoma-specific death. J Clin Oncol 2002;20(3):791–6; with permission.)

system that accounts for all of the identified prognostic variables: size, grade, metastatic status, extent of resection, and margin status.

For patients deemed at high risk for metastatic spread, systemic chemotherapy generally is administered. Two chemotherapy drugs have been reliably shown to have activity against a broad spectrum of NRSTS histologies as single agents: doxorubicin and ifosfamide [31,32]. Accordingly, current NRSTS chemotherapy regimens consist of combination therapy with these two drugs.

Because local control with radiotherapy alone is not achievable, radiation is used in combination with surgery. Radiotherapy can be administered as adjuvant or as neoadjuvant treatment to augment the efficacy of the surgery. It also can be given as adjuvant therapy for patients who have positive margins or incompletely resected tumors. The National Cancer Institute of Canada conducted a randomized trial of preoperative radiation compared with postoperative radiation in adults who had soft tissue sarcoma [33]. The preoperative dose was 5000 cGy and the postoperative dose was 6600 cGy. Patients who had positive surgical margins were given a postoperative boost of 1600 cGy. Local control was identical on the two arms, but toxicities were different: wound healing complications were more common on the preoperative radiotherapy arm, whereas late effects, such as fibrosis and joint stiffness, were increased among patients who received postoperative radiotherapy [34,35]. These radiation doses are typical of those used in standard practice. The treatment volume typically encompasses the preoperative tumor or postoperative tumor bed with 5-cm longitudinal margins and 2-cm radial margins. The longitudinal margins are reduced when boost doses are given.

Summary

Pediatric soft tissue sarcomas are rare, with fewer than 1000 new cases per year in the United States. These tumors are subdivided into RMS and the NRSTS. Surgery is a critical component of the treatment of all pediatric soft tissue sarcoma patients. There has been a series of cooperative group studies of RMS, dating back to 1972, which has continuously refined the diagnosis, risk stratification, and treatment of these patients. There is a well-established risk stratification scheme that accounts for tumor histology, location, extent of surgical resection, locoregional lymph node involvement, and the presence of distant metastases. The specifics of treatment depend on risk classification, but all patients who have RMS are treated with adjuvant chemotherapy and most also receive radiation therapy. Future work will aim at maintaining the excellent cure rate for patients who have low-risk disease while decreasing late effects of treatment and improving the outcome for high-risk patients.

In contrast, the treatment of pediatric patients who have NRSTS is less standardized. A nomogram for the prediction of sarcoma-specific death has been developed and validated for adults who have soft tissue sarcomas, but this algorithm may not be accurate for pediatric patients. A retrospective review of sarcoma patients treated at St. Jude Children's Research Hospital has led to the development of a pediatric soft tissue sarcoma risk stratification scheme, but this has not yet been validated in a national study. Although the importance of radiotherapy has been demonstrated, optimal dose and timing (pre- versus postoperative) has not been determined. Additionally, the role for chemotherapy in the treatment of children who have soft tissue sarcoma remains unclear. An ongoing cooperative group study will attempt to prospectively validate a pediatric soft tissue sarcoma risk stratification scheme and to optimize the use of chemotherapy and radiation therapy for these patients.

References

[1] Gurney J, Young JL Jr, Roffers SD, et al. Cancer incidence and survival among children and adolescents: United States SEER Program 1975–1995. Vol NIH Pub. 99-4649. Bethesda (MD): National Cancer Institute; SEER Program; 1999.

[2] Malkin D, Li FP, Strong LC, et al. Germ line p53 mutations in a familial syndrome of breast cancer, sarcomas, and other neoplasms. Science 1990;250(4985):1233–8.

[3] Pizzo PA, Poplack DG. Principles and practice of pediatric oncology. 4th edition. Philadelphia: Lippincott Williams & Wilkins; 2002.

[4] Yang P, Grufferman S, Khoury MJ, et al. Association of childhood rhabdomyosarcoma with neurofibromatosis type I and birth defects. Genet Epidemiol 1995;12(5):467–74.

[5] McDowell HP. Update on childhood rhabdomyosarcoma. Arch Dis Child 2003;88(4):354–7.

[6] Seale P, Sabourin LA, Girgis-Gabardo A, et al. Pax7 is required for the specification of myogenic satellite cells. Cell 2000;102(6):777–86.

[7] Lam PY, Sublett JE, Hollenbach AD, et al. The oncogenic potential of the Pax3-FKHR fusion protein requires the Pax3 homeodomain recognition helix but not the Pax3 paired-box DNA binding domain. Mol Cell Biol 1999;19(1):594–601.

[8] Klem ML, Grewal RK, Wexler LH, et al. PET for staging in rhabdomyosarcoma: an evaluation of PET as an adjunct to current staging tools. J Pediatr Hematol Oncol 2007;29(1):9–14.

[9] Meza JL, Anderson J, Pappo AS, et al. Analysis of prognostic factors in patients with non-metastatic rhabdomyosarcoma treated on intergroup rhabdomyosarcoma studies III and IV: the Children's Oncology Group. J Clin Oncol 2006;24(24):3844–51.

[10] Neville HL, Andrassy RJ, Lobe TE, et al. Preoperative staging, prognostic factors, and outcome for extremity rhabdomyosarcoma: a preliminary report from the Intergroup Rhabdomyosarcoma Study IV (1991–1997). J Pediatr Surg 2000;35(2):317–21.

[11] McMulkin HM, Yanchar NL, Fernandez CV, et al. Sentinel lymph node mapping and biopsy: a potentially valuable tool in the management of childhood extremity rhabdomyosarcoma. Pediatr Surg Int 2003;19(6):453–6.

[12] Godbule P, Outram A, Wilcox DT, et al. Myogenin and desmin immunohistochemistry in the assessment of post-chemotherapy genitourinary embryonal rhabdomyosarcoma: prognostic and management implications. J Urol 2006;176:1751–4.

[13] Wolden SL, Anderson JR, Crist WM, et al. Indications for radiotherapy and chemotherapy after complete resection in rhabdomyosarcoma: a report from the Intergroup Rhabdomyosarcoma Studies I to III. J Clin Oncol 1999;17(11):3468–75.

[14] Smith LM, Anderson JR, Qualman SJ, et al. Which patients with microscopic disease and rhabdomyosarcoma experience relapse after therapy? A report from the soft tissue sarcoma committee of the children's oncology group. J Clin Oncol 2001;19(20):4058–64.

[15] Donaldson SS, Meza J, Breneman JC, et al. Results from the IRS-IV randomized trial of hyperfractionated radiotherapy in children with rhabdomyosarcoma—a report from the IRSG. Int J Radiat Oncol Biol Phys 2001;51(3):718–28.

[16] Donaldson SS, Anderson JR. Rhabdomyosarcoma: many similarities, a few philosophical differences. J Clin Oncol 2005;23(12):2586–7.

[17] Stevens MC, Rey A, Bouvet N, et al. Treatment of nonmetastatic rhabdomyosarcoma in childhood and adolescence: third study of the International Society of Paediatric Oncology–SIOP Malignant Mesenchymal Tumor 89. J Clin Oncol 2005;23(12):2618–28.

[18] McArthur GA, Demetri GD, van Oosterom A, et al. Molecular and clinical analysis of locally advanced dermatofibrosarcoma protuberans treated with imatinib: Imatinib Target Exploration Consortium Study B2225. J Clin Oncol 2005;23(4):866–73.

[19] Peng F, Rabkin G, Muzik O. Use of 2-deoxy-2-[F-18]-fluoro-D-glucose positron emission tomography to monitor therapeutic response by rhabdomyosarcoma in children: report of a retrospective case study. Clin Nucl Med 2006;31(7):394–7.

[20] Volker T, Denecke T, Steffen I, et al. Positron emission tomography for staging of pediatric sarcoma patients: results of a prospective multicenter trial. J Clin Oncol 2007;25(34):5435–41.

[21] Ball AB, Fisher C, Pittam M, et al. Diagnosis of soft tissue tumours by Tru-Cut biopsy. Br J Surg 1990;77(7):756–8.

[22] Barth RJ Jr, Merino MJ, Solomon D, et al. A prospective study of the value of core needle biopsy and fine needle aspiration in the diagnosis of soft tissue masses. Surgery 1992;112(3): 536–43.

[23] Heslin MJ, Lewis JJ, Woodruff JM, et al. Core needle biopsy for diagnosis of extremity soft tissue sarcoma. Ann Surg Oncol 1997;4(5):425–31.

[24] Clark MA, Fisher C, Judson I, et al. Soft-tissue sarcomas in adults. N Engl J Med 2005; 353(7):701–11.

[25] Clark MA, Thomas JM. Amputation for soft-tissue sarcoma. Lancet Oncol 2003;4(6):335–42.

[26] Spiro IJ, Rosenberg AE, Springfield D, et al. Combined surgery and radiation therapy for limb preservation in soft tissue sarcoma of the extremity: the Massachusetts General Hospital experience. Cancer Invest 1995;13(1):86–95.

[27] Kattan MW, Leung DH, Brennan MF. Postoperative nomogram for 12-year sarcoma-specific death. J Clin Oncol 2002;20(3):791–6.

[28] Eilber FC, Brennan MF, Eilber FR, et al. Validation of the postoperative nomogram for 12-year sarcoma-specific mortality. Cancer 2004;101(10):2270–5.

[29] Ferrari A, Miceli R, Casanova M, et al. Adult-type soft tissue sarcomas in paediatric age: A nomogram-based prognostic comparison with adult sarcoma. Eur J Cancer 2007;43(18): 2691–7.

[30] Spunt SL, Hill DA, Motosue AM, et al. Clinical features and outcome of initially unresected nonmetastatic pediatric nonrhabdomyosarcoma soft tissue sarcoma. J Clin Oncol 2002; 20(15):3225–35.

[31] Edmonson JH, Ryan LM, Blum RH, et al. Randomized comparison of doxorubicin alone versus ifosfamide plus doxorubicin or mitomycin, doxorubicin, and cisplatin against advanced soft tissue sarcomas. J Clin Oncol 1993;11(7):1269–75.

[32] Verweij J, van Oosterom AT, Somers R, et al. Chemotherapy in the multidisciplinary approach to soft tissue sarcomas. EORTC Soft Tissue and Bone Sarcoma Group studies in perspective. Ann Oncol 1992;3(Suppl 2):S75–80.

[33] O'Sullivan B, Davis AM, Turcotte R, et al. Preoperative versus postoperative radiotherapy in soft-tissue sarcoma of the limbs: a randomised trial. Lancet 2002;359(9325):2235–41.

[34] Davis AM, O'Sullivan B, Bell RS, et al. Function and health status outcomes in a randomized trial comparing preoperative and postoperative radiotherapy in extremity soft tissue sarcoma. J Clin Oncol 2002;20(22):4472–7.

[35] Davis AM, O'Sullivan B, Turcotte R, et al. Late radiation morbidity following randomization to preoperative versus postoperative radiotherapy in extremity soft tissue sarcoma. Radiother Oncol 2005;75(1):48–53.

ELSEVIER
SAUNDERS

Surg Clin N Am 88 (2008) 629–646

SURGICAL
CLINICS OF
NORTH AMERICA

The Role of Radiation Therapy in the Management of Sarcomas

Aradhana Kaushal, MD[a], Deborah Citrin, MD[b],*

[a]Radiation Oncology Branch, National Cancer Center, National Cancer Institute,
Building 10, Hatfield CRC, B2-3500, 10 Center Drive, Bethesda, MD 20892, USA
[b]Section of Imaging and Molecular Therapeutics, Radiation Oncology Branch,
National Cancer Center, National Cancer Institute, Building 10, Hatfield CRC,
B2-3500, 10 Center Drive, Bethesda, MD 20892, USA

Sarcomas are a rare disease, with 9220 new soft tissue sarcomas diagnoses and 3560 deaths expected in the United States in 2007 [1]. Management of soft tissue sarcomas is complicated by the relative rarity of these tumors, the lethality of the disease, and the fact that they can occur as several histologic findings in a variety of sites in the body, each of which has different functional and anatomic considerations regarding optimal management [2]. In this article, the authors concentrate on the radiotherapeutic management of sarcomas occurring in the most common locations: the extremities, the trunk, and the retroperitoneum. An overview of the current radiotherapeutic management of soft tissue sarcoma is presented in addition to a discussion of how surgical management may affect radiotherapeutic management. Finally, the authors describe current controversies surrounding the appropriate management of sarcomas with radiotherapy and describe ongoing studies and future areas of research.

Extremity sarcoma: role of radiotherapy

Before the introduction of radiotherapy for extremity soft tissue sarcomas, amputation was the standard therapeutic procedure, often resulting in significant physical and psychologic morbidity to the patient. With this radical procedure, local failure is uncommon, but as many as 40% of patients continued to die of metastatic disease [3]. Studies completed in the 1970s and 1980s provided the first evidence that limb salvage was possible

* Corresponding author.
E-mail address: citrind@mail.nih.gov (D. Citrin).

0039-6109/08/$ - see front matter. Published by Elsevier Inc.
doi:10.1016/j.suc.2008.03.005

surgical.theclinics.com

and could provide adequate local control without significantly increasing distant failures. Since that time, refinements have been made to determine how radiotherapy can be best integrated with surgical management to maximize disease control and functional outcomes. A variety of techniques have been used to improve disease control and functional outcomes. The timing of radiotherapy for patients who have resectable extremity sarcomas, the optimal management and sequencing of therapies for large-extremity sarcomas, and the need for radiotherapy in resected low-grade lesions are areas that have been, and in some cases still are, controversial.

The first evidence that radiotherapy could be used as a method to improve functional outcomes by avoiding amputation in patients who have sarcomas was provided by a prospective randomized trial completed at the National Cancer Institute (NCI) [4]. In this series, 43 adult patients who had high-grade soft tissue sarcoma of the extremity were randomized to amputation or limb-sparing resection, followed by adjuvant radiation therapy to a total dose of 50 Gy. Patients randomized to the limb-sparing group underwent a wide local excision designed to remove gross disease and several centimeters of surrounding normal tissue. In cases in which the pseudocapsule abutted major neurovascular structures, these structures were dissected free, even if positive margins were the result. Both groups received chemotherapy (doxorubicin, cyclophosphamide, and methotrexate) after surgery. Although there were four local recurrences in the limb-sparing group, there was no significant difference in disease-free survival or overall survival between the study arms. Importantly, an association of margin status and local recurrence is not reported in this series. This study confirmed the utility of postoperative radiotherapy; however, radiotherapy did not compensate for an inadequate surgical resection, because patients with a positive margin of resection still had a high risk for local recurrence, despite the addition of radiotherapy.

A subsequent prospective randomized trial also completed at the NCI further defined the role of postoperative external beam radiotherapy (EBRT) after a limb-sparing surgical resection. In this study, patients were randomized to receive or not to receive postoperative adjuvant radiotherapy, although all patients received chemotherapy [5]. In patients receiving radiotherapy, there were no local recurrences in patients compared with a local recurrence rate of 22% in patients not receiving radiotherapy. Of additional importance, in this same study, 25 patients who had low-grade sarcoma were randomized to receive adjuvant radiotherapy. Excluding desmoid tumors and other neoplasms that did not fit the strict definition of malignant soft tissue sarcoma, there has been recurrence in 6 of the 19 patients not receiving radiotherapy and in 1 of the 22 patients receiving radiotherapy. These data suggested that a local control benefit is seen with the addition of adjuvant radiotherapy for low- and high-grade sarcomas. Additional analysis of the high- grade and low-grade groups of patients showed no difference in overall survival with the addition of radiation therapy. Similar results have been confirmed in several series, leading to the general consensus that radiotherapy delivered after a wide local excision or function-preserving surgical procedure provides a significant benefit in local disease control, although providing no benefit with respect to overall survival or the incidence of distant metastases.

Although these data support a local control benefit for the radiotherapy administered after wide local excision, additional attempts have been made to define a subgroup of patients in whom the risk for local recurrence is sufficiently low to justify avoiding radiotherapy to minimize toxicity. This remains a significant area of controversy, however. The National Comprehensive Cancer Network (NCCN) guidelines currently recommend radiation therapy for extremity sarcomas for high-grade lesions and for low-grade lesions that are larger than 5 cm or have close or positive margins. This is based on the lower risk for local recurrence for small low-grade lesions [6,7].

In some series, additional factors, such as age, seem to affect rates of local recurrence. For example, in one retrospective series analysis from Memorial Sloan Kettering Cancer Center, age greater than 50 years was identified as an independent predictor of local recurrence after conservative surgery and radiotherapy [7]. In a Princess Margaret Hospital series, younger age, less than 50 years, was predictive of better local control [8]. These were retrospective studies, and these investigators commented that these results may have been confounded by the fact that certain aggressive histologic findings may be more common in older age groups. Nevertheless, for those patients for whom local excision alone is being contemplated, age should also be taken into consideration as a possible factor for local recurrence.

Extremity sarcoma: preoperative versus postoperative radiation therapy

Although the delivery of radiotherapy in large or high-grade extremity sarcomas is considered standard, significant controversy has existed regarding the appropriate timing of delivery in relation to surgery. Preoperative therapy allows the radiation oncologist to deliver a lower radiation dose (typically 50 Gy versus 66–70 Gy delivered in the adjuvant setting) to a smaller target volume (preoperative extent with margin versus entire operative bed with margin), potentially minimizing toxicity. In addition, marginally resectable tumors may respond to the preoperative radiotherapy in a sufficient manner to allow a negative margin functional resection.

Arguments also exist supporting the use of postoperative therapy. A significant concern with the delivery of preoperative therapy is the concern for an increase in wound complications with the preoperative approach because of impaired healing in the radiotherapy field, especially when the wound repair is under tension. Although infrequent, complications that occur during radiotherapy may postpone the definitive surgical procedure. Finally, evaluation of the pathologic findings in the setting of preoperative therapy may be complicated by radiation effect.

The decision of whether to use preoperative versus postoperative radiotherapy was examined in a large randomized trial from the NCI Canada Clinical Trial Group [9]. This trial evaluated disease control and toxicity in patients who had soft tissue sarcoma of the extremity and randomized to treatment by preoperative (50 Gy) or postoperative (66 Gy) external radiation in combination with surgery. Local recurrence, locoregional recurrence, and progression-free survival were the same between the groups. Of note, 64 of 94 patients in the postoperative group had acute toxic skin effects that were grade 2 or greater compared with 32 of 88 in the preoperative group. Grade 1 and 2 bowel toxicity did not differ between the two groups, and no patient experienced grade 3 or 4 bowel toxicity. Two-year toxicity data and functional outcomes data from this series have also been reported [10,11]. In regard to late toxicity, grade 2 or greater fibrosis occurred in 48.2% of patients in the postoperative arm compared with 31.5% in the preoperative arm at 2 years. Edema and joint stiffness were more common in the postoperative arm, although this difference was not statistically significant. Patients who had fibrosis, joint stiffness, and edema had significantly lower functional scores. Taken together, these data support that preoperative radiotherapy provides equivalent disease control with better long-term functional outcomes compared with postoperative radiotherapy.

When deciding between preoperative versus postoperative radiation therapy, the type of surgical procedure to be performed, the planned type of wound closure, the amount of expected wound tension, the probable extent of the operative bed, the likelihood of obtaining a margin-negative resection, and the histologic grade of the sarcoma should all be considered. Also, a recovery period of 3 to 6 weeks is necessary after the completion of preoperative radiotherapy to allow resolution of acute radiation effects, allow improved wound healing when surgery is performed, and allow for the desired histologic response. After eventual surgical resection, a thorough examination of the pathologic specimen is critical to determine the appropriateness of an additional boost of radiation with brachytherapy or EBRT if margins are close or positive.

Radiotherapy may be delivered after surgery instead of before surgery for a variety of reasons, including the incidental diagnosis of sarcoma at surgery, upgrading after evaluation at surgery, inability to obtain a negative margin with acceptable functional outcomes, and a more extensive lesion than expected based on preoperative imaging and pathologic data. When radiotherapy is delivered after surgery, at least 5 cm of margin is used and a dose of at least 60 Gy or higher is used, because the dose of radiotherapy delivered in the postoperative setting has been shown to correlate with local control [12]. In conclusion, postoperative and preoperative radiation treatment has benefits and detriments and should be discussed on an individual basis with each patient in a multidisciplinary setting.

Brachytherapy in the treatment of soft-tissue sarcomas

In addition to EBRT, brachytherapy has been used for the treatment of sarcomas in an effort to improve the therapeutic ratio by minimizing the extent of normal tissue treated and to permit local dose escalation simultaneously to areas at highest risk. In a prospective randomized trial conducted by Memorial Sloan Kettering Cancer Center, 164 patients were randomized during surgery to receive adjuvant brachytherapy or no further treatment after resection of soft tissue sarcoma of the extremity or trunk [13]. The entire radiotherapy treatment in this series was delivered with a brachytherapy implant without external beam irradiation. The tumor bed and surrounding tissue received an iridum-192 implant that delivered 42 to 45 Gy over 4 to 6 days. With a median follow-up of 76 months, 5-year local control rates were significantly improved with brachytherapy (82% versus 69%), but this benefit seemed to be limited to patients who had high-grade lesions. Overall local control was 91%, which is comparable to local control rates in postoperative external beam treatments.

Another observation was that patients treated in this trial who had radioactive sources loaded before postoperative day 6 had an increased incidence of wound complications. Once this observation was made, efforts were made to load the catheters after postoperative day 6 so as not to interfere with the granulation phase of wound healing. After this change was made, no difference was noted between the two groups with respect to failed tissue healing and this policy was adopted as the preferred standard. As is typical for radiotherapy series for sarcoma, there was no effect on the incidence of distant metastasis or disease-specific survival in any group of patients in this series. There were more major and moderate wound complications in patients in the brachytherapy group (11 of 23 patients) compared with the unirradiated group (5 of 21 patients).

A comprehensive review of the technique of placing brachytherapy catheters, treatment planning, and treatment delivery is outside the scope of this brief review. A comprehensive guideline for the performance of brachytherapy for extremity sarcomas has been published by the American Brachytherapy Society [14]. In certain instances, brachytherapy should be strictly avoided because of potential undertreatment or foreseeable toxicity or overdosing of neurovascular structures. Brachytherapy, although an extremely effective treatment, is technically challenging for the radiation oncologist and surgeon and should be used by multidisciplinary teams with significant experience, expertise, and medical physicist support.

The radiotherapy dose delivered with brachytherapy depends on the clinical scenario and indication, although doses of 45 to 50 Gy over 4 to 6 days are often prescribed for low-dose rate radiotherapy when delivered as the only form of radiotherapy. In situations in which brachytherapy is used as a boost after a course of EBRT, doses of 15 to 25 Gy are typically selected. As mentioned previously, treatment typically commences no sooner than 5 days after wound closure. An example of a brachytherapy treatment is provided in Fig. 1.

Preoperative regimens for extensive or locally advanced sarcomas

A variety of regimens have been evaluated as preoperative therapy for extremity and truncal sarcomas to improve resectability while maximizing functional outcomes, including chemotherapy alone, radiotherapy alone, or chemoradiation. The use of chemotherapy as an adjuvant therapy in sarcomas is controversial based on the variable results achieved in regard to disease control and response rates in prospective studies and meta-analyses [15–17]. Despite the controversy in the use of adjuvant chemotherapy for sarcomas, the use of neoadjuvant chemotherapy has also been explored as a possible strategy for improving treatment of a soft tissue sarcoma. It has been proposed that the use of neoadjuvant therapy may allow a reduction in radiation volumes or allow selection of patients who respond to chemotherapy for additional adjuvant treatment.

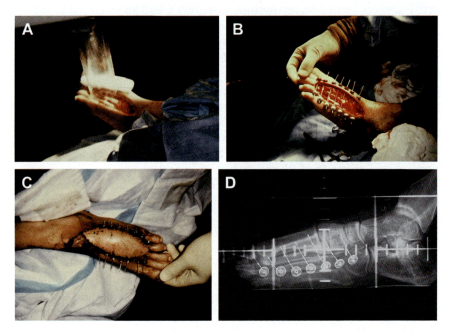

Fig. 1. Brachytherapy for extremity sarcoma. A 22-year-old man presented with a 4-cm × 1.8-cm × 1.8-cm mass on the dorsum of his left foot in a field previously irradiated for Ewing's sarcoma. A biopsy was consistent with synovial sarcoma. (A) After excision of the mass, the tumor bed was irradiated to 20 Gy during surgery with electrons by means of a specialized cone. Brachytherapy catheters were then placed across the tumor bed and secured (B) before flap placement and wound closure (C). (D) After documentation of catheter placement with treatment planning images, an additional dose of 25 Gy was delivered with an Ir-192 brachytherapy implant.

In an effort to evaluate whether neoadjuvant therapy improves outcomes for patients who have locally advanced or high-grade tumors, investigators at MD Anderson Cancer Center evaluated three cycles of preoperative doxorubicin and dacarbazine, cyclophosphamide, and doxorubicin and dacarbazine (ADIC) in patients who had stage IIIB extremity sarcoma. The disease-free survival and overall survival in patients who received three cycles of preoperative doxorubicin and dacarbazine, cyclophosphamide, and ADIC were similar to those achieved in historical studies, in which patients were randomized to postoperative chemotherapy [18]. Unfortunately, even the subset of patients classified as responders to the neoadjuvant regimen did not achieve any significant benefit in local recurrence–free survival, distant metastasis–free survival, or overall survival. A randomized trial of preoperative chemotherapy consisting of doxorubicin and ifosfamide versus local treatment alone through the European Organization for Research and Treatment of Cancer (EORTC) has been completed and final results are pending [19].

An alternative regimen to improve outcomes of soft tissue sarcoma is a combined radiation and chemotherapy approach. Perhaps the best example of this approach is a single institution series reported from Massachusetts General Hospital of a preoperative chemotherapy regimen consisting of mesna, adriamycin, ifosfamide, and dacarbazine (MAID) alternating with radiotherapy, followed by resection and postoperative chemotherapy with or without radiotherapy [20]. Patients who had high-grade extremity soft tissue sarcoma greater than 8 cm were treated with three cycles of preoperative chemotherapy combined with 44 Gy of radiotherapy, followed by surgery. For patients with positive surgical margins, 16 Gy was delivered after surgery. Five-year local control, freedom from distant metastases, disease-free survival, and overall survival were all improved compared with historical controls. Overall survival increased from 58% to 87%, which represented a significant gain in disease-free survival compared with the historical data.

Based on these promising results, this regimen was subsequently tested in a phase II Radiation Therapy Oncology Group (RTOG) trial [21]. A total of 66 patients who had a high-grade soft tissue sarcoma greater than 8 cm in diameter received three cycles of neoadjuvant MAID chemotherapy, alternating with radiotherapy and three cycles of postoperative MAID chemotherapy. Estimated 3-year rates of disease-free, distant-disease-free, and overall survival were 56.6%, 64.5%, and 75.1%, respectively, in this series. Toxicity was significant with this approach, with 84% experiencing grade 4 toxicity (78% experienced grade 4 hematologic toxicity and 19% experienced grade 4 nonhematologic toxicity). Of the five amputations in the study, two were considered to be treatment-related. The conclusion of the authors is that such an aggressive neoadjuvant regimen can be used; however, it needs to be performed in the setting of a clinical trial, given the significant toxicity.

Unresectable sarcomas

Sarcomas may be deemed unresectable at presentation for a variety of reasons. For tumors invading major neurovascular or bony structures, such as those involving the pelvic girdle or structures of the shoulder, resection may lead to unacceptable morbidity and poor functional outcomes. Additionally, complex involvement of major neurovascular structures may preclude surgical extirpation. In these situations, neoadjuvant therapy, as described previously, may be used with the hope of downsizing the tumor to facilitate resection. If the extent of disease is such that downsizing would be unlikely to result in a viable surgical option, definitive radiotherapy may be used with the hope of offering durable local control [22].

Alternatively, patients may present with medical comorbidities that preclude aggressive surgical management. For example, the option of definitive radiotherapy may provide local control after a core biopsy or in the case of a marginal excision when further surgery is contraindicated or in the case of a positive margin without re-excision [23,24]. In some instances, the burden of metastatic disease, in addition to the extent of local disease, may result in the decision to forego an aggressive local surgical procedure.

Outcomes with this approach are clearly inferior to surgically based approaches with 5-year local control rates approximating 29% to 45% in single-institution reviews [22,24–26]. Factors negatively influencing the ability to obtain local control with definitive radiotherapy in these series include increasing tumor size (<5 cm versus 5–10 cm versus >10 cm) and lower radiation dose (<63 Gy versus >63 Gy). The use of chemotherapy does not correlate with improved outcomes in this population [22].

In any situation in which definitive radiotherapy is used, care must be taken to design fields appropriately to exclude sensitive structures. The likelihood of toxicity after definitive radiotherapy depends at least partially on the size and location of the tumor, factors that affect the amount and type of normal tissue exposed to higher doses. In some series, doses in excess of 68 or 70 Gy have been associated with an increased risk for major radiotherapy complications [22,25]. The incidence of major complications that may result from radiotherapy in the definitive setting vary depending on the site treated but may include soft tissue necrosis, fibrosis, neuropathy, bone fracture, and bowel injury [22,25].

Newer technologies, such as intensity-modulated radiotherapy (IMRT), proton therapy, and helical tomotherapy, may allow delivery of effective definitive radiotherapy while reducing the risk for complications for patients who have sarcomas [27–29]. These technologies each may permit more conformal radiation delivery, allowing for effective tumor coverage with the target radiation dose while minimizing the amount of uninvolved normal tissue that is exposed to higher doses. These technologies are actively being investigated in this setting [19].

In addition to newer radiotherapy techniques, chemotherapy delivered concurrently with radiotherapy has been investigated as a mechanism to improve resectability. Although some series have found up to 25% objective responses with chemotherapy in advanced sarcomas [30], evidence that induction chemotherapy can result in downsizing sufficient to allow resection or prolonged local control is lacking. For this reason, induction chemotherapy remains investigational.

Other multimodality approaches, including such techniques as isolated limb perfusion strategies with or without radiotherapy, have been evaluated as a mechanism for increasing resectability. Limb perfusion with agents, such as doxorubicin, melphalan, and tumor necrosis factor, with or without with radiation have been reported with response rates of 53% to 85% and significant improvements in resectability [31–33]. Long-term follow-up has revealed high risks for necrosis and eventual requirement for amputation as a result of significant vascular morbidity in some series of multimodality management, including radiation with limb perfusion [34,35]. Because of the complexity of the procedure and the potential for significant morbidity, limb perfusion with or without radiotherapy is not in widespread clinical use at this time.

Retroperitoneal sarcoma

Retroperitoneal sarcomas present a unique therapeutic challenge. Because of their location, these tumors often become quite large before presenting signs and symptoms develop. In addition, these tumors are often adjacent to a several critical structures. These factors complicate surgical and radiotherapeutic management. Finally, the relative rarity of these tumors has resulted in mainly retrospective evaluations of radiotherapy in addition to surgery, precluding the ability to make definitive treatment recommendations.

Because of the relatively high likelihood of positive surgical margins and eventual local recurrence, radiotherapy has been applied in the preoperative, intraoperative, and postoperative settings. The use of radiotherapy in addition to surgical resection has achieved 5-year local control rates of 51% to 71% in several retrospective series [36–39]. Toxicity with this approach is a major concern, however, because of the proximity of these tumors to many organs and structures with relatively low radiation tolerances. Such organs as the spinal cord, kidneys, liver, and small bowel limit radiotherapy doses lower than what is typically considered appropriate for soft tissue sarcomas in the adjuvant setting (60–70 Gy). Based on these considerations, a radiotherapy dose of 45 to 50 Gy is often considered the maximal safe dose for this region of the body with conventional approaches, a dose that is considered reasonable as a preoperative dose for sarcomas.

Similar to extremity sarcomas, the timing of radiotherapy has significant implications in regard to targeting and potential toxicity. Although use of postoperative radiotherapy allows the selection of patients at highest risk for recurrence based on margin status, there are numerous reasons why preoperative therapy is preferred. In the postoperative setting, the tumor has been resected or debulked, allowing normal tissues to move into and become adhered to the tumor bed. This potentially results in a higher radiotherapy dose to some sensitive normal tissues, such as bowel, that would typically move in and out of the field of radiation if delivered in the setting of preoperative therapy. In addition, preoperative treatment volumes are often smaller because they are based on treating the tumor volume with a margin for microscopic extension, whereas postoperative therapy often includes the entire tumor bed and clips, with an additional margin. An additional theoretic benefit to preoperative therapy is the improved oxygenation of the tumor bed in the preoperative setting, a factor known to enhance sensitivity of tumors to damage caused by ionizing radiation.

Typically, preoperative radiotherapy is considered for intermediate or high-grade retroperitoneal sarcomas that are likely to be resected with positive margins. If preoperative therapy is considered, a biopsy is required to verify histology before initiating radiotherapy. Prospective trials evaluating the role of preoperative radiotherapy with intraoperative therapy or as part of multimodality regimens have found promising disease control rates [40–43]. A recent report of long-term data from patients treated in two of these prospective series found a 5-year disease-free survival rate of 46% and a 5-year survival rate of 50%. For patients in this series who completed radiotherapy and underwent a macroscopically complete resection, the 5-year local recurrence-free survival rate was 60%.

Toxicities of EBRT for retroperitoneal sarcomas may include mild to moderate acute toxicities of enteritis, nausea, and vomiting [36,37,44] and late toxicities of bleeding gastric ulcers, small bowel obstruction, strictures, and impaired wound healing [37,44]. Rates of toxicity range widely in reported series and with chosen radiation delivery method but, in general, seem to be less with preoperative approaches [45].

Retroperitoneal sarcomas remain a challenging problem, with local control rates clearly inferior to those obtained in extremity sarcomas. Attempts to improve the local control benefit obtained with radiotherapy while minimizing toxicity have led to alternative targeting methods, the use of highly conformal therapies, and alternative delivery methods. The use of local radiation dose escalation at the anticipated site of a positive margin has been explored with promising results. A single-institution series in which the entire tumor with margin was treated before surgery to a dose of 45 Gy with selective escalation with a boost to 57.5 Gy to areas expected to be at high risk for a positive margin was well tolerated, with 88% of patients undergoing a gross total resection and a resultant 2-year local control rate of 80% [46]. Studies evaluating treatment planning with highly conformal therapies, such as IMRT and helical tomotherapy, have shown the potential to reduce toxicity with these newer planning technologies by allowing avoidance of high-dose regions in organs with low radiation tolerance [47,48].

Intraoperative radiotherapy (IORT) was developed as a potential mechanism of increasing the deliverable dose while minimizing toxicity by delivering radiotherapy at the time of surgery when many sensitive normal tissues could be retracted and removed from the direct path of the radiation beam. IORT requires a specialized operating room equipped with the proper equipment to deliver the radiotherapy. This specialized equipment is currently available at a few institutions. IORT can be delivered alone or in combination with additional external radiotherapy delivered before or after surgery.

Several series of IORT for retroperitoneal sarcomas have shown favorable disease control, however, at a cost of toxicity. These toxicities are different than those typically reported for external beam radiation alone and are likely attributable to the tissues exposed to the large fraction sizes typically used and include neuropathy, ureteral fistula, hydronephrosis, and bowel obstruction [43,49,50]. Patient selection for IORT before and after surgery is critical for selecting patients who may have a lower risk for toxicity. Assessment of the total field size required, normal tissues to be included in the field, and anticipated toxicity of the therapy may lead to intraoperative determination that the therapy is inappropriate in a significant number of patients [41].

Brachytherapy is an alternative technique for delivering local tumor bed boosts. The use of brachytherapy in this setting has typically been combined with standard doses of preoperative EBRT. Toxicity in these series is significant, with reoperation rates of up to 21.5% [40,51]. There is some indication that brachytherapy to the upper abdomen may be poorly tolerated, with higher rates of late toxicity and long-term complications [40]. Early local control rates in these series are promising, but longer follow-up in larger prospective series is needed [40,51].

Planning and delivery of radiation therapy

Once the decision to use EBRT has been reached, technical aspects, such as dosage, timing, and margins, need to be considered. Radiation therapy for sarcomas can usually be delivered in the outpatient setting, with the exception of interstitial brachytherapy. The use of brachytherapy requires inpatient admission for reasons of radiation protection.

For external beam radiation treatment planning, the ability to target the areas at highest risk properly is of critical importance. Radiation oncologists typically rely on a variety of data to determine target volumes for treatment planning, including physical examination, preoperative imaging, operative reports, radiopaque clips, scars, and drain sites. CT and MRI provide complimentary information for radiotherapeutic treatment planning and should be obtained whenever possible. It is critical that the imaging obtained before surgery encompass the entire area of radiographic abnormality with margin to allow for adequate tumor targeting with radiotherapy. In addition, obtaining these images with the patient in the radiation treatment planning position (ie, treatment-planning MRI or CT) can facilitate treatment planning by allowing an acceptable fusion of these image series to the treatment planning images, significantly improving target delineation.

For radiotherapy delivered in the preoperative setting, a discussion with the surgeon who is going to perform the operation can allow avoidance of high-dose regions in areas destined to be incision or drain sites, potentially reducing wound complications. In general, radiation oncologists attempt to exclude sensitive structures from the radiation field to minimize toxicity, including uninvolved compartments, joint spaces, genitalia, and visceral organs. In addition, attempts are made to avoid treating the entire circumference of a limb because of the risk for lymphedema. Placement of surgical incisions, drain sites, and biopsy sites overlying or adjacent to these sensitive structures may result in the need to include them in the radiation field, hence increasing the risk for toxicity. A thorough discussion of the multimodality treatment plan with members of the oncology team may allow therapy to be delivered in a fashion that maximizes disease control and minimizes toxicity.

In the postoperative setting, radiopaque surgical clips placed at the time of resection can assist in delineating the tumor bed and the area at high risk. For patients with microscopically positive surgical margins in whom brachytherapy was not delivered, a postoperative external beam boost of 16 Gy may be delivered at 2.5 to 3 weeks after surgery or once wound healing is adequate. In the preoperative or postoperative setting, it is crucial to spare an uninvolved compartment of the limb from receiving a full dose to spare lymphatics. Typically, the radiation plan is also optimized to reduce the dose to poorly vascularized areas, such as the pretibial, prepatellar, and preolecranon skin. A multidisciplinary approach toward management of sarcomas can significantly improve the ability of the radiation oncologist to meet these complex dose-planning goals while minimizing toxicity. Clearly, involvement of the surgeon and radiation oncologist for planning of the surgical and radiation procedures can significantly affect the treatment plan. Representative plans from patients who have extremity and retroperitoneal sarcoma are presented in Figs. 2 and 3.

Future directions

Although significant improvements have been made in the local management of extremity sarcomas, a significant number of patients experience local failures and toxicity of therapy. The relatively few cases diagnosed in the United States further complicate matters and make conducting large trials and studies to improve management not feasible. Although

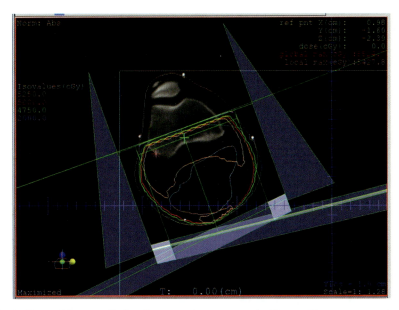

Fig. 2. External beam radiation for extremity sarcoma. A 55-year-old man presented with a popliteal mass with a core biopsy consistent with malignant fibrous histiocytoma. Neurovascular function was intact. Preoperative radiotherapy was delivered to a total dose of 50 Gy in 2-Gy daily fractions to the popliteal tumor with 5-cm margins longitudinally. Care was taken to provide an adequate circumferential margin while limiting the exposure of the knee joint and anterior tissues of the leg by using opposed lateral fields directed at the popliteal fossa. The tumor volume is outlined in pale yellow, and other colored lines represent isodose curves (*orange* = 52.5 Gy, red = 50 Gy, and *green* = 47.5 Gy). Green +, isocenter of field; pink *, local dose maximum.

management of soft tissue sarcoma of the extremity has improved greatly and there are generally accepted methods used to improve general outcomes for patients who have retroperitoneal and unresectable sarcomas, the overall prognosis remains poor for this particular subset of sarcomas. Several areas of ongoing research hope to address issues that may continue to improve outcomes in patients who have these diseases.

From a radiotherapeutic setting, the main focus of ongoing research includes improved targeting of therapy to minimize toxicity and maximize disease control. From a systemic therapy point of view, current chemotherapy regimens can be quite toxic and effects can be multiplied when used in a sandwich and concomitant setting. This toxicity has led to the manipulation of molecular targets within tumors to enhance local effects of radiation. Additional efforts have focused on identification of individual factors, such as single-nucleotide polymorphisms or gene expression patterns that may predict for toxicity from radiotherapy.

Because unresected sarcoma requires high doses of radiation therapy to achieve the best chance of local control, doses of this magnitude come with the attendant possibility of significant normal tissue toxicity. To

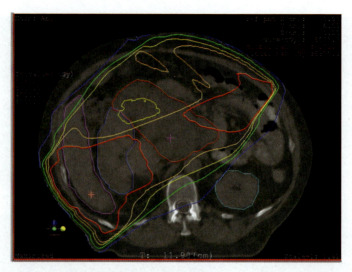

Fig. 3. External beam radiation for retroperitoneal sarcoma. A 62-year-old woman presented with increasing abdominal girth and was noted to have a large retroperitoneal mass on CT. Biopsy was consistent with high-grade liposarcoma. Preoperative radiotherapy to a total dose of 50.4 Gy in 1.8-Gy fractions was delivered, followed by margin negative resection. The tumor is outlined in dark red; other colored lines represent isodose curves (*red* = 52.5 Gy, *yellow* = 50 Gy, and *pale yellow* = 47.5 Gy). A complex beam arrangement was used to minimize the dose to the left kidney while providing an adequate tumor margin. Purple +, isocenter of field; pink *, local dose maximum.

mitigate this possibility, various other radiation therapy modalities have been investigated, such as IMRT and other forms of highly conformal therapies. The goal with these approaches is to spare as much normal tissue within the affected limb or region of the body from high-dose irradiation as possible to minimize acute and late toxicities of therapy. As discussed previously, these techniques are currently under investigation and may provide an additional method to improve the therapeutic ratio.

Using different types of particulate radiation therapy has also been of some interest because of the ability to deliver highly conformal plans with these technologies. Proton beam therapy has been increasingly used because it takes advantage of the Bragg peak and deposits little energy in tissue until near the end of the proton range, where the residual energy is lost over a short distance, ideally the span of the tumor thickness. Heavy charged particles have also been thought to be advantageous, because there is an increase in linear energy transfer (LET) and increased energy deposition in the tissue. There are some data showing that higher LET radiation is less affected by tissue oxygenation and is less sensitive to variations in the cell cycle, which may be important in sarcomas [52]. Few studies in other tumor sites have demonstrated a statistically significant benefit of neutrons over photons, however, and this approach remains investigational.

Summary

Sarcomas represent a heterogeneous, challenging, and rare group of tumors that present many management challenges. Significant progress has already been made in determining the benefit of postoperative radiotherapy; the role of preoperative versus postoperative radiotherapy; and the indications for conformal technologies, such as brachytherapy and intraoperative therapy. Refinement of surgical and radiation techniques has improved functional and disease outcomes. Several management issues, including the sequencing of therapies, the benefit of chemotherapy, defining the subset of patients who are likely to benefit from radiotherapy, and the use of radiation sensitizers to improve local control, are all active areas of research. The use of highly conformal therapies, such as IMRT, and charged particles, such as protons, is being refined as well. There are clear indications for the use of radiation therapy to improve local control. The evaluation and management of patients who have sarcoma in a multidisciplinary setting are critical so that treatment is optimized and individualized for each patient.

Acknowledgments

This research was supported in part by the Intramural Research Program of the NIH. Special thanks to Jason Duelge and Scot Fisher with their assistance in the preparation of this manuscript.

References

[1] Jemal A, Siegel R, Ward E, et al. Cancer statistics, 2007. CA Cancer J Clin 2007;57(1):43–66.

[2] Cormier JN, Pollock RE. Soft tissue sarcomas. CA Cancer J Clin 2004;54(2):94–109.

[3] Hoekstra HJ, Thijssens K, Van Ginkel RJ. Role of surgery as primary treatment and as intervention in the multidisciplinary treatment of soft tissue sarcoma. Ann Oncol 2004; 15(Suppl 4):iv181–6.

[4] Rosenberg SA, Tepper J, Glatstein E, et al. The treatment of soft-tissue sarcomas of the extremities: prospective randomized evaluations of (1) limb-sparing surgery plus radiation therapy compared with amputation and (2) the role of adjuvant chemotherapy. Ann Surg 1982;196(3):305–15.

[5] Yang JC, Chang AE, Baker AR, et al. Randomized prospective study of the benefit of adjuvant radiation therapy in the treatment of soft tissue sarcomas of the extremity. J Clin Oncol 1998;16(1):197–203.

[6] Karakousis CP, Emrich LJ, Rao U, et al. Limb salvage in soft tissue sarcomas with selective combination of modalities. Eur J Surg Oncol 1991;17(1):71–80.

[7] Geer RJ, Woodruff J, Casper ES, et al. Management of small soft-tissue sarcoma of the extremity in adults. Arch Surg 1992;127(11):1285–9.

[8] LeVay J, O'Sullivan B, Catton C, et al. Outcome and prognostic factors in soft tissue sarcoma in the adult. Int J Radiat Oncol Biol Phys 1993;27(5):1091–9.

[9] O'Sullivan B, Davis AM, Turcotte R, et al. Preoperative versus postoperative radiotherapy in soft-tissue sarcoma of the limbs: a randomised trial. Lancet 2002;359(9325): 2235–41.

[10] Davis AM, O'Sullivan B, Turcotte R, et al. Late radiation morbidity following randomization to preoperative versus postoperative radiotherapy in extremity soft tissue sarcoma. Radiother Oncol 2005;75(1):48–53.

[11] Davis AM, O'Sullivan B, Bell RS, et al. Function and health status outcomes in a randomized trial comparing preoperative and postoperative radiotherapy in extremity soft tissue sarcoma. J Clin Oncol 2002;20(22):4472–7.

[12] Fein DA, Lee WR, Lanciano RM, et al. Management of extremity soft tissue sarcomas with limb-sparing surgery and postoperative irradiation: do total dose, overall treatment time, and the surgery-radiotherapy interval impact on local control? Int J Radiat Oncol Biol Phys 1995;32(4):969–76.

[13] Pisters PW, Harrison LB, Leung DH, et al. Long-term results of a prospective randomized trial of adjuvant brachytherapy in soft tissue sarcoma. J Clin Oncol 1996;14(3):859–68.

[14] Nag S, Shasha D, Janjan N, et al. The American Brachytherapy Society recommendations for brachytherapy of soft tissue sarcomas. Int J Radiat Oncol Biol Phys 2001;49(4):1033–43.

[15] Tierney JF, Mosseri V, Stewart LA, et al. Adjuvant chemotherapy for soft-tissue sarcoma: review and meta-analysis of the published results of randomised clinical trials. Br J Cancer 1995;72(2):469–75.

[16] Bramwell V, Rouesse J, Steward W, et al. Adjuvant CYVADIC chemotherapy for adult soft tissue sarcoma—reduced local recurrence but no improvement in survival: a study of the European Organization for Research and Treatment of Cancer Soft Tissue and Bone Sarcoma Group. J Clin Oncol 1994;12(6):1137–49.

[17] Frustaci S, Gherlinzoni F, De Paoli A, et al. Adjuvant chemotherapy for adult soft tissue sarcomas of the extremities and girdles: results of the Italian randomized cooperative trial. J Clin Oncol 2001;19(5):1238–47.

[18] Pisters PW, Patel SR, Varma DG, et al. Preoperative chemotherapy for stage IIIB extremity soft tissue sarcoma: long-term results from a single institution. J Clin Oncol 1997;15(12): 3481–7.

[19] Available at: www.clinicaltrials.gov. Accessed December 1, 2007.

[20] DeLaney TF, Spiro IJ, Suit HD, et al. Neoadjuvant chemotherapy and radiotherapy for large extremity soft-tissue sarcomas. Int J Radiat Oncol Biol Phys 2003;56(4):1117–27.

[21] Kraybill WG, Harris J, Spiro IJ, et al. Phase II study of neoadjuvant chemotherapy and radiation therapy in the management of high-risk, high-grade, soft tissue sarcomas of the extremities and body wall: Radiation Therapy Oncology Group Trial 9514. J Clin Oncol 2006;24(4):619–25.

[22] Kepka L, DeLaney TF, Suit HD, et al. Results of radiation therapy for unresected soft-tissue sarcomas. Int J Radiat Oncol Biol Phys 2005;63(3):852–9.

[23] Kepka L, Suit HD, Goldberg SI, et al. Results of radiation therapy performed after unplanned surgery (without re-excision) for soft tissue sarcomas. J Surg Oncol 2005;92(1): 39–45.

[24] DeLaney TF, Kepka L, Goldberg SI, et al. Radiation therapy for control of soft-tissue sarcomas resected with positive margins. Int J Radiat Oncol Biol Phys 2007;67(5):1460–9.

[25] Slater JD, McNeese MD, Peters LJ. Radiation therapy for unresectable soft tissue sarcomas. Int J Radiat Oncol Biol Phys 1986;12(10):1729–34.

[26] Tepper JE, Suit HD. Radiation therapy alone for sarcoma of soft tissue. Cancer 1985;56(3): 475–9.

[27] DeLaney TF, Trofimov AV, Engelsman M, et al. Advanced-technology radiation therapy in the management of bone and soft tissue sarcomas. Cancer Control 2005;12(1):27–35.

[28] Alektiar KM, Hong L, Brennan MF, et al. Intensity modulated radiation therapy for primary soft tissue sarcoma of the extremity: preliminary results. Int J Radiat Oncol Biol Phys 2007;68(2):458–64.

[29] Griffin AM, Euler CI, Sharpe MB, et al. Radiation planning comparison for superficial tissue avoidance in radiotherapy for soft tissue sarcoma of the lower extremity. Int J Radiat Oncol Biol Phys 2007;67(3):847–56.

[30] Dileo P, Morgan JA, Zahrieh D, et al. Gemcitabine and vinorelbine combination chemotherapy for patients with advanced soft tissue sarcomas: results of a phase II trial. Cancer 2007; 109(9):1863–9.

[31] Hegazy MA, Kotb SZ, Sakr H, et al. Preoperative isolated limb infusion of doxorubicin and external irradiation for limb-threatening soft tissue sarcomas. Ann Surg Oncol 2007;14(2): 568–76.

[32] Hayes AJ, Neuhaus SJ, Clark MA, et al. Isolated limb perfusion with melphalan and tumor necrosis factor alpha for advanced melanoma and soft-tissue sarcoma. Ann Surg Oncol 2007;14(1):230–8.

[33] Grunhagen DJ, De Wilt JH, Graveland WJ, et al. Outcome and prognostic factor analysis of 217 consecutive isolated limb perfusions with tumor necrosis factor-alpha and melphalan for limb-threatening soft tissue sarcoma. Cancer 2006;106(8):1776–84.

[34] Hoven-Gondrie ML, Thijssens KM, Van den Dungen JJ, et al. Long-term locoregional vascular morbidity after isolated limb perfusion and external-beam radiotherapy for soft tissue sarcoma of the extremity. Ann Surg Oncol 2007;14(7):2105–12.

[35] Van Ginkel RJ, Thijssens KM, Pras E, et al. Isolated limb perfusion with tumor necrosis factor alpha and melphalan for locally advanced soft tissue sarcoma: three time periods at risk for amputation. Ann Surg Oncol 2007;14(4):1499–506.

[36] Zlotecki RA, Katz TS, Morris CG, et al. Adjuvant radiation therapy for resectable retroperitoneal soft tissue sarcoma: the University of Florida experience. Am J Clin Oncol 2005; 28(3):310–6.

[37] Feng M, Murphy J, Griffith KA, et al. Long-term outcomes after radiotherapy for retroperitoneal and deep truncal sarcoma. Int J Radiat Oncol Biol Phys 2007;69(1): 103–10.

[38] Youssef E, Fontanesi J, Mott M, et al. Long-term outcome of combined modality therapy in retroperitoneal and deep-trunk soft-tissue sarcoma: analysis of prognostic factors. Int J Radiat Oncol Biol Phys 2002;54(2):514–9.

[39] Stoeckle E, Coindre JM, Bonvalot S, et al. Prognostic factors in retroperitoneal sarcoma: a multivariate analysis of a series of 165 patients of the French Cancer Center Federation Sarcoma Group. Cancer 2001;92(2):359–68.

[40] Jones JJ, Catton CN, O'Sullivan B, et al. Initial results of a trial of preoperative external-beam radiation therapy and postoperative brachytherapy for retroperitoneal sarcoma. Ann Surg Oncol 2002;9(4):346–54.

[41] Pisters PW, Ballo MT, Fenstermacher MJ, et al. Phase I trial of preoperative concurrent doxorubicin and radiation therapy, surgical resection, and intraoperative electron-beam radiation therapy for patients with localized retroperitoneal sarcoma. J Clin Oncol 2003; 21(16):3092–7.

[42] Pawlik TM, Pisters PW, Mikula L, et al. Long-term results of two prospective trials of preoperative external beam radiotherapy for localized intermediate- or high-grade retroperitoneal soft tissue sarcoma. Ann Surg Oncol 2006;13(4):508–17.

[43] Gieschen HL, Spiro IJ, Suit HD, et al. Long-term results of intraoperative electron beam radiotherapy for primary and recurrent retroperitoneal soft tissue sarcoma. Int J Radiat Oncol Biol Phys 2001;50(1):127–31.

[44] Gilbeau L, Kantor G, Stoeckle E, et al. Surgical resection and radiotherapy for primary retroperitoneal soft tissue sarcoma. Radiother Oncol 2002;65(3):137–43.

[45] Ballo MT, Zagars GK, Pollock RE, et al. Retroperitoneal soft tissue sarcoma: an analysis of radiation and surgical treatment. Int J Radiat Oncol Biol Phys 2007;67(1):158–63.

[46] Tzeng CW, Fiveash JB, Popple RA, et al. Preoperative radiation therapy with selective dose escalation to the margin at risk for retroperitoneal sarcoma. Cancer 2006;107(2): 371–9.

[47] Pezner RD, Liu A, Han C, et al. Dosimetric comparison of helical tomotherapy treatment and step-and-shoot intensity-modulated radiotherapy of retroperitoneal sarcoma. Radiother Oncol 2006;81(1):81–7.

damaging hemorrhagic cystitis that occurs when ifosfamide is given without uroprotection [7]. Dacarbazine (DTIC) is another agent frequently used in combination regimens for the treatment of STSs; it can be used in combination with doxorubicin and ifosfamide [9] or alone as a single agent.

To improve on the response rates seen with single-agent therapies, there have been several important randomized trials of combination chemotherapy conducted by the large cooperative groups. The Eastern Cooperative Oncology Group (ECOG) conducted a series of randomized trials comparing single-agent doxorubicin with combination regimens [10,11]. Higher response rates were observed for regimens combining doxorubicin with ifosfamide and doxorubicin with DTIC. The overall response rate was 20% for doxorubicin alone, and 34% for ifosfamide and doxorubicin, with the difference between the regimens being significant ($P = .04$). The median lengths of survival were 8.8 months and 11.5 months, respectively, for the two regimens. The combination therapies offered no overall survival advantage, however, and were associated with significantly higher toxicity. The European Organization for Research and Treatment of Cancer (EORTC) performed a phase III randomized trial comparing doxorubicin (50 mg/m^2) and ifosfamide (5 g/m^2) with a higher dose of doxorubicin (75 mg/m^2) and ifosfamide (5 g/m^2) with granulocyte-macrophage colony-stimulating factor (GM-CSF) (250 μg/m^2) support. There was no apparent difference in response rate or survival [12]. In 1989, Elias and colleagues [9] performed a phase II trial evaluating doxorubicin, ifosfamide, and DTIC. The overall response rate was 47%, with a notable 10% complete response (CR) rate. It is debatable whether the addition of DTIC to the doxorubicin and ifosfamide regimens adds enough significant benefit to outweigh the added toxicity; therefore, many institutions leave this drug out of the multidrug combinations.

Beyond doxorubicin and ifosfamide

Docetaxel (Taxotere) has been evaluated and is marginally active as a single agent [13,14] in sarcomas other than angiosarcoma [15], in which it has been used with good response. Gemcitabine (Gemzar) is minimally effective as a single agent based on phase II data, with 3 (7%) of 46 patients demonstrating a partial response and 8 patients (20%) with stable disease [16]. Maki and colleagues [17,18] published results from a phase II randomized trial using gemcitabine and docetaxel as a combination therapy compared with gemcitabine alone. The combination therapy had a response evaluation criteria in solid tumors (RECIST) rate of 16%, compared with 8% in the single-agent arm. There seemed to be a slightly more favorable response in leiomyosarcomas, and particularly in uterine leiomyosarcomas. A retrospective study published by Bay and colleagues [19] examining the same regimen did not find a statistically significant difference between leiomyosarcomas and other soft tissue tumor histologic subtypes.

Facial and scalp angiosarcomas have responded favorably to paclitaxel [20], and the taxanes have generally been shown to be efficacious in case report studies in angiosarcomas at other sites, alone or in combination with other cytotoxic chemotherapies [21–23]. Furthermore, there have been published case report responses to pegylated liposomal doxorubicin (Doxil) [24] in angiosarcomas and in two phase II studies that revealed some promise in various other sarcoma subtypes [25,26]. Whether there is any utility to using these therapies in the adjuvant setting remains to be seen; unfortunately, the overall small subpatient populations make it difficult to perform appropriately powered studies.

Adjuvant chemotherapy

The role of adjuvant chemotherapy for the treatment of STS is controversial. After adequate local treatment for STS, 50% of patients invariably relapse with local or distant disease and 45% die of sarcoma within 5 years [27]. Adjuvant systemic therapy has proved benefit in several malignancies, notably breast cancer [28], and has also been used extensively in pediatric sarcomas, such as osteosarcoma and Ewing's sarcoma [29,30]. The goal of treating micrometastatic disease after addressing local disease becomes an important one, and starting in the early 1980s, investigators began to analyze whether adjuvant therapy aided in controlling sarcoma recurrences and, more importantly, overall survival. The Swedish Sarcoma Group (SSG) began an adjuvant study from 1981 to 1986 that accrued 240 patients who had high-grade STSs, randomized to four different groups based on margin status. Patients with adequate surgery received doxorubicin versus control, whereas patients with marginal surgery received adjuvant radiation and doxorubicin or radiation without doxorubicin. At a median follow-up of 40 months, the study was deemed negative because there was no significant difference between the four treatment groups in overall survival, disease-free survival, or local tumor control [31].

An interim analysis of a randomized phase III trial presented at the American Society of Clinical Oncology (ASCO) meeting in 2007 by the EORTC has thus far failed to show a survival advantage for adjuvant chemotherapy in STS [32]. This is contrasted with the 1997 meta-analysis published in *The Lancet* by the Sarcoma Meta-Analysis Collaboration, which provided evidence of statistically significant improvement in the overall recurrence-free survival and time to local and distant recurrence [33]. This study was a quantitative meta-analysis of 14 studies and examined the individual patient data of 1568 patients comparing adjuvant doxorubicin-based therapy versus no therapy in localized STS. Results of the meta-analysis provided evidence that adjuvant doxorubicin therapy significantly improved time to local recurrence and distant metastases in addition to recurrence-free survival. There was a trend toward overall survival, with an overall survival advantage of 4% ($P = .12$), and in a subset analysis of extremity sarcomas (n = 886), there was a 7% benefit in survival ($P = .029$) [33]. In a recent update of the meta-analysis presented in oral abstract form at the 2007 Connective Tissue Oncology Society, this trend was shown to be statistically significant. Four new eligible and adequately randomized trials were identified from their previously used search criteria. These trials involved a total of 385 patients, allowing for the total population to reach 1953 patients. The hazard ratio with adjuvant chemotherapy for local recurrence was 0.73 (95% confidence interval [CI], 0.56–0.95). This corresponded to a 4% absolute risk reduction (ARR). For distant recurrence, the hazard ratio was 0.65 (95% CI, 0.53–0.80), representing a 9% ARR. Finally, for overall recurrence, the hazard ratio was 0.67 (95% CI, 0.56–0.82), signifying a 10% ARR [34]. At the time the abstract was presented at the Connective Tissue Oncology Society meeting, the large EORTC adjuvant trial had not been included in the meta-analysis update. Because this is one of the largest adjuvant trials to date, and has thus far not shown a trend toward improved overall survival, this is likely to have a significant impact on the meta-analysis results. Another smaller study by the Italian Sarcoma Group examining adjuvant chemotherapy in extremity STSs reported a survival advantage in patients who had high-grade sarcomas of the extremities treated with a regimen of epidoxorubicin, ifosfamide, and mesna [35]. After a longer follow-up period with a median follow-up of 89.6 months, however, the overall disease-free survival and overall survival were not found to be statistically significant. Of note, however, compared with the original published data, the differences in median time to progression (31.2 months), median survival (not reached versus 48.6 months), and survival at 4 years (69.8% versus 52.2%) continued to suggest an advantage for the treatment group [36].

Perhaps even the small potential benefit of adjuvant chemotherapy would be worth attempting if it were not for the substantial and well-documented short-term and long-term toxicities of chemotherapy. Short-term side effects and toxicities from single-agent and combination regimens include alopecia, myelosuppression with possible infection, nausea, vomiting, diarrhea, mucositis, and neurologic compromise. The most notable long-term toxicities include cardiomyopathy, which increases with the increasing cumulative dose of anthracycline, the possibility of secondary leukemias, and nephrotoxicity.

Outside of a clinical trial, adjuvant chemotherapy in the care of STS needs to be discussed with patients on an individual basis. We await the final updated published results of the Sarcoma Meta-Analysis Collaboration and of the EORTC adjuvant trial. Despite the larger number of patients included in the adjuvant trials, however, the inclusion of such a heterogeneous group of patients within one study makes broad treatment recommendations difficult.

Neoadjuvant chemotherapy

There has been much attention given to the use of neoadjuvant therapy in the care of STS, especially in high-risk extremity STS. There are several theoretic advantages that neoadjuvant therapy could lend to patient management. First, by treating a patient who has visible disease, one has an in vivo tumor response model, using radiologic imaging and pathologic response after resection as a means to evaluate disease response. Furthermore, by potentially shrinking a tumor and enabling less morbid operations, for example, there is a better possibility of limb salvage in STSs of the extremity and less opportunity for viable tissue to spread at the time of resection. Finally, by documenting which patients respond to chemotherapy, patients who do not respond adequately are spared further cytotoxic therapy in the postoperative setting or additional chemotherapeutic agents can be added for synergistic or additive cytotoxic effects.

The theoretic disadvantage to neoadjuvant chemotherapy is the peri- and postoperative complications that could potentially be caused by chemotherapy, and the resulting myelosuppression and wound healing limitations. There has been one retrospective study evaluating this specific hypothesis by Meric and colleagues [37], in which 309 patients who presented to a single institution for definitive surgical management of primary STS were retrospectively reviewed. One hundred five patients who received neoadjuvant chemotherapy before surgery were compared with 204 patients who underwent surgery first. There was no evidence to support neoadjuvant chemotherapy increasing postoperative morbidity.

Despite evidence supporting that neoadjuvant chemotherapy does not have a negative impact during the postsurgical period, there has been little evidence to support the use of neoadjuvant chemotherapy in STSs [38–40]. A prime example of the underwhelming outcome of neoadjuvant therapy was an EORTC randomized controlled trial comparing neoadjuvant doxorubicin and ifosfamide in high-risk adult STS. This study failed to show any differences in 5-year disease-free survival (56% versus 52%) or overall survival (65% versus 64%). The study closed early because of poor patient accrual; therefore, it was underpowered [40]. Treatment-induced pathologic necrosis was examined in an interesting article by Eilber and colleagues [41] to determine whether pathologic necrosis correlated with local recurrence and overall survival in patients who received neo-adjuvant therapy for high-grade extremity sarcomas. A total of 496 patients who had intermediate- and high-grade extremity sarcomas received one of five different protocols using radiation with doxorubicin alone; doxorubicin and cisplatin; or doxorubicin, cisplatin, and ifosfamide. The 5- and 10-year local recurrence rates for patients found to have 95% or greater pathologic necrosis were significantly lower (6% and 11%, respectively) than those for the patients with less than 95% pathologic necrosis (17% and 23%, respectively). The patients who achieved 95% or greater pathologic necrosis increased to 48% with the addition of ifosfamide as compared with 13% in all other neoadjuvant protocols combined. A separate retrospective analysis evaluated the impact of neoadjuvant chemotherapy on the extent of the surgical procedure in 65 patients and the hypothesis that radiographic response to neoadjuvant chemotherapy predicts improved local control and survival. In patients who had stage II and III limb and retroperitoneal STS, only 8 patients (13%) showed a response significant enough to allow their operation to be reduced, and in another six cases (9%), there was actually disease progression, and therefore an increase in the extent of the operation. Of nine extremity sarcoma cases that were thought to require amputation before preoperative therapy, none were able to proceed with limb-sparing operations [42]. One encouraging study published by the Radiation Therapy Oncology Group (RTOG) evaluated patients who had high-grade STS 8 cm or greater in diameter of the extremities and body wall. Patients received three cycles of neoadjuvant mesna, adriamycin, ifosfamide, and DTIC (MAID), interdigitated with preoperative radiation, and then three cycles of postoperative MAID. Although only 59% of patients in this multi-institutional trial actually were able to finish all six cycles of chemotherapy, 22% of 59 assessable patients had partial responses by RECIST criteria, 64% had stable disease, and 8 patients (14%) had progressive disease. There was substantial toxicity in this trial. There were three deaths (5%) associated with treatment, and 84% of patients experienced grade 4 toxicity. The investigators concluded that outside of a clinical trial, the use of this particular regimen was not recommended [43].

New strategies

With the introduction of small-molecule inhibitors like imatinib (Gleevec) and the enormous success they have had in patients who have metastatic gastrointestinal stromal tumors (GISTs), there has been a shift away from developing further cytotoxic therapies for sarcoma or combining different cytoxic chemotherapeutics and a turn toward molecularly targeted therapies. Furthermore, in the recent GIST adjuvant trials, imatinib has thus far been quite impressive in the postoperative setting, albeit with many as of yet unanswered questions, leading investigators to explore the concept of using more molecularly targeted therapeutics for adjuvant treatment or maintenance therapy in STS [44,45].

Targeting angiogenesis

The humanized antivascular endothelial growth factor (VEGF) antibody, bevacizumab (Avastin), when used in combination with chemotherapy, has been shown to be beneficial in tumor response rates and in overall survival in metastatic colorectal cancer, breast cancer, and lung cancer [46–48]. Many STSs can overexpress VEGF [49,50]; therefore, this is thought to be a viable target and is being evaluated currently in ongoing trials. A recent article by Zhou and colleagues [51] reported on significant responses in an Ewing's sarcoma mouse xenograft model when treated with DC101 antibody, an inhibitor of VEGF-2. A phase II study evaluating doxorubicin and bevacizumab in patients who had STS found no higher rate of response beyond that seen with single-agent doxorubicin; however, 65% of patients had stable disease lasting four cycles or longer, prompting the investigators to conclude that further study is warranted. There was substantial cardiac toxicity noted in the trial, with 6 of 17 patients developing cardiac toxicity of grade 2 or more [52].

Sorafenib (Nexavar) is an effective inhibitor of several receptor tyrosine kinases involved in tumor-angiogenesis, including Raf-1, VEGFR-2 and VEGFR-3, platelet-derived growth factor receptor (PDGFR), Flt-3, and c-Kit [53]. It has recently been approved for the treatment of advanced renal cell carcinoma because of these properties, and there are several ongoing phase II studies evaluating its use in locally advanced and metastatic STSs.

Similarly, sunitinib (Sutent), which has been approved for second-line therapy in GIST, is being evaluated in several ongoing phase II studies in STSs, alone or in combination with other chemotherapeutics like ifosfamide.

Thalidomide (Thalomid), an immunomodulatory and antiangiogenic drug, has been evaluated in phase II trials of uterine leiomyosarcomas and found to have little impact on disease response and overall survival [54]. It has been used extensively and with good results in AIDS and non–AIDS-related Kaposi's sarcoma [55,56], but its use is often limited by side effects, including deep venous thrombosis.

Apo 2L/Tumor necrosis factor–related apoptosis-inducing ligand

Tumor necrosis factor–related apoptosis-inducing ligand (TRAIL) receptor 2 (TR-2) is a member of the tumor necrosis factor (TNF) gene superfamily of receptors. TRAIL is the natural ligand for TR-2, and its binding to the receptor initiates an intracellular caspase cascade and induces apoptosis through engagement of death receptors in several transformed human cell lines [57]. Ewing's sarcoma cell lines have been shown to express high levels of TR-1 and TR-2 by immunohistochemistry [58]. Furthermore, in vitro models have shown TRAIL to induce apoptosis in multiple sarcoma subtypes with activity enhanced with concurrent chemotherapy [59–61]. A phase I study evaluating Apomab, a human DR5 agonist antibody, in patients who had advanced cancer was reported in abstract form at the 2007 ASCO meeting. At the time of the presentation, there was one minor response seen in a patient who had colorectal cancer. There are several phase II trials currently evaluating these drugs in patients who have sarcoma [62].

Mammalian target of rapamycin inhibitors

Mammalian target of rapamycin (mTOR) is a member of the phosphatidylinositol $3'$ kinase-related kinase family, which can regulate protein translation, cell cycle progression, and cellular proliferation [63,64]. Rapamycin's antitumor activity is thought to occur through cell cycle arrest in the G1 phase [64]. In early phase I studies, there seemed to be demonstrable responses in patients who had sarcoma [65]. There are currently three different drugs inhibiting the mTOR pathway that are being evaluated: RAD-001 (everolimus), CCI-779 (temsirolimus), and AP23573 (deforolimus). Several phase II trials have been recently completed with results pending, and a phase III maintenance study of AP23573 is about to commence in sarcoma. An update of the phase II trial of AP23573 in patients who have advanced sarcomas was reported at ASCO 2006 meeting. Clinical best response (partial and stable disease) was reported in 30% of bone sarcomas, 36% of leiomyosarcomas, 22% of liposarcomas, and 22% of other sarcomas. For each cohort, treatment was defined as active if the proportion of patients with clinical best response for at least 16 weeks was more than 25% [66,67].

Ecteinascidin-743

Ecteinascidin-743 (ET-743 [Yondelis]) is a novel chemotherapeutic originally derived from the Caribbean sea squirt, *Ecteinascidia turbinate*, and now produced synthetically. It is a tertahydroisoquinolone alkaloid that binds the minor groove of DNA and blocks cell cycle progression in the G2 and M phases and blocks the organization and assembly of the microtubular cytoskeleton [68,69]. Preclinical studies have shown in vitro activity of ET-743, and in vivo studies have shown tumor response in a xenograft model [69–72]. A phase I trial using a continuous 24-hour infusion schedule showed promise in liposarcoma and osteosarcoma [73]. The most common toxicities included bone marrow suppression and liver function abnormalities. Two phase II studies in patients who had been pretreated with doxorubicin and ifosfamide or combination therapy reported objective response rates in 8% and 6% of patients, with an additional 35% and 50% of patients achieving stable disease for longer than 2 months [74–77]. In a phase II front-line study, one complete and five partial responses were achieved in 35 assessable patients for an overall response rate of 17.1%, with an overall clinical benefit of 20% [78]. Because of encouraging results, specifically in patients who have liposarcoma, 51 patients who had advanced pretreated myxoid liposarcomas and were treated in a compassionate use program at five separate institutions were evaluated retrospectively. ET-743 was given as a 24-hour infusion or as a 3-hour infusion every 21 days. Two patients had complete responses defined by RECIST, and 24 patients had partial responses, with an overall response rate of 51%. Median progression-free survival was 14.0 months, and progression free survival at 6 months was 88% [79].

Insulin-like growth factor-I inhibitors

Small-molecule insulin-like growth factor-1 receptor (IGF-1R) inhibitors have recently been shown to be clinically active in patients who have

Ewing's sarcoma in phase I studies and in preclinical studies [80], and there are several phase II studies being initiated at the present time to evaluate this class of drugs in sarcoma. IGF-1R is a tyrosine kinase cell surface receptor that has approximately 70% homology with the insulin receptor [81]. IGF-1R has been linked to autocrine and paracrine control of sarcoma growth, and inhibition of the receptor reduces growth, increases apoptosis of sarcoma cells in vivo and in vitro, and is thought to reduce the metastatic potential of tumors [81–85]. In a preclinical study evaluating NVP-AEW541, an IGF-1R kinase inhibitor, impairment of the IGF-1R was found to contribute substantially to control of malignancy in musculoskeletal tumors, especially in Ewing's sarcoma cell lines [86].

The future

Despite considerable attention to musculoskeletal tumors over the last 20 to 30 years, little has changed for the treatment of STS, with clinicians still reaching for doxorubicin as a front-line agent based on literature first reported in 1973 [87]. It is difficult to perform well-powered randomized controlled studies in rare tumors, and there is active interest in developing avenues by which investigators can expedite the approval of new drugs that are found to be effective in phase II trials. With continued research into the molecular biology and genetic aberrations associated with the many different subtypes of sarcoma, investigators should be able to identify new targets for therapeutic intervention. Given the recent encouraging results reported in the interim analysis of the adjuvant imatinib study in GIST at the ASCO 2007 meeting, perhaps focusing efforts on finding molecularly targeted agents that can be used in the adjuvant setting would prove more encouraging than the cytotoxic adjuvant studies performed thus far.

Summary

STSs are a heterogeneous group of connective tissue tumors, with more than 50 different subtypes. Given the heterogeneity, and the relative small numbers of patients, performing large adequately powered clinical trials in which one can glean any overall broad treatment decisions based on outcome is difficult at best. There is controversy on which chemotherapeutic agents to use in the adjuvant and metastatic settings, or even if to use chemotherapy in the adjuvant setting. In the metastatic setting, doxorubicin and ifosfamide have remained the standards of care for more than 20 years. With the introduction of what can be considered more targeted agents, however, we might be entering a new era of sarcoma management, and figuring out how to use these agents best is likely to remain a challenging therapeutic question in the years to come.

References

[1] Verweij J, Van Oosterom AT, Somers R, et al. Chemotherapy in the multidisciplinary approach to soft tissue sarcomas. EORTC Soft Tissue and Bone Sarcoma Group studies in perspective. Ann Oncol 1992;3(Suppl 2):S75–80.

[2] Borden EC, Amato DA, Edmonson JH, et al. Randomized comparison of doxorubicin and vindesine to doxorubicin for patients with metastatic soft-tissue sarcomas. Cancer 1990; 66(5):862–7.

[3] Casper ES, Gaynor JJ, Hajdu SI, et al. A prospective randomized trial of adjuvant chemotherapy with bolus versus continuous infusion of doxorubicin in patients with high-grade extremity soft tissue sarcoma and an analysis of prognostic factors. Cancer 1991;68(6): 1221–9.

[4] Benjamin RS, Wiernik PH, Bachur NR. Adriamycin: a new effective agent in the therapy of disseminated sarcomas. Med Pediatr Oncol 1975;1(1):63–76.

[5] Antman KH. Chemotherapy of advanced sarcomas of bone and soft tissue. Semin Oncol 1992;19(6 Suppl 12):13–20.

[6] Elias AD. Chemotherapy for soft-tissue sarcomas. Clin Orthop Relat Res 1993;289:94–105.

[7] Elias AD, Eder JP, Shea T, et al. High-dose ifosfamide with mesna uroprotection: a phase I study. J Clin Oncol 1990;8(1):170–8.

[8] Antman KH, Elias A. Dana-Farber Cancer Institute studies in advanced sarcoma. Semin Oncol 1990;17(1 Suppl 2):7–15.

[9] Elias A, Ryan L, Sulkes A, et al. Response to mesna, doxorubicin, ifosfamide, and dacarbazine in 108 patients with metastatic or unresectable sarcoma and no prior chemotherapy. J Clin Oncol 1989;7(9):1208–16.

[10] Blum RH, Edmonson J, Ryan L, et al. Efficacy of ifosfamide in combination with doxorubicin for the treatment of metastatic soft-tissue sarcoma. The Eastern Cooperative Oncology Group. Cancer Chemother Pharmacol 1993;31(Suppl 2):S238–40.

[11] Antman K, Crowley J, Balcerzak SP, et al. An intergroup phase III randomized study of doxorubicin and dacarbazine with or without ifosfamide and mesna in advanced soft tissue and bone sarcomas. J Clin Oncol 1993;11(7):1276–85.

[12] Le Cesne A, Judson I, Crowther D, et al. Randomized phase III study comparing conventional-dose doxorubicin plus ifosfamide versus high-dose doxorubicin plus ifosfamide plus recombinant human granulocyte-macrophage colony-stimulating factor in advanced soft tissue sarcomas: a trial of the European Organization for Research and Treatment of Cancer/Soft Tissue and Bone Sarcoma Group. J Clin Oncol 2000; 18(14):2676–84.

[13] Van Hoesel QG, Verweij J, Catimel G, et al. Phase II study with docetaxel (Taxotere) in advanced soft tissue sarcomas of the adult. EORTC Soft Tissue and Bone Sarcoma Group. Ann Oncol 1994;5(6):539–42.

[14] Edmonson JH, Ebbert LP, Nascimento AG, et al. Phase II study of docetaxel in advanced soft tissue sarcomas. Am J Clin Oncol 1996;19(6):574–6.

[15] Nagano T, Yamada Y, Ikeda T, et al. Docetaxel: a therapeutic option in the treatment of cutaneous angiosarcoma: report of 9 patients. Cancer 2007;110(3):648–51.

[16] Von Burton G, Rankin C, Zalupski MM, et al. Phase II trial of gemcitabine as first line chemotherapy in patients with metastatic or unresectable soft tissue sarcoma. Am J Clin Oncol 2006;29(1):59–61.

[17] Maki RG, Wathen JK, Patel SR, et al. Randomized phase II study of gemcitabine and docetaxel compared with gemcitabine alone in patients with metastatic soft tissue sarcomas: results of Sarcoma Alliance for Research Through Collaboration Study 002 [corrected]. J Clin Oncol 2007;25(19):2755–63.

[18] Maki RG. Gemcitabine and docetaxel in metastatic sarcoma: past, present, and future. Oncologist 2007;12(8):999–1006.

[19] Bay JO, Ray-Coquard I, Fayette J, et al. Docetaxel and gemcitabine combination in 133 advanced soft-tissue sarcomas: a retrospective analysis. Int J Cancer 2006;119(3):706–11.

[20] Fata F, O'Reilly E, Ilson D, et al. Paclitaxel in the treatment of patients with angiosarcoma of the scalp or face. Cancer 1999;86(10):2034–7.

[21] Skubitz KM, Haddad PA. Paclitaxel and pegylated-liposomal doxorubicin are both active in angiosarcoma. Cancer 2005;104(2):361–6.

[22] Yamada M, Hatta N, Mizuno M, et al. Weekly low-dose docetaxel in the treatment of lung metastases from angiosarcoma of the head. Br J Dermatol 2005;152(4):811–2.

[23] Mathew P, Vakar-Lopez F, Troncoso P. Protracted remission of metastatic epithelioid angiosarcoma with weekly infusion of doxorubicin, paclitaxel, and cisplatin. Lancet Oncol 2006;7(1):92–3.

[24] Eiling S, Lischner S, Busch JO, et al. Complete remission of a radio-resistant cutaneous angiosarcoma of the scalp by systemic treatment with liposomal doxorubicin. Br J Dermatol 2002;147(1):150–3.

[25] Judson I, Radford JA, Harris M, et al. Randomised phase II trial of pegylated liposomal doxorubicin (DOXIL/CAELYX) versus doxorubicin in the treatment of advanced or metastatic soft tissue sarcoma: a study by the EORTC Soft Tissue and Bone Sarcoma Group. Eur J Cancer 2001;37(7):870–7.

[26] Skubitz KM. Phase II trial of pegylated-liposomal doxorubicin (Doxil) in sarcoma. Cancer Invest 2003;21(2):167–76.

[27] Greene F.L., American Joint Committee on Cancer, American Cancer Society. AJCC cancer staging handbook: from the AJCC cancer staging manual. 6th edition. New York: Springer; 2002.

[28] Early Breast Cancer Trialists' Collaborative Group (EBCTCG). Effects of chemotherapy and hormonal therapy for early breast cancer on recurrence and 15-year survival: an overview of the randomised trials. Lancet 2005;365(9472):1687–717.

[29] Bramwell VH. The role of chemotherapy in the management of non-metastatic operable extremity osteosarcoma. Semin Oncol 1997;24(5):561–71.

[30] Bacci G, Picci P, Gitelis S, et al. The treatment of localized Ewing's sarcoma: the experience at the Istituto Ortopedico Rizzoli in 163 cases treated with and without adjuvant chemotherapy. Cancer 1982;49(8):1561–70.

[31] Alvegard TA, Sigurdsson H, Mouridsen H, et al. Adjuvant chemotherapy with doxorubicin in high-grade soft tissue sarcoma: a randomized trial of the Scandinavian Sarcoma Group. J Clin Oncol 1989;7(10):1504–13.

[32] Woll PJ, Van Glabbeke M, Hohenberger P, et al. Adjuvant chemotherapy with doxorubicin and ifosfamide in resected soft tissue sarcoma: interim analysis of a randomized phase III trial. Presented at American Society of Clinical Oncology 2007 Meeting. Chicago, Illinois, June 1–5, 2007.

[33] Sarcoma Meta-analysis Collaboration. Adjuvant chemotherapy for localised resectable soft-tissue sarcoma of adults: meta-analysis of individual data. Lancet 1997;350(9092):1647–54.

[34] Pervaiz N, Colterjohn N, Farrokhyar Tozer R, et al. A systematic meta-analysis of randomized controlled trials for adjuvant chemotherapy for localized resectable soft-tissue sarcoma. Presented at Connective Tissue Oncology Society Meeting. Seattle, Washington, November 1–3, 2007.

[35] Frustaci S, Gherlinzoni F, De Paoli A, et al. Adjuvant chemotherapy for adult soft tissue sarcomas of the extremities and girdles: results of the Italian Randomized Cooperative Trial. J Clin Oncol 2001;19(5):1238–47.

[36] Frustaci S, De Paoli A, Bidoli E, et al. Ifosfamide in the adjuvant therapy of soft tissue sarcomas. Oncology 2003;65(Suppl 2):80–4.

[37] Meric F, Milas M, Hunt KK, et al. Impact of neoadjuvant chemotherapy on postoperative morbidity in soft tissue sarcomas. J Clin Oncol 2000;18(19):3378–83.

[38] Pisters PW, Patel SR, Varma DG, et al. Preoperative chemotherapy for stage IIIB extremity soft tissue sarcoma: long-term results from a single institution. J Clin Oncol 1997;15(12):3481–7.

[39] Grobmyer SR, Maki RG, Demetri GD, et al. Neo-adjuvant chemotherapy for primary high-grade extremity soft tissue sarcoma. Ann Oncol 2004;15(11):1667–72.

[40] Gortzak E, Azzarelli A, Buesa J, et al. A randomised phase II study on neo-adjuvant chemotherapy for 'high-risk' adult soft-tissue sarcoma. Eur J Cancer 2001;37(9):1096–103.

[41] Eilber FC, Rosen G, Eckardt J, et al. Treatment-induced pathologic necrosis: a predictor of local recurrence and survival in patients receiving neoadjuvant therapy for high-grade extremity soft tissue sarcomas. J Clin Oncol 2001;19(13):3203–9.

[42] Meric F, Hess KR, Varma DG, et al. Radiographic response to neoadjuvant chemotherapy is a predictor of local control and survival in soft tissue sarcomas. Cancer 2002;95(5): 1120–6.

[43] Kraybill WG, Harris J, Spiro IJ, et al. Phase II study of neoadjuvant chemotherapy and radiation therapy in the management of high-risk, high-grade, soft tissue sarcomas of the extremities and body wall: Radiation Therapy Oncology Group Trial 9514. J Clin Oncol 2006;24(4):619–25.

[44] DeMatteo R. Adjuvant imatinib mesylate increases recurrence free survival (RFS) in patients with completely resected localized primary gastrointestinal stromal tumor (GIST): North American Intergroup Phase III trial ACOSOG Z9001. Presented at American Society of Clinical Oncology Annual Meeting. Chicago, Illinois, June 1–5, 2007.

[45] Zhan WH. Efficacy and safety of adjuvant post-surgical therapy with imatinib in patients with high risk of relapsing GIST. Presented at American Society of Clinical Oncology Annual Meeting. Chicago, Illinois, June 1–5, 2007.

[46] Hurwitz H, Fehrenbacher L, Novotny W, et al. Bevacizumab plus irinotecan, fluorouracil, and leucovorin for metastatic colorectal cancer. N Engl J Med 2004;350(23):2335–42.

[47] Sandler A, Gray R, Perry MC, et al. Paclitaxel-carboplatin alone or with bevacizumab for non-small-cell lung cancer. N Engl J Med 2006;355(24):2542–50.

[48] Miller KD, Chap LI, Holmes FA, et al. Randomized phase III trial of capecitabine compared with bevacizumab plus capecitabine in patients with previously treated metastatic breast cancer. J Clin Oncol 2005;23(4):792–9.

[49] Chao C, Al-Saleem T, Brooks JJ, et al. Vascular endothelial growth factor and soft tissue sarcomas: tumor expression correlates with grade. Ann Surg Oncol 2001;8(3):260–7.

[50] Potti A, Ganti AK, Tendulkar K, et al. Determination of vascular endothelial growth factor (VEGF) overexpression in soft tissue sarcomas and the role of overexpression in leiomyosarcoma. J Cancer Res Clin Oncol 2004;130(1):52–6.

[51] Zhou Z, Bolontrade MF, Reddy K, et al. Suppression of Ewing's sarcoma tumor growth, tumor vessel formation, and vasculogenesis following anti vascular endothelial growth factor receptor-2 therapy. Clin Cancer Res 2007;13(16):4867–73.

[52] D'Adamo DR, Anderson SE, Albritton K, et al. Phase II study of doxorubicin and bevacizumab for patients with metastatic soft-tissue sarcomas. J Clin Oncol 2005;23(28): 7135–42.

[53] Strumberg D. Preclinical and clinical development of the oral multikinase inhibitor sorafenib in cancer treatment. Drugs Today (Barc) 2005;41(12):773–84.

[54] McMeekin DS, Sill MW, Darcy KM, et al. A phase II trial of thalidomide in patients with refractory leiomyosarcoma of the uterus and correlation with biomarkers of angiogenesis: a Gynecologic Oncology Group study. Gynecol Oncol 2007;106(3):596–603.

[55] Rubegni P, Sbano P, De Aloe G, et al. Thalidomide in the treatment of Kaposi's sarcoma. Dermatology 2007;215(3):240–4.

[56] Cattelan AM, Trevenzoli M, Aversa SM. Recent advances in the treatment of AIDS-related Kaposi's sarcoma. Am J Clin Dermatol 2002;3(7):451–62.

[57] Kelley SK, Ashkenazi A. Targeting death receptors in cancer with Apo2L/TRAIL. Curr Opin Pharmacol 2004;4(4):333–9.

[58] Mitsiades N, Poulaki V, Mitsiades C, et al. Ewing's sarcoma family tumors are sensitive to tumor necrosis factor-related apoptosis-inducing ligand and express death receptor 4 and death receptor 5. Cancer Res 2001;61(6):2704–12.

[59] Tomek S, Koestler W, Horak P, et al. TRAIL-induced apoptosis and interaction with cytotoxic agents in soft tissue sarcoma cell lines. Eur J Cancer 2003;39(9):1318–29.

[60] Merchant MS, Yang X, Melchionda F, et al. Interferon gamma enhances the effectiveness of tumor necrosis factor-related apoptosis-inducing ligand receptor agonists in a xenograft model of Ewing's sarcoma. Cancer Res 2004;64(22):8349–56.

[61] Kontny HU, Hammerle K, Klein R, et al. Sensitivity of Ewing's sarcoma to TRAIL-induced apoptosis. Cell Death Differ 2001;8(5):506–14.

[62] Camidge D. A phase I safety and pharmacokinetic study of apomab, a human DR5 agonist antibody, in patients with advanced cancer. Presented at American Society of Clinical Oncology Annual Meeting. Chicago, Illinois, June 1–5, 2007.

[63] Schmelzle T, Hall MN. TOR, a central controller of cell growth. Cell 2000;103(2):253–62.

[64] Okuno S. Mammalian target of rapamycin inhibitors in sarcomas. Curr Opin Oncol 2006; 18(4):360–2.

[65] Hidalgo M, Rowinsky EK. The rapamycin-sensitive signal transduction pathway as a target for cancer therapy. Oncogene 2000;19(56):6680–6.

[66] Chawla SP, Tolcher AW, Staddon AP, et al. ASCO annual meeting proceedings part I. J Clin Oncol 2006;24(18S):9505.

[67] Mita MM, Tolcher AW. The role of mTOR inhibitors for treatment of sarcomas. Curr Oncol Rep 2007;9(4):316–22.

[68] Pommier Y, Kohlhagen G, Bailly C, et al. DNA sequence- and structure-selective alkylation of guanine N2 in the DNA minor groove by ecteinascidin 743, a potent antitumor compound from the Caribbean tunicate ecteinascidia turbinata. Biochemistry 1996; 35(41):13303–9.

[69] Erba E, Bergamaschi D, Bassano L, et al. Ecteinascidin-743 (ET-743), a natural marine compound, with a unique mechanism of action. Eur J Cancer 2001;37(1):97–105.

[70] Li WW, Takahashi N, Jhanwar S, et al. Sensitivity of soft tissue sarcoma cell lines to chemotherapeutic agents: identification of ecteinascidin-743 as a potent cytotoxic agent. Clin Cancer Res 2001;7(9):2908–11.

[71] Scotlandi K, Perdichizzi S, Manara MC, et al. Effectiveness of ecteinascidin-743 against drug-sensitive and -resistant bone tumor cells. Clin Cancer Res 2002;8(12):3893–903.

[72] D'Incalci M, Colombo T, Ubezio P, et al. The combination of yondelis and cisplatin is synergistic against human tumor xenografts. Eur J Cancer 2003;39(13):1920–6.

[73] Taamma A, Misset JL, Riofrio M, et al. Phase I and pharmacokinetic study of ecteinascidin-743, a new marine compound, administered as a 24-hour continuous infusion in patients with solid tumors. J Clin Oncol 2001;19(5):1256–65.

[74] Demetri GD. ET-743: the US experience in sarcomas of soft tissues. Anticancer Drugs 2002; 13(Suppl 1):S7–9.

[75] Brain EG. Safety and efficacy of ET-743: the French experience. Anticancer Drugs 2002; 13(Suppl 1):S11–4.

[76] Garcia-Carbonero R, Supko JG, Manola J, et al. Phase II and pharmacokinetic study of ecteinascidin 743 in patients with progressive sarcomas of soft tissues refractory to chemotherapy. J Clin Oncol 2004;22(8):1480–90.

[77] Yovine A, Riofrio M, Blay JY, et al. Phase II study of ecteinascidin-743 in advanced pretreated soft tissue sarcoma patients. J Clin Oncol 2004;22(5):890–9.

[78] Garcia-Carbonero R, Supko JG, Maki RG, et al. Ecteinascidin-743 (ET-743) for chemotherapy-naive patients with advanced soft tissue sarcomas: multicenter phase II and pharmacokinetic study. J Clin Oncol 2005;23(24):5484–92.

[79] Grosso F, Jones RL, Demetri GD, et al. Efficacy of trabectedin (ecteinascidin-743) in advanced pretreated myxoid liposarcomas: a retrospective study. Lancet Oncol 2007;8(7): 595–602.

[80] Manara MC, Landuzzi L, Nanni P, et al. Preclinical in vivo study of new insulin-like growth factor-I receptor–specific inhibitor in Ewing's sarcoma. Clin Cancer Res 2007;13(4): 1322–30.

[81] Baserga R. The insulin-like growth factor-I receptor as a target for cancer therapy. Expert Opin Ther Targets 2005;9(4):753–68.

[82] Toretsky JA, Kalebic T, Blakesley V, et al. The insulin-like growth factor-I receptor is required for EWS/FLI-1 transformation of fibroblasts. J Biol Chem 1997;272(49):30822–7.

[83] MacEwen EG, Pastor J, Kutzke J, et al. IGF-1 receptor contributes to the malignant phenotype in human and canine osteosarcoma. J Cell Biochem 2004;92(1):77–91.

[84] De Alava E, Panizo A, Antonescu CR, et al. Association of EWS-FLI1 type 1 fusion with lower proliferative rate in Ewing's sarcoma. Am J Pathol 2000;156(3):849–55.

[85] Scotlandi K, Benini S, Sarti M, et al. Insulin-like growth factor I receptor-mediated circuit in Ewing's sarcoma/peripheral neuroectodermal tumor: a possible therapeutic target. Cancer Res 1996;56(20):4570–4.

[86] Scotlandi K, Manara MC, Nicoletti G, et al. Antitumor activity of the insulin-like growth factor-I receptor kinase inhibitor NVP-AEW541 in musculoskeletal tumors. Cancer Res 2005;65(9):3868–76.

[87] O'Bryan RM, Luce JK, Talley RW, et al. Phase II evaluation of adriamycin in human neoplasia. Cancer 1973;32(1):1–8.

ELSEVIER
SAUNDERS

Surg Clin N Am 88 (2008) 661–672

SURGICAL
CLINICS OF
NORTH AMERICA

Multidisciplinary Management of Metastatic Sarcoma

Katherine Thornton, MD[a],*, Catherine E. Pesce, MD[b], Michael A. Choti, MD, MBA[c],*

[a]Department of Medical Oncology, The Sidney Kimmel Comprehensive Cancer Center at Johns Hopkins, 1650 Orleans Street, CRB I Room 1M88, Baltimore, MD 21231, USA
[b]Department of Surgery, The Johns Hopkins University School of Medicine, 600 North Wolfe Street, Blalock 665, Baltimore, MD 21287, USA
[c]The Johns Hopkins University School of Medicine, 600 North Wolfe Street, Blalock 665, Baltimore, MD 21287, USA

Approximately 8300 new cases of soft tissue sarcoma (STS) are diagnosed annually in the United States, yet fewer than 50% of patients receive curative treatment with current treatment modalities. Accounting for approximately 1% of all adult malignancies, STS comprise a heterogeneous group of malignancies of mesenchymal origin. Although sarcomas can arise virtually anywhere, the most common primary site is the extremity [1].

STS tend to metastasize hematogenously, with a predilection for the lungs and, less frequently, the liver and bone [2,3]. Lymphangitic spread is uncommon (<10%), except for certain histologic types such as rhabdomyosarcoma [4]. About 10% of patients present with metastatic disease, and almost one quarter of patients with localized disease develop metachronous metastases [5,6]. This percentage increases up to 70% for patients with high-grade STS [4]. As mentioned, pulmonary metastases account for the most common site of distant spread from this disease. In particular, patients with *extremity* sarcoma develop isolated pulmonary metastatic disease at some point during the course of their disease in about 20% of cases [3]. Although pulmonary metastases most commonly arise from primary tumors in the extremities, they may arise from almost any histologic variant or primary site [7].

* Corresponding author. Department of Medical Oncology, The Sidney Kimmel Comprehensive Cancer Center at Johns Hopkins, 1650 Orleans Street, CRB I Room 1M88, Baltimore, MD 21231.
  E-mail addresses: kthornt2@jhmi.edu (K. Thornton); mchoti1@jhmi.edu (M.A. Choti).

0039-6109/08/$ - see front matter © 2008 Elsevier Inc. All rights reserved.
doi:10.1016/j.suc.2008.04.002
surgical.theclinics.com

An analysis of the distribution of primary histology and grade demonstrates that, among patients in whom lung metastases develop, leiomyosarcoma is most common, followed by undifferentiated high-grade pleomorphic sarcoma, liposarcoma, and synovial sarcoma. The incidence of pulmonary metastases within each histologic group correlates with the incidence of high-grade lesions within that group. Undifferentiated sarcomas have the highest percentage with lung metastases and a significant percentage of high-grade lesions. Alveolar, synovial, and epithelioid sarcomas also represent a major proportion of high-grade lesions with high rates of pulmonary metastases. Fibrosarcoma has a low incidence of high-grade histology as well as a low frequency of pulmonary metastases [8].

The development of metastatic disease poses a major clinical problem because it is seldom amenable to a curative treatment. The efficacy of conventional chemotherapy is limited, with response rates of 30% without improvement in overall survival [9].

Surgery and metastasectomy

Surgery is the mainstay of current STS treatment. In most cases, a local recurrence can be prevented by surgery, with the addition of radiotherapy as indicated. Despite the frequent success of local tumor control, the risk that distant metastases will develop seems to depend largely on biologic characteristics of the tumor [10].

The impact of local tumor control on the prevention of systemic disease is unclear. Trovik and colleagues [11] evaluated 559 patients with localized extremity or truncal STS and concluded that the surgical margin width was not a risk factor for metastases. Contradictory results were reported in a retrospective study of 111 extremity and truncal STSs. A wide tumor-negative margin (10 mm or more) was prognostic for a prolonged disease free-survival and a reduced rate of distant failure [12]. Another study of the margin status of 2084 consecutive patients undergoing resection for primary STS showed that positive margins were linked with only a slightly higher rate of metastases, 27% versus 23% for negative margins [6].

Although developments in local treatment have reduced local failure rates, distant failure remains unaffected. The National Cancer Institute conducted a prospective randomized study in which limb-sparing surgery was compared with amputation [13]. The patients studied had intermediate or high-grade extremity STS in most cases. Despite a lower rate of local failure in the limb-sparing group, there was no difference in distant failure and overall survival between the two treatment modalities [13]. Newer limb-salvaging techniques such as hyperthermic isolated limb perfusion with tumor necrosis factor-alpha and melphalan with or without radiotherapy have local control rates equivalent to amputation but also do not affect the distant failure rate [14].

Resection is the treatment of choice for pulmonary metastases. Three-year survival rates after complete resection range from 30% to 42% [15]. A variety of prognostic factors have been reviewed in different series to predict favorable survival after pulmonary metastasectomy. These factors include the number of lesions, the presence of unilateral versus bilateral metastases, and the disease-free interval. Of all variables, the ability to resect metastatic disease completely is consistently the most significant factor in predicting survival following resection of metastatic disease [16,17].

Two large series have indicated a prognostic significance associated with the number of metastases resected. Casson and colleagues [15] demonstrated that patients with three or fewer lesions on preoperative assessment had a significantly longer survival than patients with four or more lesions. Similar findings were noted by Putnam and colleagues [18]. Patients with four or less lesions resected at operation had a longer postthoracotomy survival than patients with more than four lesions. The same group demonstrated that unilateral versus bilateral disease was not a significant indicator of prognosis. Billingsley and colleagues [8] showed similar results in that bilateral disease was not an independent negative predictor of survival; however, the number of metastases was not a significant prognostic factor either. They found that as long as the pulmonary metastases were completely resected, there was no significant difference between patients who had less than or more than four lesions resected [8].

A number of reports have demonstrated the importance of the disease-free interval in predicting long-term outcome [15,18,19]. Patients who present with stage IV disease or in whom the interval between primary therapy and appearance of metastatic disease is short have a less favorable survival compared to those in whom the metastatic disease appears years later.

Even after an apparent complete resection of sarcomatous pulmonary metastases, 40% to 80% of patients will have a recurrence in the lung [20]. Weiser and colleagues [20] reviewed data on 3149 adult inpatients with soft tissue sarcoma. Re-exploration for recurrent sarcomatous pulmonary metastases appeared beneficial for patients who could be completely re-resected. Three independent prognostic factors associated with poor outcomes determined preoperatively were (1) the presence of three or more nodules, (2) a greater than 2 cm size of the largest metastases, and (3) high-grade primary tumor histology. Patients with zero or one poor prognostic factor had a median disease-specific survival of greater than 65 months, whereas patients with three poor prognostic factors had a median disease-specific survival of 10 months. Patients who could not be completely re-resected or those with numerous large metastases and high-grade primary tumor pathology had poor outcomes.

No prospective randomized study has compared metastasectomy with no surgery. Nevertheless, pulmonary resection has been associated with low perioperative mortality rates, actuarial 3-year survival rates of 20% to 54%, and 5-year survival rates of 21% to 51%. Most studies thus far are limited by median follow-up durations of less than 3 years [16,21]. Nevertheless, pulmonary resection, when possible, has been advocated as the only potentially curative treatment in STS patients who have lung metastases [22].

Methods for local ablation have been developed in recent years with a goal of increasing the number of patients eligible for lung-directed therapy. The early experiences with metastasis ablation have been primarily with hepatic tumors. More recently, application of non-surgical percutaneous approaches to destroy pulmonary metastases have been utilized. The most common approach, radiofrequency ablation (RFA), relies on the thermal destruction of a defined area within the lung using electrical energy. Several reports in small series of patients suggest that this approach can be performed safely and with apparent satisfactory local control [23,24]. Further studies are necessary to define the role of percutaneous ablation of pulmonary STS metastases. Several small series have been reported on outcomes following resection of STS metastases of extrapulmonary sites, including brain, pancreas, and liver [25,26]. Chen and colleagues [27] observed a median survival time of 39 months in 11 patients who had undergone radical resection of liver metastases from visceral and retroperitoneal STS. Harrison and colleagues [28] reported on 25 STS patients with a median survival time of 31 months after resection of liver metastases. Only one patient was alive 5 years after surgery. Furthermore, tumor grade, tumor type, and primary site were not prognostic for survival after hepatic resection. In a more recent multi-institution series, Adam and colleagues reported on outcomes in 125 patients undergoing liver resection for sarcoma. They found in these patients 5-year survival of 31% with a median survival of 32 months; comparable to those patients with adenocarcinoma histology [29].

While adjuvant chemotherapy is often considered in patients undergoing resection of metastatic disease, the benefit is unclear [30–32]. This approach is believed by some physicians to allow more complete treatment of macroscopic and occult microscopic metastatic disease. Unfortunately, a randomized trial designed to evaluate the potential clinical benefit of metastasectomy plus chemotherapy (European Organization for Research and Treatment of Cancer [EORTC] trial 62,933) closed because of poor accrual.

Acknowledging the absence of definitive clinical trials to guide treatment decisions, Porter and colleagues [33] examined the cost-effectiveness of pulmonary resection and systemic chemotherapy in the management of metastatic soft tissue sarcoma. They found that systemic chemotherapy alone when compared with no treatment was not a cost-effective treatment strategy. Pulmonary resection alone was the most cost-effective treatment strategy evaluated. Certain patient and tumor features, such as low tumor grade, non-extremity tumor location, and a disease-free interval greater than or equal to 12 months, were associated with a greater cost-effectiveness of treatment.

Chemotherapeutic management of recurrent or metastatic sarcoma

Although surgical metastasectomy can be curative in a small proportion of patients (15%–30%) [34], the vast majority of patients in whom metastatic sarcoma develops will die of their disease, with a median survival of 12 to 18 months [35]. In attempts to palliate symptoms and prolong survival, various chemotherapeutic regimens have been evaluated in the metastatic setting with attention to outcomes such as progression-free survival and overall survival.

Doxorubicin

In 1973, the initial phase II study evaluating doxorubicin in patients with cancer was published [36]. Sarcoma patients had a 33% response rate to this single agent, with both bone and soft tissue tumors included in the sarcoma subgroup. A follow-up, dose-response study performed by the same group assigned "good-risk" patients to a doxorubicin dose of 45, 60, or 75 mg/m^2 every 3 weeks [37] and "poor-risk" patients to 50 mg/m^2 or 25 mg/m^2. The response rates for sarcoma patients were 18%, 20%, and 37% in the good-risk group and 11% and 0% in the poor-risk groups for each respective dose [37]. From that point forward, doxorubicin became the standard of care for sarcoma, with dose intensity as a therapeutic aim.

Dacarbazine

Dacarbazine (DTIC) was the next agent to have promising results in sarcoma. In a study performed in 138 sarcoma patients, 18% had a partial or complete response, with leiomyosarcomas accounting for the largest proportion of patients responding to the therapy [38]. Combination trials of doxorubicin and DTIC then ensued, with the first study combining DTIC with 60 mg/m^2 of doxorubicin. An overall response rate of 41% was demonstrated [39]. It appeared that combination chemotherapy would allow the best disease response but at the cost of added toxicity. For the first time, a survival benefit was seen, with the patients receiving combination therapy having overall survivals of 10 months compared with 6 months for those without treatment [38–41].

The Eastern Cooperative Oncology Group (ECOG) performed a randomized trial in which patients were stratified to single-agent doxorubicin in one of two different dosing schemas or doxorubicin and DTIC in combination [42]. The single-agent arms had similar response rates: 18% for the 70 mg/m^2 dose, and 16% for the 20 mg/m^2 dose on days 1, 2, and 3 and 15 mg/m^2 dose on day 8. The combination regimen had a response rate of 30% with higher toxicity profiles and no change in median survival. It was unclear after these studies whether the increased response rate outweighed the added toxicities enough to warrant using combination therapy as first-line treatment, especially given the lack of survival benefit [43].

Ifosfamide

In the 1960s, ifosfamide was introduced as an alternative to cyclophosphamide with the aim of providing more effective DNA cross-linking distance [44]. The initial promising studies were overshadowed by the dose-limiting toxicity of hemorrhagic cystitis, which would limit the drug's use until the advent of mesna in the late 1970s [45]. An early study using ifosfamide at doses of 5 to 8 g/m^2 every 3 weeks in heavily pretreated sarcoma patients reported a response rate of 38%, with 15% of patients achieving a complete response [46]. Given these encouraging results, the EORTC went on to perform a randomized study evaluating cyclophosphamide versus ifosfamide in sarcoma patients who previously had never received alkylating therapy [47]. The response rate of single-agent cyclophosphamide, which had never been evaluated in sarcoma as a single agent, was only 8%. The ifosfamide arm, on the other hand, demonstrated an 18% response rate, establishing an advantage of ifosfamide over cyclophosphamide in adult soft tissue sarcoma and creating a shift in the treatment paradigm.

Combination regimens

Given the single-agent responses seen with doxorubicin, ifosfamide, and dacarbazine, the next logical step was to discern whether a combination of these drugs was effective without adding too much toxicity. The MAID regimen was thus born, consisting of 60 mg/m^2 of doxorubicin, 7.5 mg/m^2 of ifosfamide, and 900 mg/m^2 of DTIC given over 3 days as a continuous infusion [48] in an attempt to reduce the cardiotoxic and gastrointestinal toxicity [49,50]. In a trial of chemotherapy-naïve patients, 47% of patients responded to the MAID combination, with a 10% complete response rate.

In 1993, two randomized controlled trials were published in the *Journal of Clinical Oncology* evaluating multi-agent regimens in the treatment of sarcoma. The first trial was an Intergroup study that randomized patients to either MAID (doxorubicin, 60 mg/m^2; ifosfamide, 7.5 mg/m^2; DTIC, 1000 mg/m^2 via continuous infusion) or DTIC and doxorubicin at the same doses [51]. Patients who received MAID had a higher response rate (32% versus 17%) and longer time to disease progression (6 versus 4 months); however, the more responsive group was hampered by an overall greater amount of toxicity (92% versus 55%) as well as more treatment-related deaths (4% versus 0.6%). In the second study in the same issue of the *Journal of Clinical Oncology*, the ECOG published results from a three-armed trial comparing doxorubicin alone at 80 mg/m^2 against MAI (doxorubicin, 60 mg/m^2, and bolus ifosfamide, 7.5 g/m^2) and a third regimen, MAP (mitomycin, 8 mg/m^2; doxorubicin, 40 mg/m^2; and cisplatin, 60 mg/m^2) [52], a regimen developed by the Mayo Clinic group that had some reported responses in a phase II trial [53]. The combination regimens resulted in higher response rates (MAI 34%, MAP 32%, doxorubicin 20%); however, as documented in the prior combination trials, this improvement was at the expense of greater toxicity. The development of colony-stimulating growth factors allowed investigators to dose intensify doxorubicin with ifosfamide, prompting an EORTC phase II trial that reported a higher response rate with the higher doxorubicin dose (75 mg/m^2) when filgrastim was used as a granulocyte-stimulating factor [54,55] to limit myelosuppression.

Beyond MAID

More than 20 years since the first studies evaluating doxorubicin and ifosfamide, they are still considered to be the most effective agents in the treatment of soft tissue sarcoma whether used as single agents or in combination. Many small studies have looked at newer agents, most of which have not proven very promising. One combination that has garnered some attention is gemcitabine and docetaxel. Three published trials have evaluated this combination in sarcoma. The first of these studies evaluated 34 patients with leiomyosarcomas, with the bulk of patients having uterine leiomyosarcomas [56]. Patients received 900 mg/m^2 of gemcitabine on days 1 and 8 followed by 100 mg/m^2 of docetaxel on day 8. Patients who had received prior radiotherapy received a 25% dose reduction of gemcitabine. The overall response rate in these 34 patients was 53% with complete response achieved in three patients (two of these patients had prior doxorubicin-based therapy). A 47% 6-month, progression-free rate was observed in this study.

Several theories were postulated for why the response rate in this study was so superior. It was suggested that uterine leiomyosarcomas in particular respond more effectively to this regimen than do other sarcomas, and 84% of the study population's primary tumors were uterine in origin. This suggestion seemed to correlate with the findings in a prior study performed with gemcitabine as a single agent, which also yielded higher responses in the uterine leiomyosarcoma group in particular [57]. Another theory was that the longer infusion of 90 minutes used in the study possibly contributed to a higher success rate. Lastly, it was suggested that an in vivo synergy exists with the gemcitabine and docetaxel combination. Two further studies evaluating this regimen in metastatic sarcoma included a randomized study by Maki and colleagues [58] and a single-arm French study by Bay and colleagues [59]. In the Maki study, the overall survival and progression-free survival were superior in the combination arm versus gemcitabine alone arm (17.9 versus 11.5 and 6.2 versus 3.0 months, respectively) [58]. Again, better responses were seen in the leiomyosarcoma group as well as the undifferentiated high-grade pleomorphic sarcoma group. In the French study, 114 patients were evaluable for response. An overall response rate of 18.4% was achieved, with the leiomyosarcoma response rate being 24.2% [59]. These studies helped to define a possible second-line therapy for advanced soft tissue sarcomas, performance status allowing, especially in patients with high-grade undifferentiated pleomorphic sarcoma and leiomyosarcoma.

Pegylated liposomal doxorubicin (PLD) is a formulation of liposomal doxorubicin in which the doxorubicin is contained within liposomes coated with polyethylene glycol, leading to diminished uptake in the reticuloendothial system resulting in a much longer half-life of the drug (approximately 50–60 hours) [60–62]. It has been used successfully in Kaposi's sarcoma and is approved by the US Food and Drug Administration for this indication. Three trials evaluating PLD have been performed in patients with locally advanced or metastatic sarcoma. Skubitz reported on 47 patients who received 55 mg/m^2 repeated every 28 days. Two of 46 patients obtained a complete response or partial response, and 13 of 45 were thought to have a clinically significant response (minor responses or stable disease) [63]. The EORTC published a prospective randomized trial of PLD versus doxorubicin in advanced or metastatic soft tissue sarcoma [64]. Of 94 eligible patients, 50 were treated with PLD at a dose slightly lower than in the Skubitz trial, 50 mg/m^2, and 40 patients were treated with doxorubicin at 75 mg/m^2. The response rates were similar in both arms, albeit, low in general when compared with that in prior studies (10% in the PLD arm and 9% in the doxorubicin arm). The low response rate was thought to be due in part to the relatively high proportion of gastrointestinal stromal (GIST) patients in the study.

In an effort to take advantage of the more favorable side effect profile of PLD, Nielsen and colleagues performed a phase I study evaluating the toxicity of PLD combined with ifosfamide in patients with advanced or metastatic sarcoma [65]. Although toxicity was the primary endpoint of the study and not response, an overall response rate of 9% was found, and responders were only seen at the maximum tolerated dose (the recommended dose was one level below the maximum tolerated dose). Although it was concluded that the combination of ifosfamide with PLD is feasible, most sarcoma centers still preferentially choose doxorubicin with ifosfamide if combination therapy is warranted. PLD as a single agent is a reasonable choice as second- or third-line therapy depending on the overall performance status of the patient.

Temozolomide, an oral prodrug that achieves its antitumor effects through the formation of 5-3-methyl-1-triazenolimidazole-4 carboxamide, the active metabolite of dacarbazine, has been evaluated in a phase II trial in metastatic soft tissue sarcoma. A total of 26 patients received the drug twice daily as an oral bolus of 200 mg/m^2 followed by nine doses of 90 mg/m^2 with cycles repeated every 28 days. There were two partial responses, two mixed responses, and three patients with stable disease that lasted longer than 6 months; all of the responses were in patients with leiomyosarcomas [66]. Given that many patients never receive DTIC as part of their initial chemotherapy, this is a reasonable drug to return to in the second- or third-line setting, especially in patients with leiomyosarcoma.

Summary

It has remained difficult to ascertain the best management approach for patients who have metastatic sarcoma, in part owing to the difficulties in accruing adequate amounts of patients to clinical trials given the relative rarity of sarcoma. Furthermore, the overall heterogeneity of histologic subtypes within the studies performed makes it difficult to generalize outcomes. Further studies need to be performed because many unanswered questions remain. What is the optimal way to combine systemic therapy with surgical and radiotherapy in patients with metastatic disease? Will any of the more "targeted" therapies have a role with surgery in controlling disease or providing more long-term survivals? It is hoped that as international cooperative groups focusing on sarcoma and multidisciplinary groups within sarcoma treatment centers continue to work together, the answers to these questions will come to light.

References

[1] Jemal A, Thomas A, Murray T, et al. Cancer statistics 2002. CA Cancer J Clin 2002;52: 23–47.

[2] Coindre JM, Terrier P, Bui NB, et al. Prognostic factors in adult patient with locally controlled soft tissue sarcoma: a study of 546 patients from the French Federation of Cancer Centers Sarcoma Group. J Clin Oncol 1996;14(3):869–77.

[3] Gadd MA, Casper ES, Woodruff JM, et al. Development and treatment of pulmonary metastases in adult patients with extremity soft tissue sarcoma. Ann Surg 1993;218(6):705–12.

[4] Coindre JM, Terrier P, Guillou L, et al. Predictive value of grade for metastasis development in the main histologic types of adult soft tissue sarcomas. Cancer 2001;91(10):1914–26.

[5] Pisters PW, Leung DH, Woodruff J, et al. Analysis of prognostic factors in 1041 patients with localized soft tissue sarcomas of the extremities. J Clin Oncol 1996;14(5):1679–89.

[6] Stojadinovic A, Leung DH, Hoos A, et al. Analysis of the prognostic significance of microscopic margins in 2084 localized primary adult soft tissue sarcomas. Ann Surg 2002;235(3): 424–34.

[7] Lewis JJ, Brennan MF. Soft tissue sarcomas. Curr Probl Surg 1996;33(10):817–72.

[8] Billingsley K, Burt M, Jara E, et al. Pulmonary metastases from soft tissue sarcoma: analysis of patterns of disease and postmetastasis survival. Ann Surg 1999;229(5):602–12.

[9] Sarcoma Meta-analysis Collaboration. Adjuvant chemotherapy for localized resectable soft-tissue sarcoma of adults: meta-analysis of individual data. Lancet 1997;350(9092):1647–54.

[10] Komdeur R, Hoekstra H, van den Berg E, et al. Metastasis in soft tissue saracomas: prognostic criteria and treatment perspectives. Cancer Metastasis Rev 2002;21:167–83.

[11] Trovik C, Bauer H, Alvegar T, et al. Surgical margins, local recurrence and metastasis in soft tissue sarcomas: 559 surgically treated patients from the Scandinavian Sarcoma Group Register. Eur J Cancer 2000;36(6):710–6.

[12] McKee M, Liu D, Brooks J, et al. The prognostic significance of margin width for extremity and trunk sarcoma. J Surg Oncol 2004;85(2):68–76.

[13] Rosenberg S, Tepper J, Glatstein E, et al. The treatment of soft-tissue sarcomas of the extremities: prospective randomized evaluations of (1) limb-sparing surgery plus radiation therapy compared with amputation and (2) the role of adjuvant chemotherapy. Ann Surg 1982;196(3):305–15.

[14] Olieman A, Pras E, van Ginkel R, et al. Feasibility and efficacy of external beam radiotherapy after hyperthermic isolated limb perfusion with TNF-alpha and melphalan for limb-

saving treatment in locally advanced extremity soft-tissue sarcoma. Int J Radiat Oncol Biol Phys 1998;40(4):807–14.

[15] Casson A, Putnam J, Natarajan G, et al. Five-year survival after pulmonary metastasectomy for adult soft tissue sarcoma. Cancer 1992;69(3):662–8.

[16] Verazin G, Warneke J, Driscoll D, et al. Resection of lung metastases from soft-tissue sarcomas: a multivariate analysis. Arch Surg 1992;127(12):1407–11.

[17] van Geel A, van Coevorden F, Blankensteijn J, et al. Surgical treatment of pulmonary metastases from soft tissue sarcomas: a retrospective study in The Netherlands. J Surg Oncol 1994;56(3):172–7.

[18] Putnam J Jr, Roth J, Wesley M, et al. Analysis of prognostic factors in patients undergoing resection of pulmonary metastases from soft tissue sarcomas. J Thorac Cardiovasc Surg 1984;87(2):260–8.

[19] Jablons D, Steinberg S, Roth J, et al. Metastasectomy for soft tissue sarcoma: further evidence for efficacy and prognostic indicators. J Thorac Cardiovasc Surg 1989;97(5):695–705.

[20] Weiser M, Downey R, Leung D, et al. Repeat resection of pulmonary metastases in patients with soft-tissue sarcoma. J Am Coll Surg 2000;191(3):184–90.

[21] van Geel A, Pastorino U, Jauch K, et al. Surgical treatment of lung metastases: the European Organization for the Research and Treatment of Cancer—Soft Tissue and Bone Sarcoma Group study of 255 patients. Cancer 1996;77:675–82.

[22] Temple L, Brennan M. The role of pulmonary metastasectomy in soft tissue sarcoma. Semin Thorac Cardiovasc Surg 2002;114:35–44.

[23] Laganè D, Carrafiello G, Mangini M, et al. Radiofrequency ablation of primary and metastatic lung tumors: preliminary experience with a single center device. Surg Endosc 2006;20: 1262–7.

[24] Gillams AR, Lees WR, Mangini M, et al. Radiofrequency ablation of lung metastases: factors influencing success. Eur Radiol 2008;18:672–7.

[25] Espat NJ, Bilsky M, Lewis JJ, et al. Soft tissue sarcoma brain metastases. Prevalence in a cohort of 3829 patients. Cancer 2002;94:2706–11.

[26] Pingpank JF Jr, Hoffman JP, Sigurdson ER, et al. Pancreatic resection for locally advanced primary and metastatic nonpancreatic neoplasms. Am Surg 2002;94:337–40 [discussion 340–1].

[27] Chen H, Pruitt A, Nicol T, et al. Complete hepatic resection of metastases from leiomyosarcoma prolongs survival. J Gastrointest Surg 1998;2(2):151–5.

[28] Harrison L, Brennan M, Newman E. Hepatic resection for noncolorectal, nonneuroendocrine metastases: a fifteen-year experience with ninety-six patients. Surgery 1997;121(6): 625–32.

[29] Adam R, Chiche L, Aloia T. Association Française de Chirurgie, et al. Hepatic resection for noncolorectal nonendocrine liver metastases: analysis of 1,452 patients and development of a prognostic model. Ann Surg 2006;244:524–35.

[30] Mentzer S, Antman K, Attinger C, et al. Selected benefits of thoracotomy and chemotherapy for sarcoma metastatic to the lung. J Surg Oncol 1993;53:54–9.

[31] Pastorino U. Metastasectomy for soft tissue sarcomas. In: Verweij J, Pinedo H, Suit H, editors. Soft tissue sarcomas: present achievement and future prospects. Boston: Kluwer Academic Publishers; 1997. p. 65–75.

[32] Baxter G, Alvegard T, Monge O. VIG chemotherapy in advanced soft tissue sarcoma—results of the Scandinavian Sarcoma Group SSG-X trial. Acta Orthop Scand Suppl 1995;265: 93–4.

[33] Porter G, Cantor S, Walsh G, et al. Cost-effectiveness of pulmonary resection and systemic chemotherapy in the management of metastatic soft tissue sarcoma: a combined analysis from the University of Texas M.D. Anderson and Memorial Sloan-Kettering Cancer Centers. J Thorac Cardiovasc Surg 2004;127:1366–72.

[34] Chao C, Goldberg M. Surgical treatment of metastatic pulmonary soft-tissue sarcoma. Oncology (Williston Park) 2000;14(6):835–41 [discussion: 842–4, 847].

[35] D'Adamo DR, Anderson SE, Albritton K, et al. Phase II study of doxorubicin and bevaci-zumab for patients with metastatic soft-tissue sarcomas. J Clin Oncol 2005;23(28):7135–42.

[36] O'Bryan RM, Luce JK, Talley RW, et al. Phase II evaluation of adriamycin in human neo-plasia. Cancer 1973;32(1):1–8.

[37] O'Bryan RM, Baker LH, Gottlieb JE, et al. Dose response evaluation of adriamycin in hu-man neoplasia. Cancer 1977;39(5):1940–8.

[38] Gottlieb JA, Benjamin RS, Baker LH, et al. Role of DTIC (NSC-45388) in the chemotherapy of sarcomas. Cancer Treat Rep 1976;60(2):199–203.

[39] Gottlieb JA, Baker LH, Quagliana JM, et al. Chemotherapy of sarcomas with a combination of adriamycin and dimethyl triazeno imidazole carboxamide. Cancer 1972;30(6):1632–8.

[40] Pinedo HM, Kenis Y. Chemotherapy of advanced soft-tissue sarcomas in adults. Cancer Treat Rev 1977;4(2):67–86.

[41] Gottlieb JA. Proceedings: combination chemotherapy for metastatic sarcoma. Cancer Che-mother Rep 1974;58(2):265–70.

[42] Borden EC, Amato DA, Rosenbaum C, et al. Randomized comparison of three adriamycin regimens for metastatic soft tissue sarcomas. J Clin Oncol 1987;5(6):840–50.

[43] Benjamin RS. Grade 3 nausea, vomiting, and myelosuppression or progressive, metastatic sarcoma? J Clin Oncol 1987;5(6):833–5.

[44] Bramwell VH, Mouridsen HT, Santoro A, et al. Cyclophosphamide versus ifosfamide: a ran-domized phase II trial in adult soft-tissue sarcomas. The European Organization for Re-search and Treatment of Cancer [EORTC], Soft Tissue and Bone Sarcoma Group. Cancer Chemother Pharmacol 1993;31(Suppl 2):S180–4.

[45] Scheef W, Klein HO, Brock N, et al. Controlled clinical studies with an antidote against the urotoxicity of oxazaphosphorines: preliminary results. Cancer Treat Rep 1979;63(3): 501–5.

[46] Stuart-Harris RC, Harper PG, Parsons CA, et al. High-dose alkylation therapy using ifos-famide infusion with mesna in the treatment of adult advanced soft-tissue sarcoma. Cancer Chemother Pharmacol 1983;11(2):69–72.

[47] Bramwell VH, Mouridsen HT, Santoro A, et al. Cyclophosphamide versus ifosfamide: final report of a randomized phase II trial in adult soft tissue sarcomas. Eur J Cancer Clin Oncol 1987;23(3):311–21.

[48] Elias A, Ryan L, Sulkes A, et al. Response to mesna, doxorubicin, ifosfamide, and dacarba-zine in 108 patients with metastatic or unresectable sarcoma and no prior chemotherapy. J Clin Oncol 1989;7(9):1208–16.

[49] Legha SS, Benjamin RS, Mackay B, et al. Reduction of doxorubicin cardiotoxicity by pro-longed continuous intravenous infusion. Ann Intern Med 1982;96(2):133–9.

[50] Von Burton G, Rankin C, Zalupski MM, et al. Phase II trial of gemcitabine as first line che-motherapy in patients with metastatic or unresectable soft tissue sarcoma. Am J Clin Oncol 2006;29(1):59–61.

[51] Antman K, Crowley J, Balcerzak SP, et al. An Intergroup phase III randomized study of doxorubicin and dacarbazine with or without ifosfamide and mesna in advanced soft tissue and bone sarcomas. J Clin Oncol 1993;11(7):1276–85.

[52] Edmonson JH, Ryan LM, Blum RH, et al. Randomized comparison of doxorubicin alone versus ifosfamide plus doxorubicin or mitomycin, doxorubicin, and cisplatin against ad-vanced soft tissue sarcomas. J Clin Oncol 1993;11(7):1269–75.

[53] Edmonson JH, Long HJ, Richardson RL, et al. Phase II study of a combination of mitomy-cin, doxorubicin and cisplatin in advanced sarcomas. Cancer Chemother Pharmacol 1985; 15(2):181–2.

[54] Steward WP, Verweij J, Somers R, et al. Granulocyte-macrophage colony-stimulating factor allows safe escalation of dose-intensity of chemotherapy in metastatic adult soft tissue sar-comas: a study of the European Organization for Research and Treatment of Cancer Soft Tissue and Bone Sarcoma Group. J Clin Oncol 1993;11(1):15–21.

[55] Steward WP, Verweij J, Somers R, et al. The use of recombinant human granulocyte-macrophage colony-stimulating factor with combination chemotherapy in the treatment of advanced adult soft-tissue sarcomas: early results from the EORTC Soft-Tissue and Bone Sarcoma Group. Cancer Chemother Pharmacol 1993;31(Suppl 2):S241–4.

[56] Hensley ML, Maki R, Venkatraman E, et al. Gemcitabine and docetaxel in patients with unresectable leiomyosarcoma: results of a phase II trial. J Clin Oncol 2002;20(12):2824–31.

[57] Patel SR, Gandhi V, Jenkins J, et al. Phase II clinical investigation of gemcitabine in advanced soft tissue sarcomas and window evaluation of dose rate on gemcitabine triphosphate accumulation. J Clin Oncol 2001;19(15):3483–9.

[58] Maki RG, Wathen JK, Patel SR, et al. Randomized phase II study of gemcitabine and docetaxel compared with gemcitabine alone in patients with metastatic soft tissue sarcomas: results of sarcoma alliance for research through collaboration study 002 [corrected]. J Clin Oncol 2007;25(19):2755–63.

[59] Bay JO, Ray-Coquard I, Fayette J, et al, Groupe Sarcome Français. Docetaxel and gemcitabine combination in 133 advanced soft-tissue sarcomas: a retrospective analysis. Int J Cancer 2006;119(3):706–11.

[60] Gabizon AA, Barenholz Y, Bialer M. Prolongation of the circulation time of doxorubicin encapsulated in liposomes containing a polyethylene glycol-derivatized phospholipid: pharmacokinetic studies in rodents and dogs. Pharm Res 1993;10(5):703–8.

[61] Gabizon A, Catane R, Uziely B, et al. Prolonged circulation time and enhanced accumulation in malignant exudates of doxorubicin encapsulated in polyethylene-glycol coated liposomes. Cancer Res 1994;54(4):987–92.

[62] Northfelt DW, Martin FJ, Working P, et al. Doxorubicin encapsulated in liposomes containing surface-bound polyethylene glycol: pharmacokinetics, tumor localization, and safety in patients with AIDS-related Kaposi's sarcoma. J Clin Pharmacol 1996;36(1):55–63.

[63] Skubitz KM. Phase II trial of pegylated-liposomal doxorubicin (Doxil) in sarcoma. Cancer Invest 2003;21(2):167–76.

[64] Judson I, Radford JA, Harris M, et al. Randomised phase II trial of pegylated liposomal doxorubicin (DOXIL/CAELYX) versus doxorubicin in the treatment of advanced or metastatic soft tissue sarcoma: a study by the EORTC Soft Tissue and Bone Sarcoma Group. Eur J Cancer 2001;37(7):870–7.

[65] Nielsen OS, Reichardt P, Christensen TB, et al. Phase I European Organisation for Research and Treatment of Cancer study determining safety of pegylated liposomal doxorubicin (Caelyx) in combination with ifosfamide in previously untreated adult patients with advanced or metastatic soft tissue sarcomas. Eur J Cancer 2006;42(14):2303–9.

[66] Talbot SM, Keohan ML, Hesdorffer M, et al. A phase II trial of temozolomide in patients with unresectable or metastatic soft tissue sarcoma. Cancer 2003;98(9):1942–6.

ELSEVIER
SAUNDERS

Surg Clin N Am 88 (2008) 673–680

SURGICAL
CLINICS OF
NORTH AMERICA

Index

Note: Page numbers of article titles are in **boldface** type.